Climax
By Jacqueline DeGroot

An Erotic Thriller and
A Sizzling Romance

ISBN: 0-75962-754-1

This book is printed on acid free paper.

1stBooks – rev. 5/16/01

To my husband, Bill who has been supportive and encouraging through all my endeavors, to my children who were patient when I was writing, to all my friends who have listened and advised, to my parents who are always there for me, and to my sister and brother—I love them dearly. A big thanks to all my friends who read and critiqued and to Rebecca and Gary Justice for their help with some of the research. A very special thanks to Deanna, Peggy, Jessie, Kathy, Ron, Dick, Jim, Arlene, Debi, Tammy and Chris.

Disclaimer

All characters in this book have no existence outside the imagination of the author and have no relation whatsoever to anyone bearing the same name or names. They are not even distantly inspired by any individual known or unknown to the author and all incidents are pure fiction.

Prologue

Fairfax, VA

October 23, 1989

Dr. David Sandler sat at his desk in his darkened home office, staring at the neatly arranged desktop. Even though his eyes were open, he wasn't seeing what was there, he was seeing what had been there before. It hadn't been that long ago that he had sat in this same chair, surrounded by pills of varying colors and shapes. Numb, he remembers gazing over the physicians' instruments of his patients' destruction, now, soon to be his own. Dreams of a lifetime have turned to devouring demons, obsessive and voracious. Innocently they pour from a past of strife and brilliant successes, always hiding in the edges of what David can barely see until the room seems to drown in them. Demons he had tamed with the light of reason and rationale were now coming for him. There could be no turning back.

Leaning his head back against the padded headrest he closes his eyes. He envisions the colorful pills of poison and matches betraying lies with the faces of his victims. He can still see the dark green ones that he'd planned for Liesel, the pretty purple and pink ones that had been Betsy's, the little white round ones that he'd so carefully researched for Leroy and the elongated yellow ones that had been for Donna. Among them, scattered on his shiny mahogany desk had also been the methadone syringes that went to Shawn and the nasal spray that had become Henry's. Actually, he thought—it had been a long time ago. Long enough for something to go wrong.

How had it come to this? Just how had he allowed this to happen? Thinking back in his mind he can't actually remember a conscious desire to take this course of action, yet he had just the same. And now look where it had led him. All he had ever wanted was to be the best doctor in his field and to have a wife and child who adored him. He never thought he'd have to do all this to get them and now it was too late to stop what had to happen.

Just when had his lifetime dreams become his obsession? All he wanted was within his grasp now, he was so close. Now would he even be able to do what was necessary to provide for the ones he loved? Remembering the array of medicines that had been spread out around him almost a year ago, he wondered which one he should be prescribing for himself now. Then he decided, no, there was a better way to do this.

Mechanically he sat up and looked at the list of things he must do that would end his career, his dreams—his life. "Get a coffin, pick out a plot, visit attorney, secure safety deposit box, organize office, clean out apartment." He picked up his fountain pen from the ornate holder and added, "buy a gun", in his bold script. With just the hint of a self-deprecating smile, he underlined it, twice. He'd have plenty of time to do that before he left for the airport tomorrow.

As he sat back in his chair again and ran his fingers through his hair, his mind grasped coldly for the reason everything had gone so terribly, horribly wrong. His mind unraveled, searching for the last time he had been in control of his emotions and his plans for the future, trying to ferret out the mistake that would cost him all; the moment his soul was sealed.

Jenny...It had all started with Jenny. His thoughts crowded each other as they backed up to when everything had started.

He had met her about ten trade-ins ago, nine that he actually hadn't needed, except as an excuse to see her. The first time he saw her had been the day she had approached him on the lot at Royal Pontiac and asked if she could help him. He'd been smitten then, warmed by her bubbly personality, charmed by her coy manner and utterly impressed by her knowledge of cars. She didn't flaunt her sexuality but the message came through inexplicably anyway. The ink hadn't even dried on the first of many contracts on Trans Ams before he was completely captivated by her.

Chapter 1

Vienna, VA 1976-1979

In May of 1976 Jenny joined the sales force of Royal Pontiac GMC, just as they were opening their doors for the first time. It was a very exciting time. Even though selling cars was very hard work, she loved it. Some days she knew she had to have walked at least four miles, between showing cars on the lot, retrieving keys from the key closet and going back and forth between customers and managers—all this in high heels no less. It was hot in the summer and the cars on the lot were like saunas. It was cold in the winter and she had the added enjoyment of cleaning the snow off them before a test drive. It was physically grueling some days and mentally grueling on others.

Then there were the days that were both because they were totally wasted due to breakdowns in negotiations, not being able to match a customer to a car or the dreaded credit problems of over-burdened people who didn't pay their bills on time. Those days were the pits and they made her more tired than the days when she delivered three cars. She did exactly the same work but had nothing to show for the effort, except hot, tired feet.

The economy was booming in the late seventies and the age of consumerism hadn't made all new and used car salesmen the scourge of the universe yet. She found that if she really knew her product, and the competition's as well and was honest and nice, she did quite well. In fact she soon became the one to beat in the heated competitions between the salesmen. She won Salesman of the Month, which was not known to be improper gender-typing at the time, most months of the year. By the early eighties she was well set and thoroughly entrenched in the car business.

Customers were always surprised when she greeted them. She did not look anything like the image they carried in their mind of a car salesman. She was young and beautiful, petite and curvy and had a dazzling, confident smile. She had long blonde

1

hair with the occasional help from L'Oreal and penetrating, soft green eyes. Her petal-soft, pink lips framed perfect white teeth when she captivated her customers with her engaging smile. She was cute and wholesome-looking, feminine all the way, even as she tried to be just one of the guys.

Women found her friendly and sincere while most men looked at her and noticed her body before appreciating her personality. Even though she was petite in stature, she was well-endowed under her prim bow-tied blouses and she preferred short skirts to slacks, with high heels to maximize her height. "Dy-no-mite!" was what the construction workers called out to her from the construction site of the office building being built next door to the dealership.

She met and married another car salesman who specialized in used cars at another dealership right up the road on Auto Row. He was flamboyant and charming as well as extremely good looking and she couldn't believe her good fortune. His name was Robert Jared Miller, but everyone just called him R.J.

They were very happy and very prosperous, but they hardly ever saw each other. Both of them were highly competitive and would easily sacrifice a night together to win another sales contest or some bonus trip that they would sell to another salesman instead of taking. They bought a house in Vienna, far bigger than they needed and requiring much more work than they had the time for.

Things continued this was way for several years. It was as if they were always running races but never stopping to enjoy the prize. They bought video machines when they first came on the market and a big screen television when the price was somewhat reasonable. They had an Atari game system with all the popular games, and any type of stereo component that was the new and trendy thing. They even had an Alfa Romeo sports car in the garage that R.J. was going to recondition one day. Since both of their companies provided demos for them to use, it wasn't a pressing thing for R.J. to get to it, so it sat for the better part of two years untouched. They had a lot of nice things but were rarely home to do anything but dust them off. Still it was important to R.J. to keep up with his cohorts at work and to project a very successful image. His shirts had his monogram on the cuffs, pocket or collar according to what was the current trend. His cufflinks were also monogrammed as well as his poker chips and his brief case, which carried personalized stationary, engraved Cross pens and of course personalized business cards. None of this mattered to Jenny who was beginning to think how nice it would be to have a baby.

Every time she brought the subject up she got rebuffed. It wasn't the right time. They needed to save more money. A child would be too limiting—they wouldn't be able to go anywhere. They really didn't go anywhere now. Once, they'd gone to Paradise Island in the Bahamas, courtesy of a conversion van company's sales contest and they'd had a really nice long honeymoon driving across the country. Both times had been wonderful and romantic, but really, the child could graduate high school before they would probably go anywhere again. R.J. liked to stay home when they weren't working, they really didn't socialize much with anyone. Jenny's family was always trying to get them to come to reunions and barbecues and weddings, but they always said they had to work, and usually they did. All the good stuff happens on Saturdays. In the real world and the car world, Saturdays are it.

It was a Saturday, in fact, that Jenny found herself in the ladies' room for the fourth time that day. Normally she only needed to use the facilities once in the morning and once at night no matter how much she drank. Here it was only two o'clock, what was up? She vaguely remembered her gynecologist recommending a break from the birth control pill she was on, a low dosage one because others caused blackouts. She'd been using it non-stop for many years. But R.J. didn't like the alternate method. It spoiled his fun and ruined the spontaneity for him. Boy, this was going to ruin his fun for sure!

Jenny knew that R.J. didn't want kids. He'd said it in so many ways over the years and at first she'd agreed with him, she didn't either. Now she was 27 and it seemed like such a good idea. She wanted someone to mother and to take care of. Someone little, not like R.J. A little bundle that smelled like baby powder, well...most times.

Chapter 2

1979

She was afraid to tell him she was pregnant. She knew that he would be very angry so she didn't want to be alone with him when she told him. So the following Saturday after work she asked him to meet her for a drink before they went home to prepare dinner, which they would eat on their laps in lazy-boy recliners watching "Saturday Night Live".

There, in the lounge of the Westpark Best Western Hotel, she told him what her doctor had told her. They could expect a new addition to the family in November. Since this was only the middle of March, it seemed a long time away for her. Not nearly long enough for him.

He was not only upset, he blamed her for it happening, not once acknowledging that he was the one who had refused to try a new method of contraception. He tried for days to talk her into aborting. She was adamant that that would never happen. She already felt a bond with this child and was happy to be carrying this new life inside her. Although normally a very placating person with R.J., she stood her ground even when he threatened to leave her. It was an idle threat. He was afraid she would leave him, so he stopped pushing the issue of an abortion. But he was never happy about this, and he let everyone know it. As soon as someone asked a question about her or the baby, he would sneer and make a derisive comment about the soon-to-be-arriving *brat*.

Everyone, friends and family alike, told her that as soon as he held that precious bundle in his hands, he would change. She prayed that this would be true, although she was really having her doubts.

Her pregnancy was wonderful, she was very healthy so the doctor said she could work as long as she liked. And since she'd rather be anywhere than at home with a sullen R.J., she worked long hours, careful to rest and put her feet up often. Her customers were terrific, they wouldn't even let her walk to the back storage lots to bring up cars for them. They took the keys and found the cars themselves and then came back from test drives too sympathetic not to buy. I mean really, would a waddling pregnant woman give you a bad deal? She had one of her best months ever in September, the last month she worked before delivering a month early on October 2, 1979.

R.J. refused to be with her during the delivery but he came to see her as soon as she was out of the recovery room. Jenny made sure he held the baby right away, then she waited for the big transformation. From the look on his face you'd think he was holding a blanket full of hog waste. Maybe it would have been better if the baby had been a girl instead of a boy, she thought. She named the baby Russell Martin because she loved the nicknames Russ and Rusty and she hated all the names R.J. had suggested. Really, did people actually name their children Bartholomew, Thaddeus or Geoffrey?

Chapter 3

1979-1980

Two days later when Jenny and the baby came home from the hospital, they had their first fight over the baby. Well, actually, their first fight happened before they even left the hospital parking lot. Because Rusty had arrived a month early, they really hadn't prepared the nursery or completed the layette yet. It was a mad scramble to find an infant car seat when Jenny refused to transport the baby without one. Since it was a Sunday morning none of the stores were open yet. Fortunately the hospital had a loaner program. Then, despite R.J.'s assurances while she was in the hospital that he was "working" on getting the baby's furniture ready for the homecoming, it wasn't. He had purchased a used dresser from the classifieds and stapled some vinyl-covered padding to the top to be used as a changer. Another taller dresser sat in the corner, not even matching the other piece. Thank God she'd had the forethought to buy a new crib and crib set much earlier.

It bothered her a great deal that whenever R.J. bought something for himself, it was always the best money could buy, but for his child, well...he would have to settle for used, dilapidated furniture that he'd slapped a few coats of paint on. The man's Sabatier knives could have paid for a whole new bedroom set for crying out loud. He was making it pretty obvious that this child was not welcome in his home.

Jenny was grateful that her parents were there for the first two weeks to help out. And if they hadn't been there, the arguments would have been a lot worse.

During the next few weeks and months Jenny and Rusty bonded like peanut butter and jelly. She was learning how to become a mother but forgetting how to be a wife. R.J. was being neglected due to the natural demands of the baby and he didn't like it one bit. One night he even suggested that they ship him

7

down to her parents in Florida and let them raise him. The sad part about the whole conversation was that he was dead serious. If he could only talk her into it, he would have had no problem doing exactly that.

Jenny took four months for maternity leave and was truly enjoying this time at home with the baby. She really didn't miss work all that much, but there was no chance of extending her leave of absence, R.J. was set on that. Four months to nurse and then back to work. At the end of the third month, she set out to find someone to care for Rusty. She finally found someone that she felt she could trust to watch him, but she could only watch him during the day. Jenny would have to make other arrangements for the nights she'd have to work.

So when Jenny went back to work she arranged her schedule so she worked exactly opposite her husband. That way there would always be somebody home in the evenings to take care of Rusty. R.J. was not happy about this arrangement and they argued about it constantly. He did not want to take care of the baby at all. Since he was the one forcing her to leave her baby and go back to work she thought R.J. should have an active part in Rusty's care. She also thought that if he did take care of Rusty, maybe he would become attached to the baby and they could become the happy little family that she prayed for.

It was apparent after only a few weeks that this was not going to work out. When Jenny came home late at night, she suspected that the baby had been neglected. Most of the time his diaper was soiled and he was ravenously hungry. Either that, or when she found him in his crib, it looked like he had been crying for a long time. She never came home to find him in his father's arms being rocked or fed.

Everyone, friends and family alike, knew that R.J. wasn't making the transition to papa very well at all. Whenever anyone asked how the baby was doing, he would say that the *brat* was a big waste of time and money. When her parents phoned from Florida to check on their newest grandson he would offer to parcel post him down to them. Rusty had been born on October

2nd. Jenny had gone back to work at the beginning of February. By the end of March it was obvious that something had to give.

She was exhausted trying to do everything by herself. The cooking, cleaning, laundry and 8 to10-hour workdays, as well as the sleepless nights, were beginning to take their toll, and everyone knew it, except R.J. Well, maybe he did know it. It was her punishment for getting pregnant and then going through with the delivery and bringing that *brat* home.

As far as he was concerned that kid was ruining everything. Jenny no longer had any time to spend with him and he hated the noise the baby made. The crying in the middle of the night angered R.J. as well as Jenny's subservient attitude, as she jumped up to do every little thing she could for the new obsession in her life. He felt like he was being punished and he didn't like it.

In April Jenny got some much needed assistance with the baby. Her parents decided that they missed their children in Maryland and Virginia and their new grandson, especially. They sold their new retirement home in Florida and moved back to the area they had moved from just two years earlier. Jenny's mother and father wanted to take care of the baby while Jenny worked. Things were working out after all.

Chapter 4

1980

It was during June that things came to a very dramatic conclusion for Jenny and R.J. Jenny had been unhappy about her marriage to R.J. since her pregnancy began. She was finding it hard to even like a man who wanted to do away with or give away a baby, nevertheless love him. She couldn't seem to find those old feelings of trust and devotion she used to have towards him. Maybe it was motherhood, maybe it was her eyes opening to the kind of man he really was. Fight it as she might, she started falling out of love with him. She was ambivalent about their love-making, when once she had been almost addicted to it. And she was starting to listen to the negative things people said about him. They could say them now without her getting mad, she wasn't his biggest supporter anymore.

After a particularly tiring day at work and after putting Rusty to bed, Jenny went to bed exhausted. That was the night that Rusty decided he wanted to stay up and bother Mommy. She could not figure out what was wrong with him. He didn't need changing, he had no fever, there were no pins sticking him anywhere, and he wasn't a colicky baby. What was the problem? Every time she got him back to sleep he would wake right up as she laid him down. A few times he would stay asleep for five or ten minutes, just long enough for Jenny to get back in bed and back to sleep.

R.J. kept mumbling something about "...damn kid" every time the baby cried and woke them up again. But he never got up to help. Finally around 5 o'clock in the morning she got him down and he seemed content, not fidgety. She went back to bed and noticed R.J. was in the bathroom from the light under the door. He walked out of the bathroom then went to the baby's room, opened the door wide and then slammed it as hard as he could.

Well of course that woke up the baby, and it also woke up Jenny, literally and figuratively. She knew in that moment that she didn't want to raise a baby in that kind of environment. She went to get the baby and brought him back to bed with her. R.J. threw a fit about the baby being in their bed but she completely ignored him.

When R.J. got up to get ready for work she stayed with the baby in bed instead of getting his breakfast ready. When he slammed out the back door she was ready to cash everything in and get a new life for her and her son.

Chapter 5

1980

The first thing she did after R.J. left for work was to check for her rings. She didn't wear her engagement ring unless they were going out somewhere special because she was afraid it would get damaged. It was a heart-shaped diamond,1.86 carat VVS1 quality in a platinum mounting. The insurance on it had become so expensive that they had dropped the rider from their policy. She was always fearful of slamming it into one of the shop walls at work or scratching up the platinum finish while pointing out something in a car engine. They kept it, along with an emerald and diamond cocktail ring, in a hollowed out book on one of the bookshelves in the guest room. Neither one was there. He'd beat her to them. He knew she was running.

She packed a bag for the baby and dropped him off at her parents house. She told them what was happening on the off chance that R.J. might decide to come and get the baby to make her change her mind somehow. They were very supportive of her. It helped that they never really liked R.J. to begin with and they saw this action as definitely better for Rusty.

Then Jenny went to the dealership to talk to the owner, who was her boss as well as her friend. He was someone she could trust and someone she could count on to help her. He and his family had a lot of influence in Northern Virginia. They owned over 25 dealerships within a 100 mile radius, from White Oaks, MD to Woodbridge, VA. They were king of the car companies. She called him Ron while everyone else called him Mr. Royal. He didn't mind the familiarity, they'd been through a lot together since the dealership had opened and they'd seen a lot of people come and go who couldn't handle the volatile business of selling cars.

He gave her sound advice and then called one of the corporation's attorneys. He arranged for her to be seen right away and she heard him tell the man over the phone "I don't care what happens to the bastard, just make sure she's taken care of."

Later that day when she arrived at the attorney's office she received his full attention and expert care. By four o'clock that afternoon separation papers had been drawn up and R.J. had been notified of her intentions. He was to make other arrangements for living quarters for three days to allow her time to pack up her personal belongings and those of the baby. All the major items were listed and she gave possession of them to him. She gave him her rings even though the lawyers insisted she had all rights to them. But she knew R.J. wasn't stupid, by the time she'd get them back the diamonds would be zircons. She gave him all their furnishings except those that had been hers before the marriage and she gave him all the video and audio equipment. She gave him everything he could have wanted.

All she wanted was her personal things, items that had belonged to her before the marriage, and complete 100% sole custody of Rusty. She didn't even want any child support. Now, she didn't want R.J. to have anything to do with her baby.

Jenny and Rusty moved in with her parents until things settled down and she could afford her own place. It was a great time for all of them. Jenny and her parents enjoyed watching Rusty grow in a completely loved-filled home. Rusty's grandfather, known to him as Poppy, became his very positive male influence and Rusty's grandmother, known as Nan, proceeded to make Rusty the most spoiled child in America. Life was good again.

R.J. licked his wounds for awhile but knew better than to make any trouble. He'd fared extremely well and he knew it. A few months later she heard that R.J. was dating an eighteen-year-old title clerk and it didn't bother Jenny one little bit.

Chapter 6

1980-1985

For the next few years Jenny dedicated herself to her career and her son. She lived with her parents in their house in Sterling, VA for a little over a year, which allowed her to put away enough money to buy a nice house in Herndon, VA. It was important for her to plan for Rusty's future and she wanted him to go to school in Fairfax County. It was the number one county in the nation for public schools and since it only required her to move a few blocks away from her parent's house to get into the county, that's what she did.

It had been a model home and was decorated to suit her tastes perfectly. It was a low country style with a large porch running across the front of it. It was a bit much for two people but she was hoping that one day there would be a husband and maybe even another child and anyway, it was a much better investment than a townhouse would've been.

She worked very hard to be the best salesman Royal ever had and she was. She was well known throughout the area car dealerships. She had even placed as first runner-up in a national competition held in Michigan for Best Walk Around presentations. She was among the top Pontiac salesmen in the country and was even asked to do several instructional and motivational videos for General Motors.

All her spare time was spent with her family and Rusty. He was the most beautiful child, inside and out. His hair was so blonde it was almost white, he had deep blue eyes and deep dimples when he smiled. Everyone adored him, especially his grandparents. They did everything for him and bought everything for him. Soon his playroom adjacent to the family room was overflowing with toys, books and stuffed animals. He had two sets of everything, one for each house. His room at

Jenny's house was just as crammed with stuff as his room at her parent's house was.

Jenny didn't get to spend as much time at home as she would have liked. The times she missed being away from her family were her peak times to be at work, weekends and evenings. She was always missing reunion parties, weddings, birthday parties, funerals and every kind of shower the family was having because she had to work. Rusty went to all of these and his doting grandparents enjoyed taking care of him and showing him off. Jenny was making a lot of money and even after paying her parents a generous child care allowance she was still able to save a fair amount.

When Rusty was about five years old, Jenny started thinking about having another baby. She thought about having a little girl to dress up and play with, a sweet toddler with ringlets in her hair, and later a young lady to take shopping and to share secrets with. She'd lost Rusty to her parents years ago, this one would be hers to spoil. How to accomplish this without a husband? She'd had no luck finding one, though she dated frequently. No one appealed to her. She just couldn't get that spark to get a relationship going. She'd only dated one man twice and that was because they won tickets to Wolftrap when they were on their first date together attending a charity ball for the American Heart Association that Ron Royal had bought a table for.

She briefly thought about tracking down R.J. and asking for a sperm specimen from him with no strings or child support attached. Genetically they seemed to make a pretty good baby. But that was only a fleeting thought. His new wife probably wouldn't like the idea and even if he agreed to do it she knew it would cost too much one way or another.

Over the next several months she read about conception methods and surrogate parenting. She even considered adoption. She figured there were enough married couples trying to get a baby that couldn't that she probably wouldn't stand a very good chance of getting one as a single parent. And she really did want a baby, not an older child.

She had really fond memories of Rusty as a baby. She'd loved nursing him. It had been a very special time for her even with those middle of the night feedings when she felt that no one else in the whole world was up but her. This time she would nurse as long as she liked. There would be no R.J. to tell her that "those things belong to me, get him off of them!" She had loved bathing him and putting baby lotion all over his soft, smooth skin. And the smell. Was there anything like the smell of a freshly bathed and powdered baby. And the feel. Holding a naked baby next to your naked body in the shower trying to wash you both without dropping anything, especially the baby. Or holding a baby in a soft cloth diaper, before it starts to get warm and soggy. This was what she wanted...another baby.

Chapter 7

1985

The more she thought about it, the more she liked the idea of artificial insemination. She decided to go one step further and talk with her gynecologist, Dr. JoAnne Kimber. Dr. Kimber was in her early thirties. She was spunky and outgoing and she almost always had a big smile on her rather round face. She was a bit on the heavy side even though she was constantly dieting and her black hair already had quite a few gray strands woven through it. She had a sweet motherly demeanor and everybody thought she was the greatest.

When Jenny met Joanne several years earlier she had liked her right away, it was nice to visit a doctor who didn't rush you in and out. She always took time to explain things thoroughly and cared very much about her patients and their families. Once when Jenny was there for a checkup Dr. Kimber came into the examining room with tears overflowing her eyes and running down her cheeks. The previous patient had terminal cancer which could have been detected early enough to cure if she had not waited two years to come in for a pap smear. It was apparently tearing her up to watch one of her young patients die and not be able to do anything to help her.

One day in June, Jenny went for her annual check up and broached the idea of having another baby to Dr. Kimber. Jenny was not prepared for the bubbling enthusiasm Joanne displayed. She was so excited at the prospect that you'd think she was going to be the mother. When, in fact, she would actually be the father, so to speak. They talked it all out and went over the pros and cons and costs. This was not something her health insurance would cover.

It was pretty easy really. A donor would be selected from a questionnaire she filled out. The sperm donors were generally interns, residents and other medical professionals associated with

Georgetown Medical Center who needed money for their next Mercedes payment. She could specify a lot of things: level of education, height, weight, religion, nationality, hair and eye coloring, skin coloring and even some introvert or extrovert personality traits. As an added bonus, tests were done on prospective donors so that any serious medical problems that could be passed on to the next generation would be detected. Once the sperm was obtained all Dr. Kimber had to do was inject it into Jenny. When Jenny left her office she was so excited. This was all becoming real. She could really do this.

During the next few months she charted her basal temperature every morning before getting out of bed. This would determine when she was the most fertile. The highs and lows would be examined by Dr. Kimber and these, along with a few other symptoms Jenny would pay attention to, would determine the day they would attempt to *father* a child. One of those symptoms was called "ferning", because the mucus gathering around the vagina would become more elastic and sticky and resembled a fern when looked at under the microscope. This ferning occurred a week to ten days before a woman's period, when she was the most fertile and the most bitchy. And judging by the population, the most attractive. Another reminder to Jenny that in nature's scheme of things men really were attracted to the women who treated them the worst. She sometimes felt this was why she was still single, she was just too darned nice!

Dr. Kimber determined that her next most fertile day would be August 4th. The sperm had already been ordered based on her answers to the questions. She requested her donor be college educated, tall, medium build, average weight, Christian, German or English ancestry so the baby would look a little like Rusty with his Teutonic heritage, and blonde or light brown hair with green or blue eyes to look a little like her.

Jenny decided not to tell anyone what she was planning to do. She didn't want to feel she had to give progress reports to her friends and family and she was a little afraid she might get some opposition, especially from her family—her sister in particular.

And then there was the chance this wouldn't work and everybody's hopes would have been raised for nothing.

The money she needed to pay for the procedure and the sperm bank was just sitting in her savings account. It really wouldn't get too expensive unless she had to be inseminated many times. If it came to that she could always stop for awhile until she saved more money. But she didn't even see that as a problem, business had been very good lately.

The longer she stayed at Royal the easier her job was getting. She was building up a client list of referrals and repeat customers that was the envy of all the other salesmen. She had customers that came back year after year and whole families who wouldn't even think of buying a car without her advice.

There was one family, the Cranes, who had bought their first car from her about the time Royal had opened in 1976. At the time the husband worked for Mobil Oil somewhere out by Manassas, VA. They had three children, all in middle school, so the wife stayed home to manage them. They were an adorable couple. He was very handsome and she was as cute as could be. They were devoted to each other and to their kids. They were struggling to get his career established. He had a PhD in some Geological Science having to do with petroleum discovery or something like that. Their first car from her was a badly needed station wagon, and since their only car had broken down in Manassas and had to be towed to the dealership to be used as a trade-in, she loaned them her demo until they could get a deal worked out. They never forgot how well she treated them and that she gave them a good deal without all the hassles. Over the next nine years they bought over forty cars from her. She watched their family grow and change as Dr. Crane started his own petroleum analysis company, sold it for millions a few years later, and then was hired back to run it again for millions more. She watched as they moved from a modest house in Herndon to a mansion in McLean and she saw all three kids get shipped off to top-notch colleges all over the country. They could have purchased any kind of car they wanted, but they stayed with Pontiac and her. They were just the sweetest people.

She had a lot of customers like that. It wasn't at all unusual to see the same last name on the delivery board two and three times a month as mothers and fathers, brothers and sisters, nieces, nephews, in-laws and ex-laws were sent in to see the "down-to earth, honest and extremely caring" car salesperson that their relative or friend had found. As her repeat business and referral business grew, the time she had to spend on the showroom floor taking "ups" diminished, until finally she was no longer required to wait on the new floor traffic coming in.

Jenny was really enjoying her job more and more because it was like coming to work to share her time with old friends. There was hardly any negotiating to do anymore. She was so well trusted. The most difficult days were the ones where she couldn't match up the stock on hand to the customer and had to spend hours locating the perfect car or truck and then arranging to have it brought in. There was one customer in particular that almost drove her up the wall. Royal never seemed to have the exact car he was looking for in stock...he was so picky.

Chapter 8

1985

Dr. David Sandler was driving his new Trans Am around the Beltway towards Royal Pontiac. He had noticed a slight vibration in the steering and was wondering if there might be something wrong with the tires. He had called ahead and as usual the service department was waiting for him when he pulled into the lane. After chatting a little with his service advisor he made his way to the showroom to find his salesperson.

His salesperson. Lord, he wished that were true. Over the last six years he had bought or leased ten cars from Jenny Miller and had been responsible for the sale of eight more to friends and relatives including his wife, Linda. He had gotten to know Jenny real well, in fact, he fancied himself to be secretly in love with her. He admired her very much. She had come a long way in a male-dominated business and she had accomplished it without sacrificing any of her integrity. He spotted her across the showroom floor talking with other salesmen. There was no mistaking her very shapely legs. He had dreams about them almost nightly.

When she spotted him in the doorway to her office she smiled brightly and walked across the showroom floor, the light staccato of her heels echoing in the large area.

"David! How nice to see you! You aren't having problems with that new Trans Am already are you?" He was so particular about his cars, that the shop had a penciled in appointment for him every Tuesday.

"I thought I felt a slight vibration or shimmy in the steering wheel so they're checking it out for me now. How about a cup of coffee, my treat?"

She thought about it for a moment. She hated to leave the sales area during her shift. It could cost her a sale, or at the very least, part of one should she have to split a deal with another salesman. But Dr. Sandler was one of her best customers. What the heck. "Okay, but you know the drill. I have to check out first with the up desk and the switchboard." She stepped into her office, picked up the phone and dialed the operator then she dialed the up desk, she told them both that she'd be gone for 15-20 minutes.

The only coffee they had on the premises aside from the personal pots upstairs for the general offices, was a machine. Since it didn't brew one cup at a time it was invariably too strong for anyone but the caffeine-addicted mechanics. Any frequent visitor knew that the best place to get a fresh cup of good coffee was at Angie's, a short walk across the Used Car lot to the office building next door. In the basement of the building next to a cargo loading ramp was a little deli and grocery shop run by a Korean woman and her son. Her name was Angie or at least that's what everyone called her. Angie called Jenny "Preety Lady" and always stopped what she was doing to wait on her.

While David and Jenny walked across the lot he asked about her family and her son. She told him how well Rusty was doing in a summer day camp program and that he was getting a beautiful tan from his daily swimming lessons. She asked about his wife, Linda, and he shrugged the question off, mumbling something about her finding new ways to spend money everyday. He never liked talking about his wife and she sensed that all was not well at home. So instead she asked him about his work. That brought a sparkle to his eyes and he proceeded to tell her about a convention he was asked to speak at in Orlando, Florida. He was a very prominent psychiatrist whose speciality was hypnotherapy. He had even written a few books on hypnotism that were published a few years ago.

When they walked into Angie's store, Angie was restocking shelves. She hurriedly dropped the boxes she was stacking and scampered over to the counter. With her high pitched voice she exclaimed "Preeeety Lady with very handsome man."

Being as forward as Angie always was she looked at David and said " You ask Preety Lady out for date?"

David laughed out loud while Jenny blushed deeply. Then Jenny replied, "Angie, you've seen Dr. Sandler here before. He's one of my customers and he's married. Married men are not supposed to date."

She helped herself to a cup of coffee while David grabbed two muffins and a cup of coffee for himself. He paid Angie the amount she asked for and then he gave her a five dollar tip and winked at her.

They returned to Jenny's office to enjoy their muffins and coffee and to wait for word from the service department about the status of David's car. David never tired of looking at all the awards on every wall of Jenny's office. He was very proud of her and he felt that several of the salesman of the month awards had been due to his efforts. Anytime anyone even mentioned the words "car" or "truck" he made sure they had her business card in their hand and he talked her up as if she were family.

Two years ago he had talked his wife into getting a Bonneville SSEi instead of the BMW she wanted. That had been the hardest deal he'd ever helped Jenny to get. Linda was no fool. As soon as she saw Jenny she knew that the reason her husband spent so much time and effort promoting her had nothing to to do with him finding a "truly honest car salesman." She had made that car buying experience hell for both of them. She had insisted on several test drives in all the high line cars and trucks even knowing that it would be the Bonneville she would have to settle for. Then she refused every color combination available insisting on one she had seen at her country club.

When Jenny had finally located one in Richmond and had arranged to have it driven up, she refused it when she saw it, saying it wasn't as pretty as she had remembered. Then she changed her mind about the sunroof, someone told her that they leaked, even though Jenny assured her that they did not. Finally, David told her to pick out an SSEi that was on the lot or he'd bring home a Sunbird and that would be her new car. She had promptly selected a white one with a tan leather interior and a sunroof.

The Service Director came to the door of Jenny's office and announced that David's car was ready. They had made some type of adjustment that he explained in such a way that neither one of them understood it. Entirely too technical. Something about "framping a rachetting sprocket." It sounded like nonsense to Jenny, and it was. The Service Director knew that you didn't tell your best customer that the only thing wrong with his car was the driver.

Chapter 9

Fairfax, VA. August 1985

Dr. Sandler ushered his last patient of the day out of his office, a kindly elderly gentleman who had recently killed his wife. Mr. Benton Riviera, a retired banker, had come to see Dr. Sandler five months earlier to get some relief from the insomnia he was having.

Benton Riveria could no longer stand to watch his beloved wife of 55 years linger in the throes of death in her private hospital room, so one night he had released one of her hands from the restraining straps and held it tightly in his before wrapping it around the IV tube and jerking it down causing the IV holder to fall against her breathing tube and disengage it. As he turned and took one last look at her she had managed a small smile for him and he quietly left her room, knowing that the alarm would not be heard for several minutes as the nurses station was unmanned. Everyone was at the other end of the hall watching the commotion as Santa Claus was coming off the elevator, jangling his sleigh bells and bellowing the perfunctory "Ho! Ho! Ho!"

He went home to wait for the hospital's call. There was a message on his machine when he arrived home to call them. No one ever mentioned that they all had been feeling contrite because they hadn't heard the alarm in time to save her and he didn't even ask how death had come to her. He hadn't been able to sleep at all for days. The funeral seemed to cloud his mind with doubt as to whether he had done right by his Louise. When three months had passed and he still couldn't sleep or woke with nightmares when exhaustion finally made him sleep, he decided to get some help.

Dr. Sandler had come highly recommended by his health care provider and as Benton knew, he'd have to have the confidentiality of a psychiatrist in order to come clean without being prosecuted. Dr. Sandler was using therapeutic imagery to get Mr. Riviera to visualize his wife talking to him from a cloud floating in the heavens. He had achieved this by awakening his sense of smell with her favorite perfume, L'air du Temps, which he liberally sprayed around his office just before his appointments. Having him concentrate on her presence sitting on a cloud with her feet swinging over the edges, happily swaying them back and forth, he helped him to visualize her completely at peace, grateful for his help in getting her to this wonderful place where she was just relaxing and enjoying herself while she waited for him to join her. Within two sessions he was sleeping almost normally, the hypnosis helping him to forget his dreadful deed during the blackest hours of night. A few months after his wife had passed he learned that he was terminal with colon cancer.

As Dr. Sandler put Mr. Riviera in the elevator, he bid him a peaceful night's sleep saying, "sleep with the angels."

Walking back from the elevator Dr. Sandler passed a portrait of himself and his wife, Linda, taken several years ago when things were better between them and there was still so much promise ahead for their life.

When had everything unraveled so? It wasn't just her exorbitant spending, although that was beginning to be a real problem. He was beginning to begrudge her almost every dollar she spent, after all, she wasn't doing her wifely duty at all. She had failed to become pregnant the first seven years of their marriage and now after undergoing extensive testing and trying all sorts of techniques and procedures they were not any nearer to having a child than before.

The tests had shown that he was not the problem, she was. First the doctors had believed that there was a blockage in her tubes, so she had surgery to ream them out. Then, after that didn't work, they tried inseminating some of her eggs with his sperm. They tried that three times with only a failed pregnancy and over $80,000 in medical bills to show for it. Every time there was even the slightest glimmer of hope that some new procedure would work, they tried it. Not only was it very expensive but it was very emotional, and each let down pulled them further away from each other as he came to despise her for not giving him the one thing in life he really wanted, a child of his own.

Linda could sense his disappointment and displeasure in her and felt very inadequate each time they would view a pregnancy test together and see the negative result. The one time she managed to conceive, she lost the baby in the fourth month and he blamed her for it, saying she had spent too much time on her feet out shopping for the nursery and layette.

Just last year they had arranged to have a surrogate mother inseminated with his sperm. It had taken months to talk Linda into the idea and then after all the legal details had been worked out the surrogate mother had changed her mind because she had met someone who wanted to marry her and start their own family. With each set back David grew more agitated with Linda and saw less redeeming value to her as a wife. And with each set back Linda grew more despondent because she knew she was running out of time, and so she used shopping as a balm to her wounded womanly pride.

Dr. Sandler went into his office, picked up his car keys from his desk and rode the elevator down to the garage. The new 1986 Trans Am would be out soon. He wondered if Jenny had any information on it yet. He pulled out of the garage and headed towards the traffic-clogged road that would take him to Tyson's Corner and the dealership where she worked.

Chapter 10

Tyson's Corner, VA. 1985

It was time. Her time. The most fertile time. Tomorrow morning would be the most optimal time for her to conceive. The sperm had been ordered and tomorrow Dr. Kimber would attempt to become the surrogate father of her baby. That was all well and good and very exciting until Jenny happened upon a TV blaring the six o' clock news in the dealership's lunchroom. What she heard stopped her as she neared the refrigerator and she turned to look at the set mounted in the far corner. Three women in Australia had been diagnosed with the AIDS virus contracted from artificial insemination procedures, all three had used the same donor. It had been a few weeks since Rock Hudson had died from the AIDS virus and the news media was headlining any story relating to this awful disease. Jenny couldn't believe it. It hadn't even occurred to her that it could be transmitted this way, but why not? The only thing different would be a syringe instead of a penis.

The anticipation she had experienced all day quickly turned to terror. What was she going to do now? How could she go through with it, knowing it could kill her? And what of the baby if there was one? What about Rusty? He could loose his mother because she was trying to become one again. The risk seemed too great, especially since it hadn't even been a consideration until this very moment. What was she going to do? The donor was probably at home now trying to do his part. Was he infected? Would he even know it if he was?

While all these thoughts were swirling around inside her head, she subconsciously heard the loudspeaker paging her name. A few minutes later the page was repeated, "Jenny Miller, showroom please, customer waiting." She shook off the fog that had descended over her and turned off the TV. Walking back to the showroom she told herself she would think about her dilemma later, right now she had to put a cheery smile on her face and greet one of her customers. As she turned the corner from the hallway she realized that even if this customer bought ten cars tonight, it really wouldn't cheer her up any.

Jenny scanned the showroom until she saw the familiar face inside the Trans Am grinning at her. "David, how nice to see you, what a surprise! To what may I owe the honor of this visit? I hope you're not having another problem with the Trans Am?"

He stepped out from behind the wheel and reached for her hand. It was a bit formal for them, but he so wanted to touch her. "I thought I'd drop by and see if you have any information on the '86 Trans Ams, I know mine is only a few months old, but I want to see what the changes will be."

She turned and called over her shoulder, "Follow me, we don't have the new Pontiac brochures yet, but I've got the new 'Car and Driver' and it has a write up on it, it's really sharp looking. Wait 'til you see what they've done to the front end."

They sat side by side in chairs facing the front of her desk as she had never liked having a barrier between herself and her customers. Flipping through the magazine, a thought came to her. David was a psychiatrist and apparently a very good one, judging from the cars he was always buying, maybe she could ask his opinion. She really needed someone to talk to about this and who better to pour your troubles out to than a psychiatrist?

She suggested that they take a walk around the lot to look at some of the 1986 cars that had already arrived. There were no Firebirds yet, but he could get an idea of some of the new colors available. It was a beautiful evening and the lot lights made the hoods of the cars shine and the windshields glow with an iridescence that reminded her of those very expensive champagne glasses you could buy at Bloomingdales.

While he was admiring a particularly bright red Grand Prix, she turned to him and asked, "David, would you mind if I confided a problem to you? I don't know who to talk to about this and it's just tearing me up."

"Of course not," he replied. "What is it? I'd like to help if I can."

She explained about her desire to have another child and the steps she had taken so far and then she told him about the newscast and her new-found doubts. He asked her a lot of questions about the procedure and the screening process and she answered the best she could. He asked about the sperm bank she was using and all she really knew was that it was somewhere in Silver Spring, MD. He wondered out loud how the specimen would come to be at Dr. Kimber's office by 9 o'clock in the morning and she told him that the sperm bank had a courier service that would run it over very early in the morning and leave it in the laboratory box the doctor had on the front steps to her office in a townhouse office complex off of Lee Highway in Fairfax.

After much discussion, he told her that she should call her doctor tonight and express her concerns to her and see what she had to say. Since she was an OB/GYN he knew that she would be accessible to her answering service at this late hour. Jenny agreed that would be a good idea, so they went back to her office to place the call. Fifteen minutes later they heard her paged for a phone call and David left her office to give her some privacy. He didn't go far though, just to the next office which happened to be unoccupied. Since the offices on the showroom didn't have ceilings the sound carried from one to the next, he angled his head so he could just make out what she was saying.

When he heard her hang up he came back around to her office. She looked up at him and smiled. God, she was so beautiful, he wanted so much to hold her. He cocked his eyebrow up in a questioning way and she gestured for him to take a seat across from her.

"She said that there was no easy test that could be done to determine if the donor was infected, and even if there was he's not required to take it, however she said that she was going to call the sperm bank and have them call the donor and screen him. She said that there were several pertinent questions that they could ask that would determine his vulnerability to the disease. If his answers are all negative, then the odds are greatly in our favor and she would have no qualms about going ahead with the procedure. She said she'd call me later at home once she heard back from them."

"So, what are you going to do, providing the donor checks out, of course?" he queried.

"I guess I'll go through with it. At this point I'm too emotionally involved not to," she replied. She walked with him through the showroom and then out to his car. "Thank you so much for listening to me. You don't know how much it means to me to be able to talk to somebody about this. I'll let you know what happens."

"You'd better," he replied, and then added, "maybe I'll get to be the kid's godparent."

She answered him in her best southern accent, "Why sure thing. Any ol' thing for you." She turned and walked back to the showroom in a much better frame of mind than she had the right to be in. Tomorrow could be the beginning of something or the end of something. It was time to go home and do some serious praying.

Chapter 11

That Same Evening

Sibley Hospital, Silver Spring. MD.

Dr. David Sandler entered the hospital through the emergency room doors and made his way through the long halls making all the necessary turns until he came to an office door labeled Brian Lister, M.D. right next to the laboratory department. He hadn't expected Brian to be in his office when he had called him from his car phone, but as luck would have it, he was way behind in his paperwork and was working late.

David knocked on the door and then entered. Finding Brian asleep at his desk with his head on top of his crossed arms caused him to smile. It was always like this when they had roomed together at GW. Brian always had good intentions of studying late into the night, but the tediousness of studying almost always put him out like a light. He was just not a late night person and that's probably why he chose to be a blood specialist instead of a clinical doctor doing long overnight stints.

David tapped him on his shoulder and Brian jerked upright like a student caught napping. "Wha...oh, it's you, how are ya?"

David replied, "Just fine. Things couldn't be better. Well, that's not exactly true but you know that old story. Still can't stay up past eight eh?"

"I've been working on budgets and projections and all that other garbage they make you do around here and you know how I can't handle that numbers stuff. I wish they'd just leave me alone to run the lab and hire someone else to do this mind-numbing tripe. What brings you around? I haven't seen you since last year's Heart Ball."

David pulled a chair up to the overflowing desk, shaking his head as a quiet commentary to the disorganization. "I need some help from you. What can you tell me about artificial insemination?"

"What can I tell you? You should be the expert on it by now!" Brian exclaimed.

David calmly responded in a matter of fact tone. "I know about the collecting and distributing of the sperm from the male and female aspects. What I don't know is what happens after the sperm is ejaculated into a cup and before it's injected into the vagina. Like how long can the sperm live out in the open? I'd always heard that they died with exposure to the air, but I know that's not exactly true since I've donated for Linda several times. And how is it prepared for transport? Is it refrigerated, frozen or what?" David leveled a stern look at Brian and said, " and do me a favor, don't ask why I want to know, okay? Just answer the questions."

Brian Lister sat back in his chair and started his dissertation on the collection and storage of the sperm specimen, even going so far as to retrieve several blood collection vials from the phlebotomy room for his presentation. After a few more questions and some general comments on life in general they agreed to get together soon and David rose to leave. He picked up the vials from the corner of the desk and put them in his blazer pocket, never even considering to ask if he could take them.

"Thanks Bry, good luck with the budget", he called out as he closed the door behind him. He strolled to the car, fingering the vials in his pocket.

When he got home he went straight from the elaborate foyer, up the grand staircase and down the hall to the master bedroom, closing the door behind him as he heard Linda coming out of the kitchen calling his name.

He grabbed a magazine from his nightstand drawer and went into the bathroom, locking the door behind him. He had done this many times for Linda, now he was going to do it for Jenny. Just the thought of her thighs spread to receive his seed made him quiver and the task did not require anywhere near the time that it normally did.

Very early the next morning he was sitting in his car waiting in the parking lot of the professional center where Jenny's doctor's office was. It was a group of townhouses clustered together and they all looked exactly the same on the outside except for the neat little shingles over the doors announcing which business was which.

On the stoop outside of Dr. Kimber's office was a small silver box just like the kind they used to deliver milk in years ago. He knew that the laboratory companies used these so they could pick up specimens after office hours and he was sure that this was where the sperm bank had been instructed to leave their package. He waited for the courier sent by the sperm bank to come and place a package in the box and then leave before he quickly went up the steps and opened the box.

He found a small Styrofoam box which he opened then hurriedly switched the vial nestled in the hollowed out niche with the one he had in his pocket and got back into his car. It was so early that no one else was around but he had been a little nervous about being able to make the switch before other workers arrived. He breathed a long drawn-out sigh and then drove to his office savoring the idea of having extra time to contemplate the conception of his child that would occur at 9 o'clock that morning.

Chapter 12

The Next Morning

Fairfax, VA August 1985

Jenny parked her car in front of the row of townhouses that served as offices for several medical professionals affiliated with Fairfax Hospital, just a few blocks away. She had been awake since 4 am finalizing her decision and dealing with her anxiety. Dr. Kimber had called around 11 last night and they had discussed the situation. The screening couldn't have been any better, the donor was heterosexual and had always been, there had been no blood transfusions in his past and he'd never been out of the contiguous United States. Her fears had been alleviated somewhat and she had thanked Dr. Kimber profusely for all the trouble she had put her through.

She was the first patient to sign in and actually had to wait for the doctor to arrive. After she was ushered into the examining room she put on the prerequisite gown and sat on the edge of the table. She wondered where the male counterpart to her egg was at this very moment, in the refrigerator maybe? Oh, that would be incredibly cold. She also wondered about the donor and what kind of person he might be. It had been explained to her and she had signed papers to the effect that she could never find out who he was. His identity would always be protected by the sperm bank. But she still wished she could meet him for just a few moments to see if he was the kind of guy she'd want to have a child with. Oh well, this was it, even if she chickened out now she'd still have to pay five hundred dollars for the specimen.

When she heard Dr. Kimber's knock she jumped. Dr. Kimber was all smiles and eagerness. "Good morning, Jenny. All set to conceive that baby of ours?" She sat down and produced a vial from her pocket. "Here's the Daddy!" Jenny held the vial in her hand, marveling at it's smallness. In this purple-capped tube was life, the other half of the life that she was going to provide. "Don't worry about it being cold, I'll warm the syringe in my hands. Would you like to see the actual spirochetes? I have to put some on a slide to make sure that they are still viable." "Sure," said Jenny. Dr. Kimber inserted a tiny swab into the vial, recapped it, and smeared the swab on a glass slide. She put it under the microscope, made some adjustments and then turned on the light. "Look at those suckers go!" She exclaimed. "Here, hurry before the heat kills them." Jenny jumped off the table and peered through the lens. She saw what seemed to be hundreds of little tiny tadpoles, squirming around and bumping into each other in a frantic race to find something. This was so exciting!

"Come on let's get you situated and give these guys something to go for!" While Jenny got back up on the table and positioned herself with her feet in the stirrups, Dr. Kimber got the syringe ready. "Here we go!" She called as she placed the syringe and pulled the plunger. Jenny felt a wet sensation that was similar to her monthly flow trickling down, only this was going up. She willed the sperm to swim, hoping that the absolute best one would get there first. "Survival of the fittest" had a whole new meaning to her today. Dr. Kimber instructed her to remain lying down for twenty more minutes keeping her legs elevated and her pelvis tucked under, then she could go about her day. It would be nine days before they would know if they had been successful.

Chapter 13

Fairfax, VA. September 1985

Two weeks later Jenny called David to let him know that she wasn't pregnant. Dr. Kimber felt that they had probably missed the window of opportunity by only a day. Next month they would divide the specimen and inject two days in a row. All in all she was very optimistic and tried to reassure Jenny that this was not all all unusual, in fact four to five times was more likely the norm. Jenny didn't have to tell David, but she felt she should since she had made him aware of the attempt. He seemed extremely disappointed and asked her if she was going to keep trying. She told him she could afford to try three or four more times before she'd have to wait until she could save up some more money. He made her promise to let him know exactly when she was going to try again under the auspices of praying at the precise time she was inseminated.

So, it was to be Labor Day weekend this time, how appropriate. Since the donor was scheduled to be out of town that weekend the sperm bank had to arrange to have the specimen collected Thursday evening and then frozen. Since it was to arrive frozen they delivered it Friday morning instead of Monday morning when it would be needed. Jenny had relayed all this to David Wednesday afternoon on his answering machine at work, since his secretary was off and he didn't answer the phones on Wednesdays. He didn't actually get the message until Thursday so he had to act fast. He called Brian and asked him how they froze sperm specimens for use later and ended up having to go back to Sibley to get the proper container that Brian had secured for him.

Thursday night found him back in his bathroom, book in hand, and something else in the other one, literally. He used the freezer in the garage where he kept the fish he caught on his boat. It wouldn't do for Linda to discover it. She'd probably seen enough of these specimen containers in the last few years to recognize it immediately. He wouldn't want to answer the questions that would present.

Friday, before the sun was up he was sitting in his car again, down the street from the doctor's office. He hoped he wouldn't have to do this too many more times.

Chapter 14

Ocean City, MD September 1985

Jenny decided to take Rusty away with her for the weekend. Her parents could use a break from babysitting and she desperately needed to see the Ocean. Since it was after Labor Day, the hotels had out of season rates so it wouldn't be very expensive. She packed the pregnancy test that she could have taken a day ago, but she wanted to give it a little more time, thinking that would make the difference between positive and negative. She was doing a lot of wishful thinking lately.

They arrived at The Carousel at the north end of the beach late Friday afternoon. Since Rusty had slept most of the way there he was very anxious to get down to the beach. Jenny carried the huge bag of beach toys that his grandparents had purchased for him earlier that summer and a cup full of champagne and a book for her. Her love for champagne was part of the legacy that R.J. had left her with. The irony was that now she couldn't afford the Veuve Clicquots, Mumms Cordon Rouge, Moet & Chandon White Star or Tattingers. Now it was Domaine Ste. Michelle at best, but Andre or Taylor State were more likely.

The water was delightfully warm and the vista was as calming as a mother's lullaby. Soon the stresses from work and the problems of day to day living were gone. They were taken away by the waves or the champagne, she didn't know which. She just knew she was enjoying watching her son and he was enjoying just being with her.

They had dinner in the restaurant next to the lounge and when the music got so loud they couldn't even talk, they went upstairs to their room and watched TV until Rusty fell asleep. She carried him to the full-sized bed and tucked him in. Then she finished the bottle of champagne she had started that afternoon, reasoning that if she found out tomorrow that she was pregnant, she'd just have to pour it down the drain. Sometimes when you drink the reasoning processes become very self-serving.

She woke up so early the next morning that there wasn't even a line of light showing where the draperies didn't quite meet. She fished in her suitcase for her pregnancy test, reread the directions for the sixth time and headed for the bathroom. She collected her first urine of the day, carefully applied some to the cardboard treated stick, placed everything on the counter as directed, left the bathroom and closed the door so she wouldn't be tempted to cheat and look before it was time.

Then she waited and waited and paced and paced. When it was time, she was afraid to open the door. Finally she reasoned that she'd better find out now so that if it was negative she could have her crying jag and be over and done with it before Rusty woke up. She slowly opened the door as if she'd expected someone to come out and yell, "Yes, Yes, you are, you are!" There was no sound at all just a big blue dot staring at her and it's message was loud and clear "Yes! Yes! You are! You are!"

She picked up the stick and stared at it in wonder, deliriously happy and wanting to wake up the world to share her good news. That's when it really dawned on her that that's what this was, her good news, her baby, she was on her own with this one. All the responsibility would be hers. She felt a little lonely and went to cuddle with Rusty.

Chapter 15

Herndon, VA September 1985

Jenny sat on the floor of one of the upstairs bedrooms, staring at the walls and trying to envision what the nursery should look like. This time the nursery was going to be ready long before the baby came home from the hospital. She had promised herself that while she was driving Rusty and herself home from the beach. She had called Dr. Kimber first thing that Monday morning and had been instructed to high tail it over to the Hospital lab to get a blood test.

Why was it that doctors never believed the results of over-the-counter pregnancy kits? That test was positive also and Dr. Kimber was ecstatic. She told Jenny she should change her name to Fertile Myrtle and giggled herself silly as she rummaged through a supply closet for prenatal vitamin samples to give her.

While Jenny was driving home she thought about who she should tell next, and of course, that was her parents. She drove to their home in Sterling, even though she had just left there a few hours ago when she dropped Rusty off on her way to the doctor's office. She was scheduled to work the 3 to 9 shift, so she still had plenty of time.

Her mother, Mildred, was the best homemaker you could imagine. Her house was always spotless and there was always delicious food ready to be served at the drop of a hat. She was a loving mother and a doting grandmother. Everyone just adored her. She managed to personally stay in touch with everyone on her side of the family and her husband's even though they were both from very large families and also with practically anybody she or her husband had ever worked with.

She was always sending out birthday cards, anniversary cards and get-well cards. Her Christmas card list would probably rival the White House's.

When Jenny and her siblings were growing up, Jenny's mom always had a job outside the home to supplement their income, but still the house was always clean, the food was always served on time, and on Sunday night there would always be a big family dinner that would include lots of relatives. She was a dynamo and didn't rest until all the work was done, no matter the task. It wasn't until Jenny's parents had retired and moved to Florida that she had started to run out of work long before she ran out of daytime. She was a fantastic woman. A super mom long before the words had been coined.

She loved children, all children. It didn't matter if they were smeared from head to toe in their own excrement, she would take them and hold them tight, clean them up and rock them to sleep and never want to put them down. In retrospect, she would have made a great pre-K or Kindergarten teacher, or even a neonatal nurse, but instead she followed her husband from duty station to duty station taking jobs with the local civil service offices as a clerk or secretary. She never aspired to elevate herself in any job, she knew her real jobs were wife and mother.

So Jenny knew she'd be extremely happy about this baby. The challenge would be to keep her from running for her crochet needles. She pulled into the driveway, got out the key to her parents house and walked into a kitchen that smelled of chocolate chip cookies.

"Mom, where are you?" Jenny called.

"Down in the playroom!" was the answer she heard coming back to her.

Jenny went through the kitchen to the basement door and down the stairs to what everyone referred to as "the Sterling Park annex to Toys R Us." There on the floor was her mom and Rusty amid a pile of Transformer toys. Rusty had it all, Pound Puppies, and not just one—the whole set, all the plush Sesame Street characters, balls, puzzles, books and Disney movies galore. Whatever toy fad was the rage Rusty had it as soon as it arrived in the stores.

Once, her mom had stood in line at a toy store for over three hours at Christmas time just to win a *chance* to buy a Cabbage Patch baby that Rusty had seen on TV. She still suffers back twinges from that episode.

"What are you doing home so early, forget what shift you're working?" her mom asked.

Jenny said, "No, I have to go in tonight, I just had a few errands to run this morning. Got a minute to talk?"

"Sure," her mom said and Jenny helped her get up off the floor.

"How would you feel about Rusty getting a brother or sister sometime next summer?" she asked her mom with a wide smile on her lips. Jenny watched her mother's face as it took her a few moments to understand what she was saying.

Her mom was stunned and didn't know exactly what to say. The word "Who?" came to mind but she didn't think she should ask. She just hugged her daughter tight and simply said, "a baby..." and then sighed happily.

Jenny walked upstairs with her mother and over a cup of tea she explained everything. Over the next week she would explain it several more times but not once was she prepared for the reaction she got from her sister, Jean.

They had a big family dinner on Sunday and Jenny took that opportunity to take her sister aside to tell her the news. When Jenny told Jean she was going to have a baby, Jean was quite surprised. When Jenny told her sister how the baby had been conceived, she was shocked and she even seemed to be mad at Jenny.

At first Jenny thought Jean might be a bit jealous, because she and her second husband weren't able to have a child together because of a vasectomy he'd had years before they'd even met each other. But that wasn't like Jean, she was always able to sincerely enjoy everyone else's accomplishments and good fortune.

She pressed her sister for an explanation of her rather standoffish attitude saying, "I've never seen you like this before. What is it that bothers you about me having this baby?"

Jean replied, "It's not your having the baby that bothers me, you know that. It's how the baby came to be. It's not God's will to conceive a baby that way. It is scripturally unlawful for a man to spill his seed upon the ground, which is what this donor did when he masturbated into a cup!"

Jenny just stood and stared. It took her a few moments to gather her thoughts for a rebuttal and to try not to say it in a harsh way. "God gave us the technology to do this."

"He gives us technology and the ability to do lots of things, but that still doesn't mean it's right to do them just because we know how to. We still have to search out his will for us and this is something I don't believe he sanctions. If he wanted you to have another child he would have provided you with a husband and allowed you to conceive a baby naturally, through your union as man and wife."

Jenny thought about this. "So you think I've sinned against God by taking a different avenue than the one prescribed biblically?"

"Yes," Jean replied, " I do."

"Well I haven't sinned!" she retorted, "the donor did! If anything I kept his seed from being 'spilled on the ground' and wasted!"

Jean replied softly and with great patience, "if you hadn't contracted with him for his sperm he wouldn't even have been in the position of spilling his seed into a cup. You made him sin."

Jenny's eyes filled with tears and she flippantly replied, "So now what am I supposed to do? Undo it because I did it the wrong way?" really getting mad now, despite the tears flowing down her cheeks.

Jean's eyes got wide with terror and she reached for Jenny and grabbed her around the shoulders and hugged her tightly as she rocked her gently and admonished "No, No, of course not.

44

Don't you even think that way. The baby's hairs on its head are already numbered. God loves this baby already and so do I."

From then on Jean was Jenny's most ardent supporter and long before the baby was born, Jenny had decided that Jean would be the baby's godmother. She was a bit zealous sometimes in her religious beliefs, but that was a whole lot better than having none she supposed.

Chapter 16

Fairfax, VA September 1985

The suspense was driving him crazy. David Sandler sat at his desk twirling his Mont Blanc pen between his fingers. It had been almost three weeks since the insemination and he still didn't know whether it had taken this time or not. He'd had to keep in almost daily contact with Jenny before the second procedure to make sure of the timing so he could collect and switch the sperm again. It had been difficult to keep coming up with reasons to call her and to remind her that he wanted to be remembered the day before under the ruse of praying for her. After the deed was done he didn't know how to go about approaching her for the results. He just figured she'd call him. She should know by now. Why hadn't she called? Of course, there was really no reason she should, he was just a customer in her eyes.

He could call the hospital laboratory and get the results, if she'd had a blood test there and if he could think of a reason why a psychiatrist who wasn't her doctor needed to know. He could call her OB/GYN's office, but again what reason would he give for him needing to know. No, he'd have to wait this out. Even if she didn't call him time would tell if she was. But what if she wasn't? It was getting close to the time she would try again and he needed to be prepared. He decided he would have to call and hint around if he didn't hear anything by the weekend.

When Jenny called his office two days later he could hardly breathe. This was taking quite a toll on him emotionally. He tried to keep the nervousness out of his voice and made a joke about how many rabbits had she killed lately? She didn't understand his question right away and hesitated for a second and then it dawned on her what he meant.

"Just one," she sang happily

He almost fell out of his chair when he pushed it back to stand up. "Outstanding!" he yelled. And then added, "This is terrific! Our prayers were answered! You must be thrilled beyond belief. I know I am!"

"Yes," she replied, "I am extremely delighted."

He asked her how she was feeling and she told him never better. They talked about the new Trans Am that had come in as that had been her reason for calling. He made an appointment with her to come see it over the weekend and then ended the call with, "Make sure you get plenty of rest and eat properly. We want a healthy baby come springtime!"

She assured him that he didn't need to worry about that, she was taking excellent care of herself.

As soon as he hung up the phone he sat back down in his seat and put his forehead against the coolness of his desktop and the tears just came. He watched them drip from his cheeks to the carpet by his feet as he said over and over again, "I'm going to be a father. I'm going to be a father. I'm going to be a father." Many minutes later when he was able to regain his composure, he wiped his face and called for his next patient.

When he left his office that evening he went to the toy store just around the corner from Jenny's dealership. He strolled up and down the baby aisles until he found something he thought she would like for the baby, a soft pillow shaped like a sports car with a set of plastic keys attached with velcro to a steering wheel in its center. Then he went to Clyde's Restaurant a few blocks away, sat at the bar and had a few drinks to congratulate himself before going home to Linda.

Chapter 17

Fairfax Hospital, VA June 1, 1986

Jenny's baby girl was born at 6:26 am. It was an easy and natural delivery, a perfect culmination to a wonderful pregnancy. When she was awakened by cramping so severe that she couldn't stand up straight she called her parents, and then Dr. Kimber. Since it was early on a Sunday morning, her Dad stayed at her house with Rusty while her mother drove her to the hospital. She had taken natural child birthing classes and that was a very good thing because by the time she arrived at the hospital she was too far along for any pain relievers to have had time to work before the baby was to arrive.

When Jenny had arrived at the hospital the nurses on duty examined her and called Dr. Kimber at home to report that Jenny was fully effaced and that the head was visible. Jenny's mom was sent to scrub up since she was Jenny's partner from the Lamaze classes. Meanwhile, Jenny was using several different breathing techniques trying to keep from pushing to allow Dr. Kimber time to arrive and get prepped. As it was, she just made it. Jenny delivered a beautiful baby girl just twenty-six minutes after arriving at the hospital.

As soon as the baby was placed in her arms Jenny kissed her forehead and then she and her mom examined her, marveling at her tiny perfect body. She had a birthmark at the base of her throat that was slightly red and after receiving Dr. Kimber's assurances that it was nothing to worry about Jenny stroked it lightly, thinking that it was nice to have a distinguishing mark so she'd always be able to tell her apart from all the other beautiful baby girls in the world. The slight imperfection was actually a welcome one as she remembered all the stories she'd heard over the years about babies being switched in the hospital maternity wards. She'd know if hers was, instantly.

As if on cue with her thoughts, a neonatologist arrived to whisk the baby away. She had to go to the neonatology intensive care unit because there had been some meconium in the placental waters and they wanted to make sure her lungs were not affected. So while Dr. Kimber was delivering the placenta and making sure Jenny was not having any abnormal bleeding, Jenny marveled at the beauty and completeness of nature. This remarkable process of childbirth was as timeless as the hills, but each time she had phased through it she felt like she was the only one who had ever done it in exactly that way.

Both of her childbirth experiences had been so different but so uniquely special. She knew she'd remember them always as the happiest times of her life. She looked up at her mother and smiled. Her mom squeezed her hand with one of her own and wiped at her tears with her other one.

"A precious little girl! What are we going to call her?" she asked.

Jenny replied without hesitation, she'd known almost from the beginning what the names would be for both a boy or a girl. "Paisley. I've always loved paisley designs. It's quite unique don't you think? Paisley Jean. We can call her P.J. for short if she really hates it when she's older."

Her Mom, never being one to interfere with the decisions of her adult children, just nodded her head and repeated the name several times trying to get the feel of it. "Paisley... Paisley... Paisley, okay, I like that. Paisley it is." And so it was.

Chapter 18

Fairfax Hospital, VA June 1, 1986

There she was, at long last. His daughter. His baby girl. His progeny, she was made of his flesh and blood. His seed had done this. He was in awe of her and he itched to hold her, to somehow touch her and feel her smooth soft skin with his fingertips.

How he came to be standing here outside the nursery window on the exact day of her birth was quite a fait accompli. After anguishing over how to find out about the baby's birth as soon as possible, he'd come up with a brilliant idea. Who would know about the baby's birth the soonest? Why the Grandmama, of course!

During Jenny's seventh month he'd called Mrs. Fleming, having had the phone number from a long time ago when it had been listed on one of Jenny's business cards when she'd lived with them for awhile after her divorce. He'd explained who he was, supposing Jenny had told her of one of her best customers, which indeed she had. He then conveyed his desire to surprise her with a unique baby gift. He wanted to present her with a copy of every major cities' newspaper for the exact date the child was born. Something the child could look at in years to come to see what was happening in the world on the day of its birth.

He told her that in order to do this he would need to know about the baby's birth as soon as possible so he could drive downtown to one of the newsstands that carried papers from all over the country. In the case of a late night delivery, he would need to call and order copies to be saved for him. Would she be so kind as to notify him at home or at the office as soon as the baby had arrived? She had said she'd be delighted to and wrote down all his phone numbers, including his car phone number. He swore her to secrecy and thanked her for helping him with his surprise for Jenny, his favorite car salesman.

He had received the call at 7:30 in the morning, just an hour after her birth. Linda had wanted to know who had called so early on a Sunday morning and he had replied, "Just somebody from the newspaper. I complained about it coming so late in the morning so they're going to start delivering ours first on their route starting next week. Meanwhile I guess I'd better go buy one if I want to read it with breakfast." With that said, he got out of bed and went to the bathroom to shower and dress before leaving for the newsstand.

He had already checked out the visiting hours for Fairfax Hospital and had found out that visitors would not be allowed to see the babies until 7:00 pm. So he spent the day at his office catching up on some paperwork waiting for the time to come when he could see his daughter. He wondered if she had a name yet and was sadly reminded that she would not have his name.

During Jenny's pregnancy he had tried to visit her at least once a week using some pretense or another to just show up at the dealership. His love for Jenny grew just as her belly grew and he yearned to be more than just a client or confidante. He made several awkward attempts to try to put their relationship on a more personal level but each time he suggested a date of sorts it sounded to his ears like he was interested in having a tawdry affair instead.

Jenny smiled and declined all his offers saying it wouldn't be proper for them to go out alone together, adding "What would Linda say about you taking me to a movie, when you should be taking her? I'm okay going by myself, don't worry about me," she'd say innocently not picking up on his real reasons for wanting to escort her around. The trouble was she knew all about Linda and Jenny just wasn't the type to go out with a married man and he knew it. That's when he started thinking about getting Linda out of his life.

If it weren't for Linda he was sure he and Jenny could have a wonderful life together. They could be a family, he and Jenny and their baby. He wanted her. Sometimes so much that he couldn't sleep, tossing around in his king-sized bed, trying not to so much as even brush slightly against Linda's sleeping form. They hadn't been getting along for several years and their marriage had disintegrated steadily downhill with his knowledge of Jenny's pregnancy. It was as if confirming what he'd known all along.

The fault had never been his. It had always been with Linda. She couldn't even do the one thing he'd married her for and now after years of watching other fathers with their children while he had been deprived of them, he wanted out. Out of this marriage contract that had been broken by Linda when she failed to give him the one thing he wanted more than anything on earth. Jenny was giving him what he wanted, why couldn't he just have her?

Now he was standing in front of his daughter and he had no rights to touch her, to hold her as all the other fathers were doing with their babies. The irony of the paternity of this baby was tearing him apart. He could tell no one, but he still wanted to scream "I'm a father, I'm a father, I'm a father!" and "it's a girl, it's a girl, it's a beautiful baby girl!" He looked at the sleeping baby in her bassinet and spoke softly as he gently touched the glass, "One day you'll know that you're my baby girl."

He turned and walked down the hall, got on the elevator and went to the lobby. How appropriate it was that she should be born on June 1, the anniversary of his marriage to Linda. He drove home to tell her he would be divorcing her. All these years wasted on her infertility, he could only hope that he could make them up with Jenny.

Chapter 19

McLean, VA 1986

Linda had been furious when David told her he wanted a divorce. Of course, he couldn't tell her exactly why he wanted it, divorcing on the grounds of infertility would make him seem like a real cad, so he just told her he didn't love her anymore. Which was absolutely true. He couldn't even remember the last time he even had a fond feeling towards her. He thought he had loved her when he had married her, now he was even doubting that. It must've just been the idea of being in love with somebody and wanting to share the good times of raising a family together that he had been in love with.

Linda had just fit the bill at the time, she was very attractive with good social standing in the community and she had expressed a desire to have children and be a homemaker instead of having a career of her own. That had suited David just fine. He had just finished medical school and was doing his residency in the psychiatric ward at Sibley Hospital when they decided to get married. Her family was somewhat prominent in the Chevy Chase area and they had put on a lavish affair at the Sheraton Ambassador Hotel. Linda looked like all those pictures of brides you see in the papers, radiant, polished and full of youthful promise.

For Linda, David had been a most marvelous catch. He was a Doctor! And he was very handsome. He was also thoughtful, conscientious, organized and impeccably clean. There were no lingering sparks after the initial passion died, but she reasoned, you can't have everything. This was probably as good as it was going to get for her and she knew it, so when the idea of marriage was first brought up she jumped at it, before he had really even asked her properly. Her parents had been delighted to announce all over town that their daughter was marrying a doctor. They didn't mention that he had been abandoned as a child and had been reared as a ward of the state since the age of nine.

Linda wasn't taking it very well that her seemingly perfect society marriage was breaking up. She liked her life the way it was. Sleeping in late, going to lunch with one of her girlfriends and shopping at White Flint Mall before finishing with a manicure and facial at one of the toni shops on Wisconsin Avenue. Then coming home to an elegantly decorated manor in McLean, Virginia and waiting for her husband to arrive home so she could signal the staff to serve dinner in their formal dining room. Just down the hall from his study where he would retire after dinner to read, was her sitting room where she would watch TV and talk on the phone to her friends until it was time to go to bed.

She wasn't giving all this up without a huge fight. She hired one of the best firms in Washington to contest the divorce. David was granted a divorce from Linda but Linda ultimately got what she wanted; the house, a Jaguar to replace the Bonneville she had never wanted, a share of their stock portfolio, and a whopping $10,000 a month alimony payment. David got his freedom but he'd had no idea that it would cost him as much as it had.

Chapter 20

Fairfax, VA April 1987

It was quarter past two and his patient was late. Considering the fees he charged, generally his patients were early for their appointments, not late. Benton Riveria had never been late in the almost two years David had been treating him. At first they met twice a week but as Mr. Riveria had started to improve and the sleepless nights had dwindled down to less than once or twice a month, they agreed to meet once every two weeks and then only once a month.

Dr. Sandler checked the appointment calendar on the computer screen to verify that this was the right day. Then he looked up Mr. Riveria's phone number and dialed it.

After several rings it was answered by a woman with a sweet, young, timid voice, "Hello," was all she said.

"Is Mr. Riveria at home? This is Dr. Sandler, I have an appointment with him this afternoon."

There was a long moment of silence before she replied. "I'm sorry, Dr. Sandler, my father died two weeks ago, and with all that's been happening we forgot to notify you. I am very sorry about the appointment, we should have remembered. You've been extremely kind to him and we should have remembered you, especially after all you did for him after our mother's death."

David whispered hoarsely, "No, I am the one who is sorry. He was truly a remarkable man, I'm sure you must miss him greatly. He seemed to be doing so well with the cancer. Was that what took him?"

Mr. Riveria's daughter sighed deeply as if trying to hold back tears, "He died in his sleep and since the cancer was so widespread his doctor waived an autopsy. But that's the general feeling since they only gave him six months to live when he was first diagnosed over a year and a half ago. My father said he was being made to endure the pain my mother escaped from when she accidentally killed herself and cheated death of what it was due. He said he was doing a penance for her of some sort so he hardly ever took his pain medication. We finally had to administer morphine shots to him ourselves. It has been a sad time for us, first our mother and then our father, but it's good knowing that they are no longer in pain and that they are together again in heaven."

David thanked her for her time and her graciousness and said goodbye. Then he sorted through his mail and answered some letters before preparing for his next appointment, Liesel.

Liesel Palmer was one of the most fascinating cases he had ever encountered. When she had come to him she was having severe anxiety attacks, a genuine paranoia against being left alone with strangers and she could only get dressed in her closet. She was a very pretty young woman with brunette hair cropped short, framing her face and dark sparkling eyes that said she liked to laugh. She sported an all year around tan with a sprinkling of light brown freckles over her nose and checks. Her lips were almost maroon with lipstick, the only makeup she ever wore. She was slightly taller than average due to her long legs and her slender frame was filled out with generous curves just where they were supposed to be. She was the picture of hale and hearty and happy-go-lucky all at the same time, but inside she was living with the memory of a harrowing tale.

Liesel, who was named after the eldest daughter in the movie, "The Sound of Music" by her mother, who had always loved that movie, was a free lance photographer. Liesel had finally grown into her name after years of instructing everyone to pronounce it like "diesel" with an "L." Liesel had led a very privileged life and even though it was not required of her to work, her independent streak would not let her play the society role expected of her. After graduating from Stanford, she set up her own photography business operated out of her condo. She was doing very well and had built up a loyal clientele, mostly magazines and periodicals but also a few ad agencies.

Toward the end of last summer, while working on a nature layout in a remote area of Oregon, she had been kidnapped by a lone drifter who lived on the outskirts of a small lumber camp. She had been taking pictures all day of the sun shining through the treetops and the mirror-like reflections in the lake at the base of a long primitive lumber trail. Her Jeep was parked a few miles back, closer to the highway. She had hiked through the wilderness to this remote area hoping to find a pristine environment to photograph. No beer cans or discarded cigarette packs to ruin her shots. She really wasn't aware exactly how far she had hiked into the woods. She just kept looking for a magical place without any sign of human intrusion in the peaceful serenity.

Chapter 21

Oregon August 1986

When Liesel had hiked about four miles around the perimeter of the lake and then an additional mile or two up into the timberline she found the site she had been looking for. It was breathtaking with its clarity. The spectrum of the shades of green from the forest and the shades of blue from the lake and the sky mixed to create a panorama so beautiful she couldn't take pictures fast enough. After shooting two rolls of film, she was loading another when she heard a slight rustling in the underbrush behind her. It caused her to jump and the film came off the sprocket she had been feeding it onto.

"Who's there?" she called softly, wondering if it was possible that she might have trespassed onto private property. When there was no answering call she listened for any additional noises. Hearing none she turned back to her camera in time to see a vague image of a man's face just before a fist lashed out and caught her on the jaw, just below her ear. As her world went fuzzy, then black she remembered almost instinctively not to drop the camera she still held in her hand.

She came to several hours later, groggily blinking her eyes and wondering where she was and why her face hurt so badly. She tried to put her hand to her face and that's when she realized her hands were lashed to the corner supports of a bunk house bed, her boots had been removed and her ankles were also lashed to the bed. She was filled with panic and out of her throat came a deep guttural sob that did nothing but assure her that she was at least alive. She looked around at her surroundings, the terror of what had happened to her coming back accompanied by waves of nausea that she had to swallow since couldn't turn her head enough to the side to spit it out.

The ceiling reminded her of a rustic ski lodge. She could see where the timbers and beams met in a corner and a four foot width of fieldstone began and then ended. She assumed that it must be a chimney for a fireplace. The wood looked old, it was dry and dusty and the windows on the two walls she could see were grimy with soot and dirt. There were no curtains and the only thing she could see on the walls was a set of hooks with dirty clothes hanging from them. The clothes were on the wall to her left towards the corner so she could only assume that the door to this ramshackle cabin was on the same wall as the headboard of the bed, way to her left and out of range of her peripheral vision.

She was scared to death but she was also angry. Angry at herself for not telling anyone where she would be and angry because she knew better than to get herself into a situation like this. What was she going to do now and where was the person who brought her here? Where was here? As she strained against the straps that attached her wrists to the corner uprights she saw that with a little bit of effort she might be able to inch the straps up and off of the rectangular posts. After struggling for quite some time she realized that she would never be able to slip the straps off of the posts. There wasn't enough slack in the straps attached to her ankles to allow her to move her body up hardly any at all and the foot posts were at least a foot higher than those at the top of the bed. When she realized her efforts were futile she said some prayers and tried to calm down. Her head was pounding, her jaw was throbbing and she had to go to the bathroom.

Looking out the windows she could see that evening was descending and the cabin was filling with a dusky glow replacing the bright haze of the afternoon. Straining her ears she listened for any sounds and when she heard none, she began to wonder, what would be worse? If her attacker did come back or if he didn't? The idea of starving to death didn't appeal to her and she was getting very weary of being stretched out spread eagle. Her back was killing her. At least if her attacker did return she'd have some chance for escape, as it was now she had none.

When she could no longer see anything in the cabin or out the window she started crying, and when that gave her the hiccups, she started cussing and then screaming. That's when the door burst open and she could smell her jailer as he came into the cabin.

"There ain't no use to be hollerin' like thet, ain't nobody around for miles and miles, that's why I didn't gag ya, but I will if you don't shut your trap!" He walked over towards the bed, struck a match and lit the lantern that had apparently been on a table beside the bed.

She had her first glimpse of her captor as the wick caught and the flame was turned up. It was all she could do not to gag but she did scream. There in front of her was the grizzliest, dirtiest mountain man she'd ever seen. He was covered from head to wherever she could see with something that looked like sawdust covered with sweat. He reeked with putrid body odors and he had crooked teeth that looked like they had never seen a toothbrush. He smiled down at her and she saw food encrusted in his beard and mustache.

Her panic must've shown in her eyes because he sat down on the edge of the bed and took one of her hands in his rough calloused one and said, "I know I must look pretty awful but I just haven't had a reason to get spruced up 'fore now. Now thet I gots me a woman, I guess I'd best get me a bath!"

"No! No!" she cried, "I'm not your woman! Please let me go! Please. Please. I won't tell anyone what you've done. I won't press charges, I promise. Just please let me go! You can't keep me like this, people will be looking for me!"

He just stroked her fingers and shook his head, "No, not letting you go, finders keepers, losers weepers. Never had a woman I could call my own before and never saw one so doggone pretty. I got a few chores I gotta do, then I'll come back and you can show me the rest of you." With that he got up and walked out the door.

Liesel just laid there whispering, "no, no, no", softly crying into the collar of her shirt, trying in vain to find even the smallest space to crawl into to hide herself before he came back. An hour later she heard him coming back, clanking some chains together and then dropping them on the floor at the end of the bed. There was a new terror building in her. Was he a love sick mountain man or a demonic killer and how could she escape from him? He came back to the bedside and looked down at her. She timidly looked up at him hoping to establish some kind of eye contact to show she wasn't afraid, even though she was terrified.

She was astonished at his transformation, he was much younger than she originally thought. When she'd seen him before she had thought that he was in his fifties, the sawdust making his brown hair look gray. She now thought he must be in his late thirties. He had bathed, shaved and cut his hair and although she still regarded him as repulsive it amazed her that he had gone to so much trouble for her when he knew he didn't have to. That's when she decided that she would go along with his game for the time being and see if she could plan a way out, she smiled and said, "Wow, you really clean up nice."

He blushed and shrugged his shoulders. She pressed on, "I really have to go to the bathroom and my back is killing me. Do you think you could undo me so I can relieve myself?"

He walked to the end of the bed and untied her feet, and then bent over to retrieve the chain he'd deposited there a few moments earlier. To her dismay he wrapped a length of it around her waist and secured it with a padlock, putting the key in his pocket. Then he untied her hands admonishing her as he did so that if she struck out at him he'd have to tie her back up again. He helped her off the bed rubbing the small of her back as he led her out the door with the extra length of the chain used as a leash to tether her. He told her where to go to relieve herself as he wove a piece of the leather into the end of the chain to use as a grip. She had about ten feet of slack and although she didn't like the idea of him being so close while she was eliminating, she had no choice. She found a bush to hide behind and took care of matters.

As she was adjusting her shirt back into her jeans she looked all around. This was pretty much just a cabin in the woods, if it hadn't been for the circumstances she might even have enjoyed the view. It was clear that they were a long way from anywhere. Where would the closest help be? Where was it that he had gone to clean up? Were there any neighbors around here? And just where had he gone after depositing her in his bed? She had a lot of questions but no answers. She felt a gentle yank on the chain.

"Ain't ya done yet?" He called.

"Yeah, I'm coming," she mumbled.

"I brought us some dinner from the mill. I took some extra sandwiches from the mess line at lunchtime. It ain't much but you won't starve."

He led her back to the cabin and sat her down on the bed. She cringed at the slovenliness of it. There were no sheets, just a thin blanket stained in several places atop a mattress that she was glad she couldn't see. He handed her a sandwich that he had taken from the pocket of his grimy flannel jacket and if she hadn't been as hungry as she was she would have declined the offer. The condition of his jacket was bad enough but the sandwich itself looked pretty unappetizing on its own. Dried up ham and cheese on stale bread. She thought about the breakfast she should have had that morning at the hotel and regretted her haste to get out early.

While he put some logs into the fireplace she nibbled around the edges of the side that had been wrapped tightly. She was looking for a chance to flee. Her heart plummeted when he took the end of the chain and threaded it through an iron ring sunk into the fireplace. Attached to it was a bracket that was used for moving a kettle over the flame. He produced another padlock and locked the chain to itself.

"I'll be back shortly. I have to lay in some more wood. Sometimes it gets a mite chilly at night up here in the mountains even though it's still summertime. By the way, my name's Jake. What's yours?"

When she didn't answer him, he shrugged his shoulders and went outside.

A few minutes later he returned and dropped the wood onto the hearth, brushed his hands off on his already soiled jeans and turned to face her. "I think I would like to see you naked now," he said as if he was commenting on the weather.

She got up and ran towards the door, not actually getting any further than a few feet from the bed before he grabbed her and pushed her back onto the bed. He took both of her hands and started rubbing them between his.

"Since you won't tell me your name, I'm gonna call you Anna. I like that name Anna. Now Anna, I'm not going to hurt you unless you make me. I don't want to hurt you none, I just want to see all your womanly parts, and then I'll decide if'n I'm gonna court ya. I don't sees any reason for us to rush things none, it's not like you're gonna up an' go anywhere for awhile. So let's just get to know each other, one step at a time, sorta like we was datin'. Now don't be afraid. I won't hurt ya none. I'm not like that at all. I'm not the type that likes to beat on his woman. I want to take care of you proper but you gotta do what I tells you to do. All right?"

He looked down at her tear-streaked face and tilted her chin up. "Now do what I tell you and take your clothes off before I have to do it for you."

"Please don't make me do this" she sobbed. "Please. My parents are wealthy. I can call them and get you money. They'd pay you a lot of money to get me back."

He sneered at her and replied, "I don't need any money, I need a woman. I'm tired of livin' without a woman. You ain't goin' back!"

He leaned over to stroke her cheek and she turned her head away from his hand. His face turned red with anger and he yelled, "Unbutton your shirt and take it off! Now!"

She slowly moved her hand resignedly to her shirt front and with shaking fingers began to undo the buttons. She slowly inched the shirttail out of her jeans. He stared at her intently and when she hesitated he said, "go on, take it off."

She opened her shirt and eased if off her shoulders, hugging it in front of her chest. "Now the bra," he said.

Tears started cascading down her face as she reached behind her and undid the clasp, then let each strap slide off of her shoulders. He grabbed the bra and shirt from her clasped hands in front of her and tossed them aside.

When her breasts were completely exposed to his view she hung her head down letting the tears fall into her lap. He put his fingers under her chin and lifted it saying, "You've got nothing to be ashamed about darlin', your tits are beautiful. Just beautiful." He reached out to touch them and she shrank away from his touch.

He pushed her down on the bed and she screamed at him as she pounded against his chest, "No! No! Don't do this! Don't touch me, you bastard!"

He roughly rolled her over onto her stomach and straddled her just below the waist. She bucked upwards trying to get him off of her. Then his hands started massaging her lower back, working in small circles and then progressing into larger ones encompassing her whole back. He was being incredibly gentle, trying to soothe her aching back and to calm her down at the same time. The tenseness was leaving her shoulders and she was actually relaxing her muscles as he continued his slow ministrations up and down her back.

"I want to give you pleasure and I want you to be happy here with me, you'll see, it'll just take time."

He massaged her for a long time before he eased himself off of her and turned her over onto her back. He put his hands on both sides of her throat and her eyes filled with panic but all he did was stroke the sides of her neck and then her collarbones. Gradually he worked his way down to her chest, grabbing whole handfuls of her breasts and gently squeezing them and pushing them together. He rubbed his thumbs back and forth across her nipples. He savored the feel of them, enjoying himself immensely. When it seemed that he didn't want to stop his fondling of her breasts and he wasn't trying to progress any lower she opened her eyes and looked at his face. He looked deliriously happy, his face was in a full grin and he looked so content that Liesel wondered if this might be the first time he'd touched a woman's breasts.

His calloused and roughened hands felt like sandpaper rubbing her breasts. It had felt good on her back but her nipples were getting sore from the pressure of his thumbs and fingers tweaking and pulling on them.

She didn't want to say anything for fear that he'd continue on with the next part of his agenda which would be a whole lot worse for her. But then an idea came to her, "Jake", she said, saying his name in a soft sultry voice. "You're right about giving me pleasure, you've surprised me. But I am starting to get a little chafed with your rough hands and all. I think that's enough courting for tonight. Maybe we could do some more tomorrow if you're up to it."

He looked into her eyes and she kept hers steady. "All right, I did say we needed to take our time with this and your skin is awfully soft and tender and all." He moved away from her and she sat up and reached for her shirt.

He took it from her hands and said to her in a testing way, "Okay we'll stop, just gimme one more look at ya. Pose for me. Put your arms behind your head and stick your titties out for me, like a pin-up model on a calendar."

She glared at him for a second but did as he asked, knowing that if she didn't, it might anger him and cause him to want her to do more. She hated herself for succumbing to this degrading pose while he just stared at her with a wild lust in his eyes. After a few moments it became apparent to her that he would ogle her like this as long as she let him, so she put her arms down and snatched her shirt from his hands. He hadn't had his fill of looking at her but he didn't seem to mind her covering up. He was already looking forward to the pleasures tomorrow would bring.

He allowed her to sleep alone in the narrow bed. After all they were just beginning their courtship, weren't they? He gathered some old moth-eaten blankets from a drawer in a dilapidated chest against the wall, on the other side of the cabin. He made a makeshift bed on the floor by the fireplace and then covered her with a tattered quilt he had found in the bottom drawer of the same dresser.

He said, "Good night, Anna," as he leaned down to stroke her cheek. She pretended to be asleep already.

As soon as she heard him snoring she started her escape plan. All she needed to do was get the key for the lock around her waist from his shirt pocket and then she could sneak out the door before he heard her and woke up. Sounded easy, but she had a sinking feeling that it wouldn't be.

She was right. He heard her as soon as she put her feet on the floor. "Anna?" he called out. "What are you doing out of bed? What's the matter?"

Leisel expelled a long drawn out sigh and then said, "I'm thirsty, don't you have any water around here?"

Jake got up and went out the door. She heard him open and close a wooden box and then return with a glass jug filled with water. As he handed it to her he said, "I hope you weren't tryin' to get away 'cause that would hurt my feelings. I'm a very light sleeper unless I'm drunk. Besides there ain't nothin' around for miles and miles, 'cept the mill."

She took the jug from him and after wiping it off the best she could with her shirttail she took a few deep gulps. "Is that where you work?" she asked as casually as she could.

"Yep," he replied. "Been there just about two whole years now, should be gettin' a raise here pretty soon. Then we can fix up this place a little to make it a bit more suitable for a woman such as yourself." He took the water bottle from her and returned it to the box on the porch. Then he laid back down on the floor in front of the fire. " 'Nite Anna."

As she sunk back down on the bed she wondered which way the mill was. It couldn't be too far from here, Jake didn't seem to have a car. At least she hadn't seen one anywhere. Tomorrow was Thursday so there was a pretty good chance that he'd have to go to work. That meant he'd be leaving her alone all day again. She had to figure out how to get away from here.

Chapter 22

Oregon

Leisel woke to the sounds of birds singing in the trees outside the cabin but as she stretched her long body on the narrow bed she gave a start as she remembered where she was. She looked down on the floor to see where Jake was and all she saw was a pile of disheveled bed clothes. The fire in the fireplace had long since died out and there was an eerie silence that at first scared her and then cheered her for she realized that Jake had gone to the mill.

As she jumped out of bed she was reminded by the cumbersome weight of the chain that she was still imprisoned, but at least she wasn't lashed down on the bed all splayed out. She looked down at the padlock around her waist. Surely she could find something to open this with. First things first though and she saw the bucket Jake had left for her to use knowing the chain wouldn't reach for her to go outside.

She spent the better part of the morning trying to pick at the lock with a piece of wire she found coiled in the mattress. When that didn't work, she used a piece of firewood to try to bash the lock attached to the chain at the hearth. Of course, that didn't work either. She broke off a piece of one of the dresser drawer handles and tried using that to scrape away at the iron ring's mooring in the fieldstone. This seemed to have some promise and she worked at this steadily until she was unexpectantly surprised by Jake's return.

When he saw what she had been up to he was furious. The anger she saw in his eyes was not borne of violence she sensed, but of rejection. But still, it was being unleashed upon her as he dragged her away from the hearth and threw her on the bed. He held her legs down by the sheer weight of his body upon hers as he struggled to get her wrists secured to the leather straps at each corner of the bed.

68

She used her nails to dig into his flesh as he tried to tie one hand down. He cursed, "You goddamn bitch!" as he snatched back his hand and smacked her hard against her cheek.

She was temporarily stunned and he was able to get her hands secured. He released one of her legs out from under his weight and he was ready when she moved to kick out at him with it. Keeping his weight on one leg he secured the other and then lifted off of her to walk around the bed to take care of the other. When she was again lashed down and splayed spread eagle on the bed, he took care of his bleeding hand with a handkerchief and glared down at her.

"You ungrateful bitch! I was trying to be nice to you and treat you like a lady, but no more. No. No more!" With that he leaned down and took both of her cheeks in one hand, squeezing her lips into a pucker and kissed her full on the mouth so hard that his teeth hit against hers. He moved his lips back and forth across hers and then sucked on her lower lip before releasing her abruptly. He stomped out of the cabin and didn't return until it was dark. He had the stench of sawdust and perspiration with him again only this time it was also accompanied by the odor of belched beer.

He lit the lantern and untied one of her hands as he said, "Well, if it isn't the lady of the house, and how was your day m'dear?" He tossed her a cold hamburger wrapped in foil and said, "It was warm when I brought it home to you for lunch."

She unwrapped the burger by holding it against her side for leverage. "I can't eat lying down. Aren't you going to untie me?" she asked.

"No." He said simply. He wadded a blanket up and stuck it behind her back to prop her up a bit. "There try that."

She realized that this afternoon's rejection was still bothering him and that unless she smoothed it over, she was going to have to remain in this punishing position. "I'm sorry about today", she murmured, "I just don't like being cooped up all day. That's why I have a job that lets me be outside. It wasn't against you personally. I simply don't like being caged up like this."

"Do I look like a moron to you? You don't fool me any. I know you can't stand the sight of me! Girls like you are all the same, they want a man who's captain of the football team, tall, dark and handsome," he sneered "I'll bet you were popular in high school too, maybe even a cheerleader."

When she averted her eyes from his he knew he had guessed right. "Well now the cheerleader's gonna show the class drop out her pussy!"

She blanched not only at his crudity but at what he meant. Instinctively she tried to put her thighs together. He laughed at her reaction and told her to finish eating. He went out to the porch and brought in a six pack of beer, he handed her one and chuckled, "maybe this'll loosen you up, baby!"

She took small bites of her burger and little sips of the beer trying to stall him for as long as she could. His mood had not improved at all since this afternoon and she found herself hoping that he wasn't a mean drunk. She eyed the remaining four beers and wondered how many it took for him to get rip-roaring, passing out drunk. He probably hadn't brought that many home. "Why don't you have a girlfriend?" she asked, knowing full well what the answer was. Maybe if she could just get him talking that would distract him for awhile.

"Oh, I don't know," he retorted. Then added sarcastically, "Probably has to do with the fact that I'm not good lookin', I'm not rich, and I've got a dead end job!" He sat down on the hearth and looked at the floor. After a few minutes he said in a low voice. "I had a girlfriend once, but she never let me touch her. She said she was saving herself for the man she was going to marry. Then I found out she was givin' it out to everybody on the football team. I tried out for the team a coupla times but I could never make the cut. Never had another girlfriend, but I've had a few whores."

He got up and retied her hand, removed her socks and untied one ankle. Then he started massaging her foot. It actually felt wonderful to her. He lavished and adored it like it was a prized trophy. Then he returned it to the leather strap and did the same for the other one. When he was finished massaging it, he leaned up and undid the button on her jeans and unzipped the zipper.

"Please don't," she said softly.

But he paid her no mind, he tugged them down until he had them totally off of one leg and all bunched up around the bottom of the other. She trembled at his touch as he lightly stroked her legs, first one and then the other, running his hands up and down her inner and outer thighs, down one way and then up the other. When he put his thumbs under the elastic of her underwear she squirmed away and sobbed, "Oh, God, please no! Don't do this, please I'm begging you."

He looked up at her face and the look in his eyes told her that she was doing exactly as he wanted her to. He wanted her to beg, he wanted her to know who had the control. She squeezed her eyes shut as he slowly drew her underpants down to join the jeans already around her ankle. Then he retied that leg so that he could completely remove her pants and panties from the other. When he was done, he stood back to admire the view. He'd never seen a woman displayed like this and he was totally enthralled by the triangle between her legs. He put his head down between her legs and his hands around the outside of her thighs with his thumbs pressing firmly against the inside. He pushed up, achieving a much more exposed view of her.

As she lay there shaking and crying piteously he just stared completely transfixed by a sight he'd never seen before. After what seemed like an eternity he removed a hand from one thigh and tentatively touched the lips of her labia. She screamed and gyrated trying to shake off his hand. He responded by grabbing her harshly with both hands on the upper most part of her thighs gripping her where her pubic hair began.

"Hold still!" he hissed. Then he wriggled his way up and moved his face closer, putting his lips on her, sending an electric shock through her that made her cry out like she was in pain.

71

He continued ministering to her with his lips and his tongue, licking her all over. At first she squirmed continuously but finally she gave up the fight and relaxed allowing him to indulge himself as he pleased. He sat back to look at her some more and while that unnerved her greatly, she couldn't help the tingling sensations that were making her feel warm and liquid all over. He started probing her with his fingers all the while watching her contract and open up to his explorations. When he thrust two fingers deep inside her and began moving them in and out she started moaning and joining in with his rhythmic strokes.

She was so worked up into a frenzy by the time he removed his fingers that she almost protested their departure. He quickly started lapping and sucking in the area where her clitoris was and within seconds she climaxed violently right into his mouth. He laved her lightly soothing the aftershocks until she was no longer responsive. Then he got up on his knees and kissed her lightly on the mouth, saying "you are deeelicious!"

He got up to get another beer and went to sit on the hearth angling his head so he had a clear view of the area he had just satiated. He remained, admiring the view for a long time, then got up for another beer and offered it to her. When she nodded he untied her hands and handed it to her.

He stroked her brows and said,"I'm gonna make you so happy, you just wait and see." With that he untied her legs and secured the chain around her waist before throwing a blanket over her, dousing the lantern and settling himself in by the fireplace. Within a few minutes he was asleep.

She looked around for something to knock him out with but there was nothing. The extra firewood was piled over in a far corner and to get to the smoldering logs in the fireplace, she'd have to step right on him. The only thing within her reach was the lantern and that would probably only make him mad.

As she sat there sipping her beer in the dark, she pondered the strangeness of this man. He had taken quite a few liberties with her but he hadn't raped her. He hadn't satisfied himself in any way at all that she could see. How long was this to go on she wondered. No one probably even knew that she was missing yet.

Tomorrow was Friday, she wouldn't be missed until Saturday night when she was expected to attend her father's birthday party.

Chapter 23

Oregon

The far off sound of an engine idling woke her. She strained her ears trying to determine how far away it was. Not close, but closer than a mile. And then it was gone. There must be a road somewhere close by. Jake had thoughtfully left buckets of water by the hearth for her to use to wash up. The water was crystal clear but incredibly cold. She thought about heating it up in the fireplace but could find no way to light the wood. She looked toward the night stand where the lantern sat and saw a book of matches. Maybe she could catch the cabin on fire and then someone would see it and come rescue her.

But what if they didn't and she burned to death attached to the hearth? She'd taken many pictures of rural houses that had burned to the ground and somehow the chimney had always managed to survive, maybe she could crawl up inside it. She quickly discarded that idea when she remembered the basic principles of cooking and how most pizzas are made, baked in a hot brick oven.

Well at least she could have a warm sponge bath. She went to retrieve the matches.

"Hey," she said aloud " Maybe I can drag the mattress outside and the smoke from it burning might bring somebody."

Then again, it might not and Jake would probably not take it too kindly if she ruined his old musty, stained mattress. She picked up the match book and with great dismay realized that there were no matches under the cover. All her ideas were academic now and a cold sponge bath was to be the highlight of her day it seemed.

She filled her afternoon with little naps and some yoga exercises she remembered from classes she had taken a few years ago. Every once in awhile she would look out the window to see the lushness of the trees and the birds flitting from one branch to another. It reminded her that there was another world waiting for her return and her determination to get back to it soared.

She heard that real low, far off engine idling sound again and about twenty minutes later she heard Jake coming up the porch steps. Was someone picking him up and dropping him off from work? That made sense since obviously he didn't have his own transportation anywhere around here. Jake had said there was nothing around here for miles and miles so whoever it was must work at the mill also.

When Jake returned to the cabin the sun was already below the trees and the last rays of sunlight were making long shadows of her silhouette as she paced back and forth trying to exercise her body and relax her mind. On top of everything else she was going stir crazy. The chain only let her go as far as the door so she couldn't even see the outside world unless she looked out the windows and she had already memorized the vistas out of both. Trees and sky. Trees and sky.

Apparently Friday was pay day for Jake as he entered the cabin with a partially full grocery bag. He smiled at her and unloaded the items on the hearth.

"We're gonna have a decent meal tonight. I hope you like steak and baked potatoes. There's an old brick BBQ out back I can use to do the cookin', but first I'm gonna get cleaned up for you," and with that he grabbed her around the waist and twirled her around, then threading the fingers of one hand through her short hair he leaned up and kissed her.

She jumped back and slapped him hard across the face. As he rubbed his cheek with one hand he grabbed the chain with the other and jerked her towards him.

With his face only inches from hers he snarled, "So that's how it's gonna be huh? I'll show you who's boss missy!" And with that he grabbed her shirt by the front pocket and pulled. It ripped right off of her, buttons scattering everywhere. She started clawing at him and he quickly jerked the chain and wrapped it around her neck. As she struggled to breathe, he unhooked her bra and slid it off her shoulders. When she slumped to the floor, blacking out from the lack of air, he removed the rest of her clothing. Then he used a cool wet cloth on her face to revive her.

When she finally caught her breath, she glared at him with hatred in her eyes and said, "I am not your woman! I don't want to be here with you! You repulse me!"

He grew red with fury and he jerked her to a standing position. He lecherously eyed her naked body up and down, feasting on the sight of her as her chest heaved in and out. "Well, you don't repulse me! So I'm gonna keep ya! Even if I have to keep you chained up until you're fifty! And there ain't nothin' you can do 'bout it, so just quit fightin' me!" He picked up the bag containing the steaks and potatoes and grabbed a six-pack of beer and then he went outside, pulling her behind him.

"Wait, I'm not dressed!", she hollered.

"Just the way I like you best", he replied, and led her around the side of the cabin toward the back where the BBQ was.

She felt totally humiliated and very uncomfortable with her body exposed as she was in front of him outside in the cool night air. "I'm cold!" she complained, as she tried to cover herself with her hands.

"Suffer," was his only reply.

She started feeling mosquitoes biting her and she swatted at them. "I'm getting eaten alive!" she protested.

He said nothing as he continued preparing the fire and gulping down a second beer. After he placed the potatoes and steaks on the grill, he returned his attention to her. Admiringly, he watched the way the moonlight gave her body a pearly white glow. He backed her up against a tree and wound the entire length of chain around her midriff and hips, pinning her arms at her side. Then he stood back to look at her. He rubbed his hands over her shoulders and down her arms, never taking his eyes off of her breasts with their dusky nipples fully erect from the chill of the air on them.

He leaned over and cupped one with his hand and hefted it to feel the weight of it. "You have marvelous tits," he murmured before he put his mouth on the tip of it and began to lightly suckle it. She flinched and stiffened to his touch but that only made him suck harder.

That night they ate well, even though they did it without utensils. Liesel's face and hands were greasy from eating the steak with her bare hands. She felt barbaric, much like the cave women from ages ago must have felt. Then he took her for a walk through the woods like one would walk a dog. As he held her on the leash he observed the way her breasts jiggled up and down. Then he made her walk in front of him so he could watch her buttocks as she walked.

When she made a remark about having to go to the bathroom, hoping to have a few moments of privacy from his feasting eyes, he surprised her by sneaking back to watch her as she relieved herself. She had never felt so shamed in her life and she wondered if this was how animals felt when their owners walked them. He was being demeaning and he was loving it. She would not give him the satisfaction of complaining.

He wouldn't let her go to sleep that night, insisting that she pose this way and that way, assuring himself that he had explored every inch of her before he attached the chain back to the hearth and passed out on the floor by the fireplace.

After a few moments of listening to his even breathing, she gingerly sat up and accustomed her eyes to the dark cabin. Liesel didn't know how much more she could take of this. She had to get away from this brute! As she leaned over his sleeping form she tried to remember which pocket he'd put the key in.

As it turned out, he was sleeping on his stomach with the key safely pressed beneath the bulk of his body. She tried to reach under him and then she tried to turn him over, both futile efforts because he was so heavy and she was afraid of waking him. Then she found what remained of her clothes and put them on enjoying the feeling of warmth they gave her. Crying into her hands, she sat on the edge of the bed until she was exhausted, then she slept.

When they woke up it was late Saturday afternoon. She thought about her father's birthday party and how she should be getting ready to help him celebrate. A part of her was glad that he didn't know what was happening to his little girl way up here in the wilderness. Tomorrow they would start looking for her. They would find her Jeep and eventually, she hoped, they would find her.

This man was odd, even though he had made her do many vile things, he really hadn't seemed to get any gratification for himself. She was sure that it would only be a matter of time before he did the ultimate violation of her and allowed himself the pleasure she felt sure he had been denied all his life. The way he adored her body and the fact that he was absolutely fascinated with the sight and feel of her made her believe that he had never been with a woman, regardless of what he had said about the whores. But he had obviously seen some dirty pictures somewhere because the positions he had placed her in for his perusal last night were right out of those sleazy pornographic magazines you could buy almost anywhere.

She tried to sound friendly and cheerful when he came back from eliminating all of last night's beer. She wanted to find out more about the road and the mill. "So you don't have to work today, huh?" she asked.

"Nope, I get the weekends off even though the mill is still open today," he replied.

"What do you do with all your free time, you don't seem to watch much TV," she joked.

"Oh, sometimes I do. There's a bar a ways down the road that I go to to watch some football games with the guys, I might even go there some tonight."

"Guys?" she asked.

"Yeah, there's a bunch of fellows from the mill that git together every once in awhile. None of us are married or anything so we kinda hang out together if there's nothin' goin' on."

"I really could use a bath or a shower. Is there around that I could get one?" She asked coyly.

"No place I trust ya to take ya," he said flatly. "C'n show you where I go to get cleaned up. Maybe we can together," he said with a leer.

She could've kicked herself. Now what had she done? unlocked the chain from the hearth.

"Leave your clothes here, no sense in takin' 'em down there and gettin' 'em all wet 'n all."

She glared at him as he helped her out of her pants. "Do you have a towel or soap?"

"Got some soap, but you'll just have to air dry," he snickered.

He led her down a deep ravine to a small rippling brook about six or seven feet wide. The water wasn't more than a foot deep and it was so clear that she could see the little spots on the smooth round stones at the bottom. The water was flowing rapidly downhill but no so fast that you had to worry about being swept away, however keeping a grip on the soap would be another matter. He sat at the edge while she tested the water.

"Brrr, this'll wake me up", she said with a slight smile. "Do you think you could unchain me so I can bathe?"

He gave her a skeptical look and she chided, "Where am I going to run to like this?" she gestured with her hand to her nakedness. He got up off of a rock and removed the key from his pocket and unlocked the padlock from around her waist. There were a few chafe marks where it had rubbed against her bare skin. He put his fingers to them and lightly stroked her there. He opened a knapsack that he had grabbed off of the porch on their way out of the cabin.

"I've got some soap, a little shampoo and a razor if you want."

"Just some soap and shampoo will be fine," she called.

Why did she care if her legs were unshaven for him? As she used the soap, she noticed him watching her lather up so she hurriedly finished and rinsed. He certainly didn't need any more

shampooed and rinsed her hair twice
oo in the little hotel courtesy bottle.
next week to regret that, but she
hair was this dirty. She moved to

he said, "I'm comin' in too."
she thought to herself. She turned her back so
see him undress. She sat down in the water enjoying
the current was trying to push her over. She could hear
washing and she hoped he would use plenty of soap. There
were times the smell of him made her cringe.

She looked around trying to see if there was anywhere she could escape to that he couldn't quickly track her down. As far as she could see there was nothing but woods. And unless she had a good head start on him she doubted if she could outrun him for long.

"Don't you want to see what your man looks like?" he called out.

"No, I don't have a man and I don't want one, thank you," she replied.

He chuckled and came over and pulled her to her feet, forcing her to look at his chest, which was massive and covered with lots of dark brown hair. She looked up at his face, preferring that way instead of the other and he smiled at her. He held one of her hands in his and grabbed the length of chain with the other and led her back to the cabin, both of them shivering quite a bit.

He didn't move to chain her up right away and for that she was grateful. While he was bending over to put his pants on she did notice that his manhood was not at all in a state of arousal and that in its flaccid state it wasn't at all impressive. The rest of him wasn't all that bad but he sure could stand to loose a few pounds and visit a dentist.

She looked around for her clothes and as she started to put them on he said, "Just put the shirt on, no pants or panties."

"Why?" she stammered.

He went out on the porch and returned with her camera bag. Her eyes became wild with alarm. What was he doing with her camera? "Seems like the boys I told you about don't believe that I gots me a little woman of my own, so I thought we'd take a few pictures for them."

She was aghast. "Absolutely not! No way! Nobody takes dirty pictures of me! Ever!" she screamed.

"C'mon Anna," he said as he came over and stroked the top of her breast. "For the first time in my life, I've actually got a woman of my own, and now nobody believes me. It's important to me that they believe me."

"I don't care and my name's not Anna!" she screamed.

He threw her onto the bed and tied her down avoiding her clawing hands and kicking feet but not avoiding her teeth. She had bitten him hard on his arm. There was a deep gash where the flesh had been torn. He gave her an icy glare as he massaged his arm and found a piece of cloth to bandage it with.

He bundled up some bedding from the floor and tucked it behind her back, saying, "I want your titties to stick out in the photos, not be all flattened out like they get when you lay down."

Then he roughly shoved the shirt off of her shoulders exposing her breasts, the nipples still puckered from the cold water of the stream. He turned to get the camera ready. She screamed as loud as she could. He didn't even turn around. To her it was deafening. Why couldn't anybody hear that?

"Scream as loud as you like. There's no one around to hear you," he said.

"You're just saying that," she yelled at him. "How do I know that's true?" And with that she let out a series of screams each one a little less energetic than the last. When she had finally exhausted herself she sobbed heartbrokenly.

After removing the camera from the case he whistled, "This is some camera, must 'a cost a pretty penny! Never used one this fancy before, but I think I can get the hang of it. I know I gotta remove this thing," he said as he removed the lens cover.

He came over to the bed with the camera positioned at his eye. "Please," she implored. "Don't do this. I'll meet your friends. We could go together tonight. I'll tell them I'm your woman. I promise I will. Please, please." She could not believe that this was happening to her. When was she going to wake up from this nightmare?

"I know you. As soon as we get into the bar you'll scream your bloody head off. No deal. This is the way we're doin' it!"

With that he aimed the camera at her chest and took a picture. The whirr of the film advancing had always been a pleasant sound to her. Now each whirring noise caused her to shrivel inside. As he moved around the room he looked through the lens then came to adjust something on her, a wisp of hair, a flap of the shirt, once he pinched her nipple saying, "It was a little puckered." Then he'd step back and click off a series of shots. When he came to the foot of the bed for an all over shot she turned her head and squeezed her eyes shut.

"Honey, don't worry so much," he chided, "they're not going to be looking at your face." He took another picture, then put the camera down and found two lengths of cloth, and came over to look at her. What was he going to use those for? she wondered.

When he pulled one of her knees out towards the edge of the bed, she hollered, "No! No!No!" over and over again until her mouth was so dry she made no sound.

He wrapped the cloth around the area just above her knee and pulled the cloth over the edge of the mattress and secured it to a slat. Then he went to the other side of the bed and did the same thing to her other leg. He went back to the foot of the bed and surveyed his work. He liked what he saw. And now he wanted everyone to see it too. He picked up the camera and used up the rest of the roll taking full frontal shots and then a few close-ups of her most deliciously displayed genitalia.

She cried herself to sleep that night not even noticing that he hadn't chained her up or tied her down in any way. She had been humiliated in the worst way a woman could be to her way of thinking and she was determined to make him pay. She'd get away from him and he'd go to jail for a long, long time. She'd see to it.

When she awoke the next morning her eyes were almost swollen shut, but her first thought was a happy one. Today they would start looking for her. When Jake came over and sat on the edge of the bed and stroked her cheek, she turned her head from his hand. She was sullen and she was determined that she wasn't even going to speak to him again. He stroked the side of her neck and then removed her shirt and rolled her over onto her stomach. He straddled her buttocks and massaged her back and neck, then moved down to massage her buttocks. He was very thorough in his labors and despite herself she found herself letting out a moan every now and then.

He moved farther down her legs only straddling one now. He spread her legs wide and leaned back to examine her from this angle. He stroked her inner thighs with the lightest of touches and she found herself involuntarily opening her thighs wider to accommodate his hands. Very slowly he eased his way up her thighs until he could feel her springy pubic hairs. He gently tugged on a few causing her to gyrate her pelvis into the mattress. He eased a finger into her silky slit and gently probed the warm, moist area around her vagina with his thumb. He picked up the tempo when she started moving against his finger and then joined in with yet another finger.

With his other hand he reached up under her and found her nipple and rubbed it between his fingers. Then he started kissing the back of her neck all the while removing and replacing his fingers in accompaniment to her body's frenzied gyrations. Suddenly she arched against his hand and he felt her shudder from inside where his fingers were rubbing against the front of her clitoris. After she spent herself all over his fingers, he gently cupped her with his whole hand and squeezed her lightly as if to say, "You're okay. I can always make you okay."

Before he moved off of her she rubbed her leg between his to confirm what she had thought she had known before. He wasn't even hard. Shouldn't he have had an erection with all this going on? How was it that this man could be so loving and so attentive and then be so hateful and mean? She was starting to suspect that maybe he was impotent. That would explain the source of a lot of his frustrations and his anger at her rejections. And it would also explain his reasons for wanting to show the world that he could *have* a woman.

Chapter 24

Oregon

When she woke up early Sunday morning she was immediately aware of a wet stickiness between her thighs. A feeling of dread overcame her as she tried frantically to remember what had happened last night. Had she been ravished by him and if so why couldn't she remember? She put her hand down to investigate and brought a hand smeared with blood back up to her face. With relief she realized that she had started her period. It was a rare thing to be pleased by the arrival of her *friend* but she was ecstatic that it had come early for her. Maybe now he would leave her alone, she could only hope that he was the type of person that was totally sickened by the sight of blood. She smeared as much as she could on the bed covers so he'd be sure to notice.

When he awoke, she started feigning misery from cramping. After a few hours of her tossing about on the bed moaning, he left, but not before attaching the chain to her waist and then to the hearth.

When he returned many hours later he was stone drunk and about as smelly as she could imagine a man could possibly be. It seemed he had managed to vomit all over the front of himself. Because of that he removed his shirt and threw it out the front door, along with the keys to the padlocks and the best chance she'd had to escape since he'd kidnapped her.

She sat Indian style on the bed and beat her fists on the mattress. Her stomach was growling and she realized she hadn't eaten since the steak BBQ on Friday night. Pretty soon she'd be able to wriggle out of the chain secured around her waist, if he didn't cinch it in any further.

Monday Jake was too sick to mess with her. He struggled to get himself up for work and just managed to clear the doorway of the cabin when she heard the low rumble of an engine. She heard him as he started running, crunching rocks under his feet. A few minutes later she heard the honk of a horn and she prayed that he would catch his ride before they left without him.

Liesel spent the day sleeping off and on as she really did have some cramping. When she went to the bucket to wipe off the blood encrusted on her thighs she spotted the broken drawer handle that Jake had taken from her that day. It was under the bed partially hidden by a dust ball. She got down on her stomach and shimmied under the bed to retrieve it. Then she sat on the hearth holding it against her chest as if it was a very treasured, long-lost heirloom. Quickly she got to work rubbing it back and forth across the ridge of mortar surrounding the iron ring. She was careful to listen for the sounds of Jake's return and kept sweeping the hearth with her shirttail to remove any traces of cement dust.

She really hadn't made much progress when she heard the engine noise again, but just having something to do that was working towards her freedom had improved her mood immensely.

Jake brought home a bag of doughnuts for dinner, and even though she would have preferred something with more nutritional value, she scarfed them down one right after the other until the bag was empty.

As it turned out Jake was very squeamish about bloody things. As soon as Liesel picked up on this she started keeping a bloodied cloth between her legs and doubling over with imagined pain every so often. If she ever made it to heaven she was going to ask God a few things. One of them being why women get the periods and the labor process and the menopause while the men get to be the ones who have the orgasm each and every time. Except for Jake.

Her *curse* had been a godsend. He avoided her as if she had a plague of some kind, almost neglecting her in fact. Every morning he asked her if it was over yet and every morning she said no. By Friday morning he insisted on inspecting her for himself and when he did he discovered her ruse.

He shook his finger in her face and hissed through his yellowed teeth, "You just wait 'til I get home tonight. I'm going to make you sorry you did that!"

With that he spun her around onto her stomach and spanked her as hard as he could while she kicked and thrashed trying to get away. He stopped only because his hand had started to throb. Then he stormed out the door. She could hear his footsteps diminishing as he got further away. Scrambling to her feet she reached for the drawer handle hidden under the mattress. If she knew what was good for her, she'd better get this done today.

All day long she worked on the mortar, stopping only to massage her cramped fingers and to rub her sore bottom. She had to keep readjusting the piece of cloth she was using to cover her knuckles to keep them from getting all scraped up by the fieldstone. To her dismay the iron ring wasn't budging even the slightest amount even though there was now a perceptible groove worn into the mortar around the fieldstone.

How far did the end of this iron ring go into the chimney, anyway? She faced the fact that she was not going to get free before Jake came home to punish her and she started trembling so badly that she couldn't work any longer. She cleaned up and replaced the drawer handle, that was now worn smooth, in its hiding place.

Jake came through the cabin door like a man obsessed. He was stomping his feet and hitting his fist against the walls. She cowered in the bed, sitting up against the wall.

"What's wrong?" she asked timidly, halfway afraid to hear what the answer might be.

"What's wrong? What's wrong? This is what's wrong!" and he flung a photo developing envelope at her.

Her heart stood still as she realized what this must be and she didn't even want to touch it.

"They didn't turn out! Not a single one of them!" he hollered.

It took her a moment to realize what he had said and then she let out a long sigh, realizing too late that she had angered him even more by doing that. He turned to face her and grabbed her by the hair with one hand and by the breast with the other.

"This isn't over yet, baby, not by a long shot!" He squeezed her breast hard and jerked her head back, his heated glaze boring into her.

"We'll just have to show them in person now, won't we?" he spat out at her.

As the realization of what he meant dawned on her, her eyes widened with fear. He just laughed and roughly released her. Then he went out onto the porch and she heard him open up a can of beer.

She picked up the envelope, noticing the drugstore's comments about over exposed film and the customary waiver of any charges. She opened it and only negatives slid out. Negatives with nothing on them. It was only then that she remembered that she had been startled by a noise while loading her camera and when he had come upon her she had fallen with it. Obviously the film had never engaged onto the spool so there had never been any film in front of the amperature opening when he had been clicking away. One of life's big favors, thank you, God!

It was then that she knew she was going to get out of this. She just didn't know how yet. When he came back inside he handed her a Styrofoam food container and went out again. She opened it and saw a half eaten slab of meatloaf and a cold glob of mashed potatoes along with six or seven wilted string beans. The fork he had apparently been using was still in the box. She never thought she would stoop to eating someone else's cold leftovers but she ate with abandon stopping short of licking the inside of the box. After awhile Jake came back into the cabin with a peculiar looking grin on his face. She was in dread of what he was up to now.

He removed her shirt and lashed her wrists to the bed posts. When she fought him as he tried to remove her pants, he straddled her legs and took something from his pant's pocket. Before she had a chance to see what he had in his hand he reached out and pinched one of her nipples so tightly that she winced with the pain. Then he quickly produced a clothespin and snapped it onto the nubbin of her nipple. The pain was excruciating and she flailed with her confined arms and bucked with her hips trying to find a way to remove it.

"Oh, God, that hurts! Please take it off!" she screamed.

He just laughed and repeated the same torture to the other nipple. The pain was unbearable, she'd heard of kinky people doing this, even knew that they made special nipple clips for this express purpose. But she had no idea how painful it was.

Her whole mind was focused on that area of her body, frantically searching for a release from the pain. She looked down at her chest and saw the clothespins hanging there. Shaking her breasts back and forth, she tried to remove them. That hurt even more, if that was possible. He watched the show with appreciative eyes and when she realized that they were gripped too strongly to be shaken off, she stopped and looked into his amused eyes.

"Please take them off, it hurts, it hurts, it hurts."

Never taking his eyes off of her breasts he said, "If you're a good girl and do what I tell you, I'll take them off."

"Yes, yes," she readily agreed.

He got up off of her hips and pulled her pants off and said, "Spread your legs for me and show me your pussy like I was your doctor."

She gasped at this command, but she knew she had no choice, the pain was searing and burning into her brain. She would do anything to get rid of it. She opened her legs and bent them at the knees offering him an unencumbered view of her womanhood.

This wasn't good enough for him and he put his hands on her ankles and shoved them up almost to her hips. There was no part of her hidden from his penetrating gaze and she shivered from the embarrassment of knowing exactly where his eyes were.

"How many men have seen you like this before?" He asked.

When she didn't answer he asked, "Do you want those clips off or not?"

She replied, "Two."

"Including your doctor?" he countered. "Okay, three," she amended.

"How long did they examine you like this?" He queried, still focusing on her gaping labia.

"They didn't!" she retorted, "well, except of course for the doctor, they were trying to pleasure me, not humiliate me!"

"How were they trying to pleasure you? With their mouths?" he asked.

"Yes," she demurred.

He put his hands on both of her inner thighs and leaned down to press a penetrating kiss in the area of her clitoris. Then he leaned up and took something else out of his pocket. He waived it in front of her face.

"Do you know what this is?" He asked.

She saw him waiving a wooden handled Phillips head screwdriver back and forth in front of her by the tool end.

"Yesss," she stammered.

God help her, what did he plan to do with that!

"What is it?" he prodded.

"A Phillips screwdriver," she timidly replied keeping her eyes focused on it.

"No," he said, "it's not. It's my penis. And it wants you."

She gave him a questioning look and he elaborated.

"You may have noticed that I have a little problem in that area. I thought we could work on a solution together," he said.

"H-h-how?" she stammered.

He used one hand to spread her nether lips while he stuck the wooden handle of the screwdriver way up into her vagina. Only the gleaming silver shaft of the tool was visible coming out of her body.

She gasped and said "Oh!" from the surprise of it entering her.

"How does that feel?" he asked softly.

"Awful," she gritted out in anger. "Take it out!"

It didn't hurt but it did give her a very full feeling and she found herself contracting involuntarily around it. He noticed the tool moving in and out slightly due to her manipulations so he proceeded to thrust it in and out of her very gently and slowly at first and then picked up the pace when he saw her lifting her buttocks up to meet his thrusts. With his other hand he massaged her clitoris. When she came it was explosive and it shook her to her core. As she slumped in the aftermath of her convulsions she felt an intense shame and actually hated herself for deriving any pleasure from the sadistic exploitations of this monster.

"Could you please remove the clips now?" she implored, realizing that the pain was diminished only due to numbness.

"Just one more thing and I will," he said.

Untying her hands, he flipped her over onto her stomach. He retied her hands before she had a chance to use them to remove the clips. Then he lifted her bottom up in the air and spread the cheeks of her ass with his hands. Before she knew what had happened, he had removed the screwdriver from her vagina and inserted it into her anal opening, completely up to the hilt. She screamed so loud that it hurt her ears and his. He swacked her hard on one of her exposed reddened cheeks as punishment. She started crying and sobbing so loudly that he finally started to get an erection.

He quickly jumped off the bed, chained her around the waist, and then untied her hands. "C'mon," he said "we're going for a walk."

She turned her head to look at him, tears running down her face, neck and breasts then dripping off the end of her nipples onto the mattress. "How am I supposed to walk like this?" she asked, absolutely incredulous with her predicament.

"You'll manage," he said gruffly and he jerked the chain so hard that she stumbled off the bed barely catching herself with her weakened legs before falling onto the floor.

He led her outside and as she accustomed herself to walking with the protrusion coming from her bottom she reached for the clips with her hands. "Don't touch them!" he barked.

She knew from his tone that this was not a command to disobey and she lowered her hands to her sides. "Walk in front of me," he ordered her brusquely, "I want to watch you."

As she walked down the path she stumbled over branches and rocks, trying to keep her balance in her bare feet. What kind of man was this? He must truly hate women to get any enjoyment out of this type of suffering and humiliation. She felt a slackening in the chain and turned to see what was causing it just in time to see him reach for the screwdriver.

"No!" she hollered as he grabbed the silver shaft and jammed it even further up into her.

She fell to her hands and knees and sobbed her heart out. He quickly unzipped his pants and stared at her while she was on all fours with the screwdriver sticking out of her asshole and the clothes pins attached to her hanging breasts. He masturbated until he came a few seconds later.

Jake was leaning up against a tree when Liesel noticed what he was doing. As she watched, a look of agony came over his face and he jettisoned his sperm into his hand. She stared in ghoulish fascination as it ran off of his hand and dripped to the ground. His ejaculation was accompanied by a guttural animal-like sound.

After a few quiet moments he put himself back together and walked over to her. He gently removed the screwdriver, and using the shaft end, he hurled it deep into the woods. He removed the clothespins and let them drop where they were. Then he helped her up and walked her back to the cabin.

She was exhausted. As she fell onto the bed to go to sleep, he gently rolled her onto her stomach and massaged her back, buttocks and legs until she fell asleep.

When she awoke the next morning he was gone and she was sore in places she'd never been sore before. She noticed her nipples were purple with bruising and they refused to let her forget their presence, their throbbing almost incessant. What had those whores, if there had ever been any, taught him? The depravity of this man was enormous. She shivered with repulsion as she went over the events of the last night in her head trying to figure out what it was that had finally allowed him to achieve some sort of sexual satisfaction.

Obviously he had some sadomasochistic tendencies— probably derived from his many rejections from women. Maybe he had seen his mother being badly treated. When she was at the height of her discomfort and humiliation he had finally been able to gratify himself. She wished she had paid more attention to those psychology classes in college. She was glad that she hadn't been raped by him, but she wasn't so sure now that it wouldn't eventually happen. She now knew that he could rape her as long as he was hurting her. The thought caused her to tremble and just when she thought that things couldn't possibly get worse she realized she was no longer on her birth control pills. They had been left at her hotel and God, what kind of diseases might this man have?

Chapter 25

Oregon—Saturday Afternoon

Daniel Hoffman sat at the bar watching the evening wrap up of the college football scores. But his mind really wasn't on football right now. It had been three months since he had settled into this little burg and he felt even more like an outsider now than he had then. His buddies at the mill were still a bit too crude for him and he longed for a little of the sophistication he had left behind in Baltimore.

Sure, he had run away from a lot of problems, but he hadn't meant to run away from the theater and the galleries and the malls. He had meant to trade his life in the city for a life in the country, far away from the sounds of sirens screaming in the night.

Only a short while ago Daniel had been a firefighter for the City of Baltimore. It was a grueling job. There was always too much work but he had derived a certain amount of satisfaction from it. He'd had a few other jobs when he was younger. He'd been a cowboy in Montana and had worked on an oil platform in the ocean off the gulf coast but none had given him the feeling of accomplishment like fire fighting had.

The results of a job well done were immediate and the rewards of compensation were more than adequate to allow him to marry and settle down. When he found out that his wife of two years had aborted his baby without his knowledge he divorced her and concentrated on his career.

Five months ago, during a particularly bad fire at a huge garden apartment complex, he'd made the wrong choice about which stairwell to enter to search for victims. Because of it five children had died in the next one over. Deep down he knew it wasn't really his fault. Fate had played its hand and he had only cooperated. But a month later when it was determined that the children's mother had deliberately set the fire in hopes of collecting some insurance money, he threw in the towel. The Department had urged him to seek counseling but he really couldn't see how talking to a shrink was going to help him cope with all these women killing their babies. When it came right down to it, he didn't want to get over the revulsion he was feeling. To get over it would be to say that it didn't matter, and it did.

He'd packed up his meager belongings and threw them into the back of his old pickup truck, his one true friend. He could have afforded a new truck at almost anytime, but "Trusty Rusty" had seen him through many a scrape since leaving college and who wanted to have a new truck in the city anyway?

He hadn't really known where he was headed. He just knew that now he'd like to try being a lumberjack and Oregon seemed to be the place to do that. Now as he sat in Clancy's Bar and Grill and surveyed his new found friends he wondered if he had anything in common with anyone in the whole state of Oregon. Certainly the absolute worst candidate for that would have to be Jake Tuttle.

He watched Jake swagger around the pool table trying to show off a talent for the game that he really didn't have. This was a ne'er-do-well if he'd ever seen one. According to the gossipers he'd been fired from the local service station for stealing money and then he was fired from the local high school janitorial service because of complaints of suggestive and lewd behavior he'd exhibited in front of some girls. He was a little below medium height and quite stocky and he had breath that would kill a mule.

Several times Daniel had been tempted to just drive on by when he passed the little dirt road that came down the hill from Jake's cabin. The smell of his body odors and breath combined came downright close to giving him nausea first thing in the morning. But Daniel couldn't stand to see anyone put out if he could help it so he continued to give him rides both to the mill and to town.

Curiously, he hadn't smelled quite so bad lately. A few guys came to sit at the bar with him and he ordered a round for all of them. The talk seemed to revolve around Jake and the ribbing they were giving him for lying to them yet again. The man didn't know how to tell the truth. He embellished everything, and for someone who had never really amounted to much of anything, he sure had a lot of tales to tell.

This one was about "his woman", who was beautiful, well-endowed and waiting for him every night when he came home. The guys laughed and guffawed as they drank their beer. The more they laughed the madder he got.

"It's true I tell ya, she's there now," he said, slurring his words.

"Yeah? What's her name?" someone yelled out.

"Anna," he replied without hesitation. Everyone turned their heads to look at him.

"Anna, huh?" said Clifford Baines, one of the foremen at the mill. "Where'd ya meet her?"

"Down by the lake, she was takin' pictures." Jake replied. His answers were quick and off the cuff and everyone was starting to give him a little credence.

"What's she see in you, you old buzzard?" Roger Shemple asked, and everyone howled.

"Well she just got tired of city blokes and had to have a taste of a frontiersman," Jake bragged.

Again everyone laughed. John Cane wiped a tear from his eye as he rallied with, "So what's she doin' with you?"

Jake was starting to get really ticked off. He knew they were messin' with him but that didn't bother him as much as knowing that they didn't believe him. All week he'd been trying to convince them about his woman.

"You come over tomorrow night after the game and you'll see. I'll show you Anna. In fact, I'll show you all of Anna!" Jake challenged.

"OoooohWhoooo" they catcalled at the mention of a stripped down woman. And then it was decided that everyone there at the bar would come and see his woman called "Anna" tomorrow after the football game. For once they thought they'd call him on his lies. Maybe then they wouldn't have to listen to them anymore.

Daniel dropped Jake off at the usual place and continued on up the road to his cabin about three miles away. He stopped at his mailbox and got the mail before getting back in his truck and pulling up into his driveway.

Sitting in his easy chair in front of the fireplace he looked through the assortment of catalogues and bills. When he saw the copy of "USA Today" he picked it up and sat back to thumb through it. He read the national news and the sports news and then read the page that has the news for each state.

When he got to Oregon he started reading about a woman photographer who had been missing for over a week. Her name was Liesel Palmer and her parents, who were society patrons in Seattle, were frantic with worry. She had supposedly been out taking pictures for a magazine layout and hadn't been seen since the previous Wednesday. There was a $50,000 reward for her safe return.

Daniel dropped the paper onto the floor and drummed his fingers on the edge of the recliner. Nah. This couldn't be Jake's "Anna" could it? It would explain him bringing food home and being relatively clean as of late. No harm checking it out, he thought, I guess I'll go over with the guys after the game to see this latest figment of Jake's imagination.

Chapter 26

Oregon—Saturday Night

When Jake returned to the cabin he seemed angry about something so Liesel pretended to be asleep. Maybe he'd leave her alone. He sat down on the hearth and opened a beer. Then he sat back and watched her sleep. After he had downed two more beers he came over to sit on the edge of the bed and rolled her over onto her back.

He pulled up her shirt exposing her full breasts. He reached over to the lantern on the table and turned the wick up so he'd have a better view. He noticed that her nipples were bruised and he bent over to lightly kiss them. She kept her eyes closed, hoping he would let her sleep if he thought she already was asleep. He rubbed his hands all over her chest and stomach savoring the feel of her. As he did he murmured, "Those guys are gonna like what they see tomorrow."

Her eyes popped wide open and she stammered, "Whaat? What did you say?"

Not stopping his attentions, he said, "I invited my friends to come over to see you after tomorrow's first football game. You're going to be the halftime entertainment for us. They think you're a figment of my imagination, but you're going to show them that they're wrong."

She didn't understand what it was he was trying to tell her, "Show them what?" she asked. "That I exist?" Would this be the opportunity she had been looking for, a chance to be rescued by his cronies.

"Nah," he said. "Not just that, but that you've got great tits and a sweet juicy pussy, just like I've been tellin' 'em all week. They don't believe that you're my love slave and that I own you."

She was appalled! He expected her to bare all for his buddies? Was he nuts? Of course he was nuts! That was sure a stupid question on her part. Didn't he have an inkling that she would tell his friends he was holding her against her will? Didn't he realize that she couldn't wait to get away from him?

She knew she shouldn't try to talk him out of this but she couldn't help herself, the words just rushed out, "I am not your love slave and you don't own me! I hate what you do to me and I certainly won't let you do it to me in front of them!"

He smiled at her and winked, "From the reactions I get from you I don't think you *hate* what I do to you. I think you love it and you're gonna love it when I show ya off or you'll be sorry."

"What's that supposed to mean? How can I be any sorrier than I am now, locked up by a man I can't stand?"

His face turned red and his eyes blazed. He leaned down and hissed at her through his dirty crooked teeth, "These friends of mine are not Sunday school teachers. They'll be happy to take ya on, one right after the other if I say they can. So if ya know what's good for ya you'll tell 'em that you're my woman and give 'em the eyeful they're comin' here for or I'll let 'em have ya as many times as they want to!"

He was serious. He wasn't at all afraid that she'd be found out and freed. What kind of back hills men were these? The thought crossed her mind that they might be similar to those men she remembered from the film "Deliverance", no morals, no sense of right from wrong, and no girlfriends. She was beginning to get the picture he was trying to show her.

These guys were coming by for a girlie show. They wouldn't care if the girl didn't belong here. They wouldn't be all that concerned for her welfare as long as they had their fun. But why? Why? If she was supposed to be his woman why wasn't he more protective of her? Jealous, even? She decided to gamble and ask.

"Tell me why you want 'your' woman enticing 'your' friends? Aren't you at all possessive of me? Don't you want to keep me to yourself?"

He put his opened palms flat on her breasts and rotated them around and around in little circles. "Nah," he said. "Guys like to share their toys. They like to show off when they got somethin' real special that don't nobody else have. It's braggin' rights to have a looker like you for my very own and I want everyone I've ever known to know it. Just wish the kids in high school could see me now."

He whisked the bed covers off her and looked down the length of her. "Sure will be mighty proud to be showing the likes of you off, you look as good as any picture in any magazine I ever did see."

And with that he cupped her firmly with his hand and she shivered, not just from his touch but also at the thought of what tomorrow would bring if she didn't get that ring loose before the first game was over.

Chapter 27

Oregon—Sunday

Daniel went into town early Sunday morning to see if he could find out any more about the missing woman. He picked up a local paper at the drug store and went over to the counter to pay for it. The kindly widow who owned the store knew everybody's habits and commented to Daniel about his purchase, she'd never known him to buy a paper before.

"This sure is a week for people doing all different kinda things."

Daniel looked up from the paper that he'd started reading and asked, "What do you mean?"

She said, "First Jake's been takin' pictures and now you're readin' the Gazette."

"Jake's been takin' pictures?" he asked with a look of puzzlement in his face.

"Yup, only they didn't turn out and he was madder'n a wet hen. Guess he needs to find out how to work that fancy camera he found out near Buck's Pond last week."

"Yeah," he said as he put down the money and walked out the door.

On the last page of the local section was a two column article about Liesel Palmer. They had found her jeep just two days ago, about ten miles south of here. She had apparently taken her camera and started out hiking from there. There didn't appear to be any signs of struggle around the jeep and nothing appeared to have been taken.

The keys were still in the ignition and her wallet was in the console. It was assumed that she had lost her way and was somewhere within a fifty mile radius as it was well known by her family and friends that she could easily hike twenty-five miles a day if she wanted to. There had been search parties combing the area around the Jeep since they had found it a few miles from Buck's Pond.

If Jake had Liesel, where had he found her and when? She had been last seen Wednesday morning of the previous week when she had packed up her Jeep before heading out to take some pictures of the local terrain. Where had Jake been last Wednesday? Hadn't he been working? Daniel searched his brain trying to remember and then it came to him. He had loaned Jake his pickup truck for the afternoon to lay in firewood for them both.

The mill allowed employees to gather firewood from different sites throughout the year as a way of clearing out the small sections of wood left after the logging trucks were finished in the area. The area currently supplying firewood was close to Buck's Pond. It was possible that Jake could have come across her. But why would she go with him?

It was too early to go to Clancy's yet, so he headed back home. While he was driving it occurred to Daniel that if Anna was Liesel she would have to be a dog to see anything in Jake. Why would she change her name, unless maybe she was trying not to be found. Then all of a sudden he remembered some of the gossip he'd heard about Jake.

He'd been fired from the high school because of some kind of sexual harassment, some lewd comments and propositions as he recalled it. Could he be holding Liesel against her will? Changing her name to Anna so no one would connect her to the missing photographer? If he'd been developing pictures for her wouldn't she have taken them correctly? Things were jumbling up in his head so fast that thoughts were running into each other, all the loose connections trying to find ends to connect to.

He decided to drop in at Jake's unexpectantly to see this "Anna" for himself. He turned onto the dirt road leading to Jake's cabin. It had started to drizzle and since he had never been up this road before he shifted ol' Trusty Rusty into low gear. The road was really no more than a dirt path in the woods and after driving almost a half mile, he had to stop and go the rest of the way by foot as the path narrowed to only about four feet. He hiked up the hill and went around a curve. There, about fifty feet away, was the cabin.

Chapter 28

Oregon—Sunday

Jake woke Liesel up early Sunday morning and dragged her down to the little brook so that she could wash up and prepare for his friends' visit. He had already instructed her on what he expected and what he would do if she disobeyed, or rather what he would allow them to do to her if she disobeyed. She was itching to have him gone so she could work on the mortar around the iron ring so she hurriedly washed up and let him lead her back up the hill. While she was fluffing her hair and eating the stale biscuits he had given her he said, " C'mere," and beckoned her over to the bed.

She eyed him uneasily and stayed where she was so he dragged her over to the bed, pushing her down on the edge. He removed her recently donned shirt and panties and said, "Lie back," as he pushed her down. He stood on her bare feet to keep her from kicking him and straddled her hips as he tied her hands to the bedposts on the opposite side of the bed, the ones that were the furthest apart from each other instead of the two at the top. In order to do this he'd had to lengthen the straps with some rope.

Then he strapped her ankles to the two bedposts closest to the door. These straps had also been lengthened to accommodate the spread of her legs. which couldn't even begin to come close to the posts, even when fully extended wide open. He told her that in this way he was hoping to use the larger area of the bed to display her more openly but also there would be no foot board obstructing his friends' view. He had grinned wickedly when he told her that sweet spot of hers would be the first thing they saw when they came through the door.

Liesel started protesting right away. She realized that if he left her that way she wouldn't be able to work on the ring. "They won't be here for hours. Why can't I be comfortable until then?

This position is even harder on my back and on my arms and legs. Please. You can always tell them to wait on the porch till you get me ready when you come back."

He thought about it and it made sense to him so he nodded. He looked down at her and smiled, "So you agree, this is how I should introduce you?"

She bit her lip and said, "Yes, if this is the way you want it. I'll be good, I'll do it. But you won't let them stay long will you?" She was trying very hard to say the things she thought he'd want to hear so he would just untie her and leave.

"Nah," he said "I want to get you alone so we can try a few new things I read about." Just then they heard the sound of feet crunching outside on the path. Jake ran to the door and threw it open. Daniel was just coming up the porch steps.

"Danny, my boy, what a surprise to see you!" Jake said enthusiastically.

Daniel said, "I had some spare time before the game, thought I'd come pick you up early and see if I could get a sneak-peak at this 'Anna' of yours."

Jake grinned from ear to ear. "Sure, c'mon in." And with that he ushered Daniel into the cabin.

As Daniel went through the door he was assailed by the foul stench of the place but as soon as he turned his head he forgot entirely about his nose. There on the bed, tied to the posts was the most beautiful woman he'd ever seen and he hadn't even seen her face yet. His eyes were riveted to the triangle in the middle of her body. It was displayed most prominently, gaping so widely open that he could see all the way into the pink lips framing her vagina.

His eyes traveled upwards to her chest and, although she was flat on her back, he could see her delicious white mounds crested with coral colored nipples that were tipped with purple bruises. His eyes traveled further up past her long neck to her face. His eyes met hers and he knew that he had found Liesel, and she was not a dog, not by a long shot.

As his eyes searched hers he found his voice. "Anna, how very nice to meet you." Stay cool, he was trying to tell her with his eyes. "Jake has told us so much about you, and I can see that it was all true." He looked down the length of her, noting the leather thongs attached to her incredibly long legs.

"Jake," he said "How 'bout a beer for your buddy while I feast my eyes on your beautiful woman?"

"Sure," Jake said, strutting as proudly as a peacock as he quickly went out to the porch to retrieve one.

As soon as Jake had passed the doorjamb, Daniel stepped forward and bent over her as he motioned with his finger to his lips, and whispered softly,"Liesel, don't worry, I'll be back real soon." She made a loud sobbing sound that just about broke his heart.

When Jake came back through the door he handed the beer to Daniel and said, "I tol' ya'll, she's a looker ain't she?"

Daniel took a swig of his beer and stared Liesel in the face, trying with every fiber in his being not to let his eyes rove any lower, even though he very much wanted to. "That she is," he said and then quickly averted his eyes to his beer.

Over in the corner on the floor behind where Jake was standing were some rumpled bedclothes covered with blood and sticking out from under them was a very expensive looking camera case. Jake picked up a basin filled with soapy water and a razor and walked towards Liesel. "I was just fixin' to shave her up a bit. Some guys like that you know, a nice, smooth, hairless pussy."

Liesel's eyes grew wide with fear. Daniel put his hand out to stop Jake from advancing any closer. "And some guys don't. I prefer the natural look." With that Jake turned and put the basin and razor on the side table.

"Whatever you say, Dan. If that's the way you want it, that's the way it'll stay." It was obvious to Liesel that Jake thought very highly of this man and would take his advice on just about anything.

106

Jake turned to Daniel and asked, " What's your favorite part of a woman?"

"Oh, I don't know," Daniel replied, "I like it all."

Jake pressed, "Well if you could kiss just one part what would it be?"

Daniel thought this was going to turn into an invitation to do just that, so he said softly, "The part of the neck just below the ear where you can smell her essence and feel her hair on your face."

Jake gave him a strange look like he thought Daniel was out of his mind, but he said, "Well, go ahead, have at it, everybody'll get one taste of her, you can have yours now."

Daniel leaned over the bed and placed one hand on each side of her head, piercing her eyes with his, then he slowly lifted his left hand and turned her face to the left, he bent lower and placed a kiss just below her ear, whispering softly against her warm flesh, "Liesel, just a little bit longer and it'll be all over, I promise."

She shivered from the tingling sensation his kiss had caused, the spot where his lips had touched her still warm from his caress.

Then he straightened up and said "Jake, you wanna go grab a bite to eat before the game, my treat?"

"Sure," said Jake, "let's go, but first I'd better make Anna a little more comfortable. Would ya mind waiting for me at the truck?"

"Okay. Nice meetin' you Anna. See you again after the game," Daniel called out as he turned to go. He met her gaze and winked at her, mindful to keep his eyes only on hers. He noticed that her eyes were filling with tears before he turned away and walked out the door.

Jake was beside himself with glee. "Anna, ya did real good. Danny was quite taken, don't you agree?" Liesel was still dealing with her mortification to make any comment so she just lay there while Jake removed her leather straps and attached the chain to her waist.

"I'll be back in a few hours and we'll get you ready for the rest of the gang, and as a reward I'll bring you some food back from the bar. You like french fries?" When she didn't answer him, he just shrugged and walked out the door closing it behind him.

After he left she sat on the floor and cried and cried. She didn't think she'd ever run out of tears. She had never been so ashamed and felt so helpless in all her life. That man "Danny", whose very first view of her was of the most private part of her body, was not what she had expected one of Jake's friends to be like.

He had an air of sophistication about him. He wasn't from around here that was for sure. And he'd almost been gentlemanly about his perusal of her, like he hadn't felt it was his due to continue viewing all the charms she was displaying for all to see. And that kiss, it had caused a thrill deep inside her, somewhere she hadn't known existed.

He said he'd be back, what did that mean? With the others? Oh God, the others! She hopped up so fast it made her dizzy. Quickly she found the tool she'd been using and went to work scraping at the mortar around the ring. She pulled on the ring. It wasn't even jiggling, not even a little bit. Her despair was almost complete when the door burst open.

Chapter 29

Oregon—Sunday

There, framed by the doorway, was the man Jake had called "Danny". He had looked tall when she had been lying down and now she saw that he really was. His broad shoulders filled almost the entire space of the doorway. With his plaid flannel shirt opened to the center of his chest, showing a muscled expanse covered with thick curly black hair, she was reminded of a dark-haired Paul Bunyan.

His eyes were a deep sapphire blue and she remembered how they had spoken to hers not so very long ago. The cut of his jaw was square and it was outlined by the shadow of a beard grown over the weekend. He stepped into the cabin and closed the door behind him. She felt an immense feeling of dread, was he here to claim her also? She shrank back, moving closer to the hearth.

He picked up on her distress and the reason for it right away. "I'm not here to hurt you. I'm here to help you get away. My name is Daniel Hoffman. I used to be a firefighter in Baltimore and I just read about you in the paper last night. I left Jake with the others watching the game in the bar so we don't have a lot of time. Let's get out of here. Are you hurt?"

"No, I'm not hurt," she said. "But I am chained to this wall."

He crossed the cabin in three long strides. He looked at the chain in the hearth and then followed it with his eyes to her waist. She was wearing a shirt with no buttons, tied at the bottom and her lacy panties, that's all. He picked up the padlock at her waist and tugged on it a few times, then pulled at the chain attached to the ring.

Even with his superior physique exuding his brute strength, it didn't budge. "I'll be right back," he said and turned to leave.

"No, don't go! Don't leave me!" she cried.

He walked back to her and put his hands on her shoulders. "I'm just going back to my truck. It's at the bottom of the hill. It shouldn't take but a few minutes. Trust me, I'm going to get you out of here." With that he dropped his hands, turned and walked out the door. She could hear him running down the road.

True to his word he was only gone a few minutes. When he returned he was carrying an axe with a red handle. He wrapped her up in the mattress and positioned her as far away from the hearth as the chain would reach, drawing it taut against the fieldstone, then he brought the axe back behind his shoulder with both hands and swung it forward into the outstretched chain, severing it into two pieces like it was a twig. The force of the separation threw her to the floor but the mattress cushioned her fall.

"Knew this ol' fire axe would come in handy one day."

Walking over to where the rest of the chain was at the iron ring he brought the axe back to his shoulder again and hit just to the right of the ring, it took four tries before the mortar crumbled around the ring and then both the ring and the chain fell to the floor. He picked them up and walked over to her.

"This will make Jake think you escaped on your own." He looked down at her. Her breasts were barely covered in that shirt and he could feel his loins clenching. Her very slim and incredibly long legs were noticeably bare and he asked, "Do you have any pants anywhere or shoes?"

"He tore my jeans into strips to use to tie me up against the trees. I think my boots might be over here in the corner." She walked over and looked under a pile of bloody bed clothes. The boots were there with her socks beside them. She sat on the bed to put them on.

Daniel gestured towards the bloody bedding piled in two corners, "Did he cut you?"

"No." she said.

"Then what's all the blood from?", he asked.

"From my period," she replied sheepishly, "I was trying to make it look worse than it was, and it worked. He left me alone while he thought I was having it."

He took her by the arm and led her out of the cabin. She stopped, picked up her camera bag and shifted it onto her shoulder. He took it from her shoulder and put it on his and together they walked down the hill to his truck. He helped her into the passenger seat, watching her tuck her legs under her. She was going to need some counseling right away. She was already sinking into a shell and he could tell when he looked into her eyes that the sparkle had gone out.

He drove to his cabin to get her some clothes. He knew she wouldn't want to go into another man's cabin after her experiences in Jake's, so he left her in the truck while he went inside to get her a shirt and some pants. Then he went around to his shed and found his big bolt cutters. Back at the pick up, Daniel lifted Liesel out and propped her up beside the truck. He used the bolt cutters to cut through the chain around her waist and handed her the clothes. She just stared at them with unseeing eyes.

Now that the danger was over it appeared that she was going into shock. He sat her on the edge of the seat and held open the pants for her to step into. She slid off the seat into the pants and then fell against his chest when she lost her balance. He was momentarily stunned by the softness of her and struggled to upright her. His pants were so large on her that her whole body was almost swallowed up in them.

Then he put one of his oversized shirts on over hers and buttoned it. Keeping her standing up against the truck he bent over and tied her boots. He threw the chain and the bolt cutters in the bed of the pickup with the other length of chain and the axe.

When Daniel turned back to her he bent down and lightly stroked her cheek and lifted her chin with his fingers until they were eye to eye. "Liesel, you have to make some decisions now. Where do you want me to take you?"

When she just looked up at him he smiled down at her and said, "I can't help you with this. You have to tell me where to take you. Do you want to go to the Police station? Do you want to go to a hospital? Do you want to call home? If you're going to press charges it would probably be better to go to the Police station and then we can take you to get a check-up so they'll have the evidence they'll need to prosecute."

"He didn't rape me," she said matter-of-factly.

This shocked him but when no further explanation was forthcoming he said, "Well, he still kidnapped you and held you against your will, even if you did have consensual sex."

This brought the sparkle back to her eyes and with an explosive burst of energy she pushed against his chest and screamed, "Consensual sex! Are you out of your mind? Nothing he made me do was consensual! I loathed the touch of that despicable man! He should rot in hell for all his vile perversions!"

Well, he thought, now they were getting somewhere. She was coming back to life. Now let's see if we can get her to face the real world after all this. "Okay. Let's go to the police." With that he lifted her back into the truck and went around to the driver's side and got in.

As he was maneuvering down and around the mountain roads, she spoke. "Could you please take me to my hotel first? I don't think I can face the police now with your clothes on looking like I do.

"You look fine," he said softly, then added, "but I'll be glad to." He looked at her out of the corner of his eye. She did look fine. She looked fantastically better than fine. Her short brunette hair was tousled with curls everywhere and her skin was tawny colored from the sun. She had a look of playfulness about her that shone through even now when she had to be at her absolute worst.

He looked at the clock on the dashboard and suddenly a thought occurred to him and he laughed outloud. She looked over at him. He had a great laugh, but what was so funny? He looked at her and laughed again. She gave him a questioning look and he chided, "You really don't want to know."

"Yes, yes I do." She said.

So he told her "I was just thinking the football game is over now and Jake's taking everybody back to his cabin to meet you. They'll never believe anything he says ever again!" They both laughed heartily at the thought of Jake standing there with his friends trying to figure out where she'd gone to.

When they arrived at the hotel they were told that her parents had taken her things and her Jeep back home to Seattle with them. Since the search parties were still out looking for her, she used the hotel phone to call her parents and then the police. They were so relieved to hear her voice. She told them she had somehow managed to get lost and a wonderful lumberjack had found her. They were going to come get her but she told them it wasn't necessary, Daniel had insisted on driving her to her parents' home himself.

Then she called the local sheriff's office and told them she had gotten lost in the dense forests and had finally managed to run into somebody who could help her. She felt like a coward as Daniel stood beside her listening to her lies. After hanging up she looked up at him with tears in her eyes. Liesel explained that she would not be pressing any charges. The publicity and subsequent trial would ruin her parents in the social circles that were their life now. She just couldn't do that to them. She didn't want them to know what had really happened to her. It would kill them to know.

They found a nearby Walmart and Daniel bought her some clothes and toiletries. Then they found a Western Sizzlin' Restaurant and Daniel watched her eat her fill. Hopping back into the pickup, he drove her straight to her parents' home in Seattle. She curled up in her corner, leaning against the door, and slept while he drove.

Of course, her parents were so excited to see her that Daniel was forgotten in the background for awhile. When things had settled down a bit her father took him into his study and gave him the reward check for $50,000. Daniel very graciously declined, saying that he hadn't done anything that wouldn't have been expected of him.

He said his goodbyes to her after they'd had a late celebratory dinner and then he headed back to his cabin in Oregon. He hadn't even driven twenty miles when he realized that he missed her. He made it home in time to get a few hours sleep before getting up to go to work.

A very agitated Jake was waiting for him at their usual pickup spot the next morning. "Where'd you go during the game yesterday?" He asked him suspiciously.

Daniel winced and replied, "Got a real bad chili dog there at Clancy's so I went home to spend the whole afternoon and most of the night in my bathroom. How'd it go during halftime with Anna and the guys?" He asked innocently.

It was all Daniel could do not to laugh in his face as Jake bellyached about how Anna had picked the absolute worst time to go visit her mama. When Jake asked him to vouch for him to all the guys that he really did have a woman named Anna, Daniel just looked at him with an exaggerated questioning look. "What are you talkin' about? I never saw your Anna. I'm not going to lie for you! And I certainly don't appreciate you asking me to! You can find your own way to and from work from now on. We are no longer friends!" He pulled into the parking lot at the mill and pushed him out of his truck with a whole lot less force than he would have liked to have used.

That night when Daniel got home he called Liesel. She was sticking to her decision not to press any charges because she didn't want her parents to find out about the ordeal that she had really been through. He admired her for that, even though he knew it wasn't really the right thing for her to do for herself or for the next unsuspecting woman that Jake might happen upon. Daniel was the only person other than Jake who knew what had really happened and she knew her secrets were safe with him.

He called her almost every day. They talked for hours, long into the night. Liesel found it easy to talk to Daniel about

114

everything that had happened to her as long as they were on the phone. She was able to vent all her anger over the things Jake had done to her with Daniel quietly listening and encouraging her to keep talking. But when they were face-to-face, she became shy and withdrawn. Over the next few weeks he visited whenever he was invited and it became harder and harder to leave her each time. When she accepted a job offer from the National Wildlife Federation in McLean, Virginia, he was devastated and felt like he was being torn in two.

He had insisted she go to counseling and so far she was doing what he asked. When she moved to Virginia he had already lined up a new doctor for her to see—Dr. David Sandler. He'd heard he was the best from his friends in Baltimore. And so it was that Liesel Palmer became David Sandler's most fascinating case.

Chapter 30

Fairfax, VA June 1987

Things were not going as planned for David Sandler. Due to the terms of his divorce agreement with Linda, and the additional costs of setting up housekeeping on his own, he found that it was a struggle to keep up his former lifestyle. He could see that the days of trading in cars every six months were over for awhile. So were the $1200 Hart, Shaffner & Marx suits and Rockports in every style and color.

He was pulling in the reins on his spending, but he was hating it. Each time he denied himself something he thought he should easily be able to afford, he thought of Linda, and his contempt for her grew. The one exception to his new found frugalness was where Jenny, Paisley and Rusty were concerned. He was constantly bringing them gifts or taking them somewhere and it was always first class all the way. He did not want Jenny to suspect that he was having any problems with money.

Since Paisley had been born he found many ways to lavish gifts on her. So much so, that Jenny had had to curtail him. It just wasn't appropriate to her way of thinking for him to spend so much money on them. And even though he often included Rusty in his generosity, it was obvious to all that Paisley had a special place in his heart.

David managed to win her parents over with his quiet charm and warm concern for Jenny and her children but it was curious to them how he was working his way into Jenny's life without Jenny seeming to be working her way into his. Jenny started to wonder herself at the relationship they were developing. That he might have romantic designs on her was a little unsettling and at the same time a little exciting. In light of his recent divorce, she certainly didn't want to accept the idea that she might have played an unwitting part in it.

As Paisley developed and changed from a tiny infant to a small toddler, David had been there for almost all her significant achievements. He came over on weekends when Jenny had to work and took her and Rusty to the park while Nan did her grocery shopping. On week nights when Jenny was off, the four of them would go to Fuddrucker's or Friday's where everyone was tolerant of little children or David would bring over a carry-out dinner that he had picked up along with a Disney video.

It was the night they watched Pinocchio that Jenny decided their relationship needed some defining. Although they laughed and enjoyed the antics of the kids and talked about everything you could think of, there was no connection, no looking into each other's eyes and getting all jittery. They had never held hands or hugged or said anything that would indicate to one or the other that they were dating. Were they?

He was very protective of her and the children and as polite and thoughtful as an English gentleman could be but he had never made a move on her and up until now she had been comfortable with that. However, Jenny knew that if she were to go out with someone else that he would be very hurt, but she didn't quite know why.

After both children were read to and tucked into their beds, Jenny straightened up the kitchen and David rewound the video tape. Then she carried a tray of wine and cheese and crackers into the family room and set them on the coffee table.

"How about a game of chess?" she asked. They both fancied themselves to be better than the other at the strategy and always had a fierce competitive game.

"Sure, but this time maybe we should set a time limit for your turn!" he teased.

He brought the chess set over to the table from the built-in book shelf beside the fireplace and poured them each a glass of wine. Jenny decided that now would be a good time to ask her question.

Looking down at the chess set and pretending to examine the board for her next move she said, "David, where do you see this going with us?"

He looked over at her and took her chin in his hand and raised her face upwards until their eyes met. His eyes were a soft, warm brown, reminding her of the rich milk chocolate bars she melted to make fudge. The dark piercing pupils stared deeply into hers as he stroked her chin with his thumb and he softly murmured, "I see us getting married some day. You are a beautiful woman that I would like to have as my wife. It's your move."

Stunned by this revelation of his, she sat back and just stared at him. Finally she was able to whisper, "What? What did you say?"

"You heard me, c'mon and play."

"How can you think of chess right now after you've come out with that?"

"Simple, I've known it all along. It's just new to you." Then he added, "We really are going to have to give you a time limit."

Needless to say, she lost that game rather badly, as she couldn't even begin to concentrate on it. When it was over he stood up and pulled her to her feet. Holding both of her hands in his, he said, "We are going very, very slowly because this is what you need. You need to trust me before you can love me and I don't want you to think of me as one of your admirers who only wants the woman he sees on the outside. Although I like the outside very much, it's the woman inside I like the most. I have already developed strong feelings for you. I'll just have to wait for you to catch up."

With that he bent down slightly and brushed his lips lightly over hers. He straightened and looked down at her. With a smile on his face he said,"Good night" and then walked to the door and let himself out.

She put her fingertips to her lips and held them there for a moment trying to corral her thoughts. As she put away the wine and cheese she relived the last few moments in her mind. He was planning on marrying her? He had strong feelings for her? What did that mean? She locked the deadbolt on the front door and climbed the steps to the upstairs bedrooms. She looked in on Rusty and Paisley sleeping so peacefully in their beds.

Paisley's bed was an old fashioned Jenny Lind crib and she had to go all the way into the room to check on her because the side bumpers obscured the mattress from the doorway. She was as beautiful as an angel, one sweet cheek lying on the mattress with her hand tucked just under her chin. She stroked the other cheek, marveling at its velvet softness. God had been especially good to her when he'd helped her conceive this warm bundle of joy.

Rusty lay on his side with his favorite Transformer toy beside him on the pillow. One could just imagine the wild dreams he was having playing some sort of super hero. Judging from his expression he had just won the battle and was being carried triumphantly away to the next adventure. Yes, she was very blessed, indeed.

Putting on her nightgown she thought about David again. How did he fit into their plans? Since Paisley had been born she hadn't really thought seriously about marrying again. In all her thoughts about the children and their future, she envisioned herself as a single mom. And she knew why that was. After all, how many men would want to say "I do" to an instant family of four? She also knew something quirky about herself. Something she had known about herself since she had been a teenager. That *something* was something she was not going to compromise on. The doorway into her heart and soul.

As she removed the carefully placed mound of decorative pillows from the bed she started to reminisce. It had started right from the beginning, from the very first kiss way back in junior high school. She had known that kiss had not been right. It didn't feel right. It didn't taste good and she hadn't wanted to do it again, at least not with the same person. Maybe it would be different with somebody else. And thus the great search had been on.

She knew that there had to be somebody placed on this earth whose kiss would make her want more of the same. The kisses she'd read about in romance novels had been earth-shattering, heart-rending, blood-tingling and toe-curling. The kisses she'd seen at the movies had caused fireworks to light up the sky or caused a man and a woman to fall to the sand clutching at each other as the waves rushed over them.

Why did the kisses she got make her want to wipe her tongue and lips on sandpaper to get rid of the taste and feel of them? Sooner or later she'd find the right kiss, but really, how many wrong ones would she have to endure first?

So far as she knew, nobody else felt this way. The girls she talked to about kissing, seemed to like it with everybody. She tried to learn some of their techniques, thinking she was doing it wrong, but that didn't help. It wasn't a technique thing, it had more to do with the touch and connection.

It wasn't until almost two years later that she chanced to kiss a G.I. at the roller skating rink in Frankfurt, Germany where her father had been stationed. And it really was an unexpected kiss. She'd come around the corner in her skates into the snack bar lounge just as he was coming out and they'd collided. He had grabbed her around the waist to keep her from falling and when she had managed to stand upright he was looking down into her eyes and smiling.

The next thing she knew he had pressed his lips against hers. He moved them over hers causing hers to part and then he eased his tongue inside and rimmed the inside of her lips with his tongue before thrusting it deeply in to meet up with hers. The sudden delight she felt caused her to close her eyes to savor it and it was then that she saw the stars. When he pulled away from her she was looking up at him with the most amazed look on her face.

Just then an older girl pulled his arm away from her and said, "What are you doing? You're here with me!" and she pulled him out onto the rink for a couples skate.

When he turned to look back at her she had her fingers to her lips rubbing them lightly back and forth trying to figure out if that kiss had really happened or if she had imagined the whole thing. Her eyes followed him around the rink several times, but she stopped when she realized that the girl he was holding in his arms was staring at her with a savagely jealous look. Jenny wanted him to come back to her and to kiss her again so she could see if he was the one she was supposed to find but the girl he was with was pulling his face around to hers quite possessively.

As the immature teenager that she was, she dreamed about this mystery man and went back to the skating rink at every opportunity, hoping to see him again. Several months later he appeared again but he was with the same girl. None of her friends knew who he was, but a few did know who the girl was, Debbie Beacons, a senior at the high school. Apparently they had been going steady for the better part of a year, although it was continually on and off as Debbie was very jealous and he was very *friendly*. Somebody thought his name was Dusty.

It was almost two years before the opportunity presented itself for her to get another chance at a kiss from him. He and Debbie had broken up, this time from their engagement. Over the span of two years Jenny and Dusty had occasionally spotted each other at various skating sessions. He would wink at her and she would smile at him and then they both would continue whatever skating maneuver they had been attempting.

When Jenny arrived early for an evening session, a friend of hers handed her a note. It was from him. He was asking her out on a date. A double date. When she asked her parents if she could go out with him they said, "No, he's too old for you." They didn't like the idea of her going out with a G.I. She was only sixteen at the time. So she did something that she had never done before. She bold-faced lied to her parents and arranged to spend the night at her friend Samantha's but instead met Dusty for a date.

They went for a drive in a big white Oldsmobile convertible. Since it was a double date and it wasn't Dusty's car, they sat in the back. They went up towards the Taurnus mountains and found a secluded apple orchard to pull into. It was then that she finally got her second real kiss. And third. And fourth. And fifth.

And oh, oh, suddenly he wanted to do more than that. And she definitely did not. Even though everything he was doing really did feel pleasing, she knew she could not. At sixteen she had already decided that she would be a virgin on her wedding night and she wasn't going to waiver even though his kisses were melting her bones. He wasn't at all happy when she stopped him so he tried to start all over again. When he reached for her bra strap again, she was ready to go home and she told him so.

On the way out of the orchard they gathered a few apples to eat on the way home. When Dusty took a bite out of one, he instantly realized it was sour and wormy and threw it away. Too late he realized that his two false front teeth were embedded in it and all four of them spent the next two hours on their hands and knees trying to find the apple that he had bitten into among all the rotten apples on the ground. It was to no avail. So much for a good night kiss, without his teeth he wouldn't even face her.

When they finally tried to take Jenny to her friend's house, where she was supposed to be spending the night, they got lost. It wasn't until after 2 a.m. that Jenny timidly knocked at Samantha's door and Samantha's mother answered. When everything was sorted out, Sam's mother called her father and he drove out to get her.

She was put on restriction for the last two months of their tour in Germany and she never got to see Dusty again. But oh, those kisses. Someday she would find someone who could kiss her like that again. Over the years many a relationship had died a quick death because of the *kiss*. She had determined that this part of a relationship had to be right, the rest you could work on.

She found she either rushed the first date kiss or she delayed it, depending on whether she wanted her test to pass or fail.

When she really liked someone it was truly hard to back away from a slimy, thick-tongued, sloppy kiss. To her a kiss was something to savor not something to put up with. It just had to be right.

The difference between a moderately dry, gently probing tongue and a groping, thrusting, slobbering, lizard-like appendage in her mouth was the difference between the likelihood of a second date or a permanently busy schedule. Unfortunately she found most men lacking in the kissing department. They were either too eager, too wet, too rough or in too much of a hurry. When she had finally allowed R.J. to kiss her it was after they had been out on several dates.

They were in the front seat of his Cadillac demo when he gathered her into his arms and asked for her permission as if he knew that the significance of this moment would affect their future. When she granted it, he took his time and lowered his lips ever so slowly to hers. When their lips made contact it was like having an electric shock pulse through her.

She was amazed that she had finally found someone with some finesse, and a wonderful set of lips who knew how to use them. That night she enjoyed many more of his kisses and that might have been the reason that she said "yes" to his proposal only a few weeks later.

Jenny tried to remember David's kiss. It had been so fleeting that it really hadn't impressed her one way or another. And this was something she really needed to know about. His kiss. Because if the kiss is right...

Chapter 31

July 1987

It was not David Sandler's custom to go through his mail but his receptionist was away on family leave and it was beginning to pile up on her desk. So after lunch one day he started sorting through the mail. Most of it was junk mail. The rest were business statements until he came across an envelope whose return address was that of a noted local attorney.

His first thought was that Linda was taking some new type of legal action against him with a really big hitter but when he unfolded the letter and a check fell out onto his desk, he knew that wasn't the case. He picked up the check and focused on the typed dollar amount . He sucked in his breath as he read it. It was for $50,000. He put the check aside and read the letter. Six times.

The letter was from the attorney handling the estate of Benton Riveria. Shortly before he died he had added a codicil to his will endowing $50,000 to Dr. David Sandler's practice. It was given so that it could be used for the treatment of patients with psychiatric problems that he thought Dr. Sandler could help. Mr. Riveria had been so impressed with Dr. Sandler's hypnotic technique that he felt more people should be able to benefit from it. To that end he had donated $50,000.

David was stunned. This was incredible. Just when he was scrambling around trying to make ends meet that were nowhere near to even touching, a patient bequeathed money to him. He was ecstatic. Then his conscience came into play and he thought about what the money had been intended for. It would be difficult to justify using this money for anything personal. Yet, how could he not? He needed it. Quite badly, in fact.

On his way home he stopped at his bank and set up a special account. He opened it under the name of "The David L. Sandler Foundation," he endorsed the check and deposited it. Then he took the new checkbook home and paid a few bills that were long overdue. He felt so much better about everything now. He told himself that when he got back on track financially he would replace the money that belonged to the Foundation.

That night, while Jenny was still pondering the significance of David's kiss from the evening before and wondering in which direction their relationship was heading, David was unwittingly steering it in a different direction than he wanted.

The next morning when David met his first patient of the day, he was in a truly good mood for the first time in months. The money he had received from Benton Riveria had removed the oppressive, nagging thoughts that had constantly been on his mind about his accounts. He was able to give Jessica Tyler his full time and attention, which she surely deserved since her father was paying a bundle for her treatments.

Jessica was the daughter of a congressman and had taken to shoplifting as a means of dealing with her daily bouts of depression. Naturally, this was not the kind of attention her father wanted or expected from his socialite daughter. She was supposed to be attending charity balls or volunteering to help museums and art galleries with their funding problems, not waiting downtown at the police station for her father's attorney to bail her out of jail. When she had been unceremoniously dumped by her gold-bricking husband as soon as he'd found a younger woman with an even richer family, she'd gone a little crazy.

Jessica was a pretty woman but her vanity couldn't deal with the humiliation of her husband's rejection. She hadn't known that all of their friends were more his friends than hers. The thought that they were all laughing behind her back while he was nuzzling his new paramour made her cringe inside. She couldn't stand the separation from all that she had known and the loneliness it was causing. In her own way, the shoplifting had been a call for help. She enjoyed the attention her father had given her even though it was very clear that he was extremely disappointed with her.

After a few weeks David could see that his hypnotic suggestions were getting through. He had been trying to reassure her and boost her confidence while at the same time reprogramming her to deal with her inner tantrums in a less destructive way. She wasn't shoplifting anymore so far as he could tell, however, now she was drinking heavily and doing the night club scene. She came in for her Wednesday morning appointment reeking of liquor and dressed like quite the tramp.

Her brunette hair had been teased high on her head and had some sort of chopstick-looking thing stuck in it. Her lipstick and eye shadow had been smudged as if she'd just lifted her head off of a pillow. The black leather skirt she was wearing was so short that he could see the bottom clips of her black garter belt as they held her stockings up.

When she removed a feathery over wrap of some sort he nearly fell back into his seat. She was wearing a completely sheer black blouse with a sheer lacy bra underneath. The front clip was undone and her breasts were right up against the fabric of the shirt. Had she been naked she wouldn't have been any more exposed.

"Jessica! My, God woman! That isn't the way you go out at night is it?" he exclaimed as he reached for her wrap to cover her.

She looked down at herself and saw what had happened and quickly fumbled through the material to resnap the front of her bra, mumbling something he couldn't even begin to make out.

"Where have you been dressed like that this morning?" he asked.

"I spent the night in Georgetown and by the time I woke up I only had time to just get here. I had no time to go home and change. I hope you don't mind too much, but I didn't want to miss our session. Daddy would get mad, you know."

They spent the session talking about her drinking and where she thought this was going to lead her. Then Dr. Sandler used a relaxation technique to put her in a state where she would be receptive to comments he was making, telling her that she had worth, all the while trying not to stare at her voluptuous breasts getting ready to pop the snap on her lacy bra again.

Chapter 32

Tyson's Corner

The following evening Jenny had to work late so David went over to the dealership to visit and to look at the cars. He was very careful not to stop by too often, since he didn't want her friends at work to get any ideas about them until Jenny was ready for that. He came about an hour before closing time, hoping she wouldn't be tied up with another customer. As it turned out she was just finishing a delivery when he pulled into the lot and got out of his car.

He watched her as she knelt down at the back of the new car and screwed the license plate on. She was such an independent person and she wanted to carry her own against the men so much that she wouldn't even think of letting anyone help her. She relished the idea of being "just one of the guys" so much that she insisted on being referred to as a salesman, not a salesperson.

As he stood towering over her he smiled and asked, "First or second one of the day?"

"Third," she replied, and moved around to the front of the car to attach the front plate. When they walked back into the dealership together she asked how his day had been. He just shook his head and said she wouldn't believe it, even if he could tell her about it.

She laughed, "Hey, I'm in the car business, nothing surprises me!" But that wasn't really true, she was surprised all the time. "Let me assure you, that behind every car deal is a story just as there is for each of your patients."

After she finished with her customer David invited her to go to Carnegie's, a little deli just around the corner for a bite to eat before going home. She accepted and got her things together. They drove over in separate cars so she could leave to go home right from there. The little cafe had only two other customers so they had no trouble getting served. The sandwiches were enormous there so they ordered a Reuben to share, along with a beer for him and a glass of white wine for her. When the waiter left to take care of their order, David leaned over and took her hand.

"So tell me, what were the stories behind your car deals tonight?"

"You don't really want to know do you? Won't that be boring for you? Besides, I have to protect the confidentiality of my clients just as you do yours!" She flashed a bright smile to him.

"Touché," he replied and winked at her. "Have you been thinking about me lately?" he asked.

She smiled over at him and teasingly replied, "Oh yeah, of course."

"No, seriously, have you?"

"Well, I have been wondering about our friendship for quite awhile, ever since I asked your advice about Paisley's conception, things have changed between us. We don't really have the same business relationship anymore and I'm unsure about our friendship."

He just sat there and looked at her for a moment before saying, "I kind of feel like I'm her father since I was in on her conception, you know what I mean? I never had a child of my own and I'm fascinated with her. She's so cute and cuddly and getting to be so smart. I really enjoy watching her grow. Each day when she discovers something new it's a new surprise for me too. I'm seeing the wonder in the simplest things through her reactions to them."

"She really is a special baby," Jenny agreed, "I just love it when she wakes up in the morning, all smiles and giggles. She has such a good disposition, always eager to get up and get out of that crib, not whinny and impatient. She allows me the time I need to acquaint myself with the morning before making any demands. And you're right she does get pleasure out of everything, especially a mound of mashed potatoes!"

"What do you think about taking them to the beach? I'd just love to see her reaction to the waves and sand. Rusty could use a few more swimming lessons, too. I've got a time share condo at Ocean City. We could pack them up and drive there for a weekend."

"Oh, I don't think you're ready for a four or five hour drive with these two! It's all Mom and Dad and I can do to get them to Carolina Beach each summer for vacation and we usually drive at night while they're sleeping. It's no fun, believe me. It does help that I can take one of the conversion vans with the video player, but even with a box of Disney tapes the kids are restless and anxious to get out of their car seats long before we're there."

"Ocean City isn't quite as far as Carolina Beach, geez! That's past Wilmington!" he countered.

"It's still too far to go for just a weekend," she said, even though she was really thinking, "I can't go away for a weekend with you, we hardly know each other." And how improper would that be? Her mother would have a fit. She saw his frown and knew that she had disappointed him with her refusal.

"But we could go to Breezy Point for the day. That's only an hour and a half from here. We could manage that with the kids." She had effectively turned a weekend trip with three days and two long, leisurely nights into a one-day picnic excursion trip.

He wasn't happy about it, but he guessed he should grab at it and hope that they would just keep progressing as they were. Eventually, things would end up where he wanted them. Which was both of them walking with hands about each other's waists from their master bedroom suite to Paisley's nursery room each morning to watch her greet the day after they'd thoroughly enjoyed the night.

"All right, that we can do. Do you want to go on Sunday, when you're already off or do you want to go on another day?" he asked.

She tilted her head as if thinking it through, "Sunday's good. We could leave early and have breakfast and lunch at the beach and then come home after we cook dinner at the beach. The kids will be exhausted by then and we can watch a movie."

It never seemed to bother David that they couldn't go out to dinner or to the movies. He seemed to be a homebody just like her. Neither of them had time after their busy career days to do the party or bar scene and it wasn't missed since it wasn't something either of them had ever really been into in the first place. Quiet evenings at home playing with the children were what they both looked forward to.

"Then it's all settled. I'll pick everyone up early Sunday morning and we'll be off to the Eastern Shore. I'll get a picnic basket from Sutton Gourmet on Saturday so you won't have to worry about the food when you get home from work Saturday night," he volunteered.

"I think I'd better get a van for the trip. We'll never fit the kids and all the stuff we'll need into your firebird." That was a big benefit of working for a car dealership and being one of their best car salesmen. She had a new demo of her choosing every three months and whenever she had a special need for a different type of car or truck, she just took it off the line. It was like owning a fleet of cars of her own.

Generally, she chose the top of the line sports car which was a Trans Am, but maneuvering Paisley's car seat in and out of the back seat proved to be too hard on her back, so she'd switched to a Bonneville shortly after Paisley's birth. Their sandwich arrived and while they each attempted to finish just half of it, they discussed all the things they would need to pack. Traveling with kids was like going on a Safari.

After David had paid the bill, he escorted her to her car and opened her door for her. Just as she turned to get in, he put his hand on her shoulder and turned her back to him. "Good night," he said.

Then he put his fingers lightly on her cheek and stroked it from her temple to her chin, looking down into her eyes and deepening his gaze. His lips curved into a soft half smile and then he lowered his head to hers and lightly brushed his lips over hers. He moved them back and forth trying to feel the shape of her lips under his. When he ran his tongue over the bottom edge of her top lip trying to gain access to the moist interior of her mouth, she backed away, leaving him licking his own top lip and looking at her questioningly.

"Good night," she said. "Thank you for the late dinner. See you at my house around seven Sunday morning, okay?"

"Yeah," he replied and walked slowly over to his car. He watched her put her seat belt on and start the car, then pull out of the parking space and drive off. She was not showing the passion that he knew she had in her, and he wondered at that.

On Jenny's drive home she did little else than analyze her feelings about his kiss. As she mechanically maneuvered the Bonneville onto Route 7 and then onto the Dulles Toll Road she licked her lips and knew a feeling that brought her low. His kiss was not right, she hadn't enjoyed it at all. To be fair, it hadn't really been a complete kiss, she'd stopped him just as he was getting going. She knew she was being too quick to judge his amorous qualities, but she couldn't help it. The kiss had not been excitable to her. It had been pretty blaise until he'd limned her lips with his tongue, and then it had instantly become repugnant and she'd wanted no more of it.

"Now what?" she asked herself outloud. She hoped that whenever he realized that their relationship would go no further romantically that it wouldn't cost her his friendship, or Paisley a devoted babysitter.

Chapter 33

Fairfax, VA

The next day at the office was a busy one for David. Wednesdays usually were since that was the day his receptionist chose to take off, along with Saturdays and Sundays. If she hadn't been with him so long he might have considered letting her go when she had made this demand. But he really didn't want to train anyone else and he truly did understand her wanting to spend one day a week looking after her new grandson while her daughter worked.

He tried to schedule no more than three appointments each afternoon, but it didn't seem to work out on Wednesdays. There always seemed to be four or five. He was so busy on this particular Wednesday that he had no extra time to dwell on Jenny's reaction to his kiss or to thoughts of their upcoming outing this weekend.

He had dismissed her rejection of his advances as prudishness, suspecting that, other than her marriage, she was very inexperienced with the sexual aspects of men. He eagerly awaited acquainting her to his sexual aspect, but was constantly reminding himself to go slow so he wouldn't scare her off.

His last appointment of the day was with Donna Bristol. Donna had been a patient of his for almost three years, and despite the confidence he had in his skills, he had to acknowledge that she hadn't made any headway whatsoever.

Donna was in her mid-thirties, a very attractive woman with short curly brunette hair, a pixieish nose and a smattering of freckles on her checks. She probably could have passed for a teenager if it weren't for her clothing. She had a collegiate look to her. She wore a dark blue sweater over a short straight plaid skirt, navy blue stockings covered her shapely legs, ending with a shiny pair of Bass Wejuns on her feet.

She was not quite five feet. She had beautiful white teeth behind her coral colored lips. David had only seen her smile a handful of times, but it had lit up her whole face. His challenge had been to make her smile at least once each session but he hadn't been nearly as successful at that as he would have liked.

Donna had a sadness to her that was deeply seated. Try as she might she couldn't shake it. Therapy hadn't helped, pills hadn't helped, even a divorce hadn't helped. She felt like she had lost her best friend and truth be told she had.

It had all started seven years ago when Donna and her husband Kevin had moved to a new neighborhood in Reston, Virginia. It was just fate that settled them into a townhouse right next to Trace and Janine Taylor. Janine and Donna hit it off right from the start, they were about the same age and since neither had any children they spent a lot of time together shopping and decorating their new homes.

Donna was a school teacher and Janine worked as a waitress in a little diner that was only open for breakfast and lunch so they had their evenings and weekends free to help each other wallpaper and stencil and pot plants for their adjoining patios.

Kevin and Trace took a little longer to warm up to each other, Trace being an avid hands-on sportsman and Kevin preferring to be a sideline sports spectator. But after a few months, they found themselves fast friends also.

Saturday nights would be reserved for dinner and card or board games together. They didn't even use the front doors any more. They just wandered back and forth through their patio doors. It was not uncommon for one of the girls to be cooking dinner in the other's kitchen and they usually settled down to eat wherever the boys had decided to watch TV.

Trace was trying to get Kevin to accompany him on his hunting and fishing expeditions, but so far Kevin had only agreed to go to his archery club outings with him. The four of them took line dancing lessons together and even went on a weekend excursion to Las Vegas during the Christmas holidays.

Although Donna and Janine were very different, Janine was a little on the wild side where Donna was quite the conservative, they really had a good friendship. Donna didn't particularly care that much for Trace though. She found him to be somewhat arrogant and a bully at times.

She often wondered if the dark circles Janine sometimes had under her eyes could be attributed to him. Once when Janine was on her patio sunning in a bathing suit, Donna noticed some bruises on her upper arms and thighs. When she asked Janine about them she just shrugged and said "I'm so clumsy, I'm always walking into things."

Trace always flirted with Donna, just as she'd noticed Kevin flirted with Janine. It always seemed to be good natured and Donna didn't let it bother her too much, but she certainly didn't lead Trace on or encourage his attentions as she could barely stand to have him close to her.

One Saturday, just before Donna and Kevin were due to come over for a game of Trivial Pursuit, Trace took Janine into their bedroom. "Look," he said as he pulled her around to face him, "I'm not getting anywhere with Donna. If I'm ever gonna have her, Kevin's gonna have to help with it. Tonight, during the game, find a way to get him into the kitchen. Then show him your titties. That ought to get him movin' on you. You do have a marvelous set of 'em, use 'em. I want him in your pants by next week."

"What if I don't want to?", she whined.

He reached out and pinched her nipples hard through the fabric of her sweater. "Oh, you want to all right, or I'll see to it that you'll want to."

They heard Donna and Kevin slide open the patio door. With that he spun her around and smacked her on her ass. "Be a bad girl for me tonight, okay, babe?" But it really wasn't a question at all.

Later on, during a lull in the game when Kevin went into the kitchen to get another beer, Janine pushed her chair out and got up and followed him. When Kevin turned around from the refrigerator, beer in hand, he saw Janine not three feet away, facing him with her sweater pulled up over her breasts. She wasn't wearing a bra. She didn't even own one. Kevin just stared.

Her chest was heaving and flushed but magnificent by all means. He saw that her nipples were very large and distended. They also appeared to have a slight bluish tinge around the aureole area. Open-mouthed he gaped at her for quite a few moments before managing to stammer, "Jesus, Janine, what're ya doin'?"

He looked to the door and then quickly back at her. She sidled up to him and took his hand off the refrigerator door and put it on her breast, "I've been waitin' all night for you to come in here alone. I've wanted to be with you from the very first day we met, couldn't you tell that?"

Donna called from the dining room, "Kevin, it's your turn."

Janine stood on her tiptoes, put her arms around Kevin's neck and pulled him down for a deep kiss. Kevin felt fire raging through his veins and felt like his head was going to explode before she broke it off saying, "Find some time to come see me this week when the others are away." With that she moved away, pulled down her sweater and went back to the game. Kevin stood all alone in the kitchen holding his beer can to his forehead.

Three weeks later Trace decided it was time to let Kevin know that he knew what was going on between him and his wife. Kevin was so scared. He thought at first that Trace was going to dismantle him. Trace had arranged with Janine to catch them in the act one afternoon and so there was Kevin naked and trembling while Janine hid behind him naked and acting as if she was scared also.

Trace screamed at her, "Get in the bathroom and put some clothes on! I'll take care of you later!"

Kevin reached for his clothes but Trace stopped him. He put his hand around his throat and lifted him off the floor then dropped him on the carpet beside his clothes. "Get your clothes on," he snarled, "and then we're gonna go huntin'!"

"Please, Trace, don't hurt me," he sobbed as he scrambled into his clothes.

"Why should I take pity on you? You've been screwing my wife!" he bellowed.

"I"m so sorry, Trace, I know I shouldna let it happen, please, please don't hurt me."

"Well, since you've been screwin' my wife, I wanna screw yours!" Trace let just the beginning of a crooked smile come over his face. "Yeah, that's it, tit for tat, or should I say tit for tit?" He laughed at his own joke.

Kevin looked at him with a puzzled expression on his face. "How are you gonna do that? She won't let you." Of that he was fairly certain. First of all he knew Donna just barely tolerated Trace because she liked Janine and secondly, Donna was not the type to fool around. She'd only been with one other guy besides him and that had been her high school sweetheart of three years.

"She won't know it," Trace replied. When Kevin sent him a thoroughly confused look, Trace continued. "And you're gonna help me accomplish it, ol' buddy boy, pal-o-mine, my cuckolding friend."

As Kevin listened to Trace's scheme Kevin turned white with fear. He was aghast at the deviousness of his friend's imagination. And, he was appalled with the whole idea of helping someone rape his wife. When he told Trace he wasn't going to do it, Trace told him the two things he needed to hear that would change his mind.

First, was that maybe Donna would like to know how he'd been spending his afternoons when Donna thought he was working and second was his assurance that he would see to it that Kevin had a hunting *accident*, even if he had to knock him out and drag him into the woods first.

And so it was arranged. With Kevin's help, Trace would ravish an unsuspecting Donna, and just to keep Kevin in the game, Trace allowed Kevin and Janine to resume their passions for each other, provided Trace got to watch. Pretty soon Kevin started getting indoctrinated into the swinging couples theme

Trace was constantly pitching to him. In his mind he was beginning to believe that maybe the four of them would somehow survive all this and switch partners back and forth.

It didn't matter that they couldn't even coax Donna into a friendly game of strip Uno. Trace and Janine were coaching him into a new awareness of his sexuality and the tricks and devices they used were slowly turning him into a sex junkie. His perspective was changing. What would have shamed him before he now found tantalizing and he was convinced that Donna would be converted as easily as he had been. Kevin was spending all his free time and using all his sick leave to satisfy his carnal needs with Janine with Trace coaching and critiquing them and once even filming them.

About a month after Trace *caught* Kevin and Janine together, Trace decided it was time to take Donna. He'd been eager for her for so long and planning it in great detail had made it just as exciting as a hunt. He couldn't wait to overtake his quarry. Every time he thought about himself poised over her shoving his cock into her he swelled to painful proportions.

As Kevin was gradually introduced to new sexual orientations, he timidly introduced some of the new techniques to Donna during their lovemaking sessions. Trace had said it would be important to their plan to have her amenable to trying a few new things.

Kevin had been awkward at first in attempting some bondage themes with Donna but had been amazed at her enthusiasm. It was a time in their lives together that things were starting to get pretty stale between them and she welcomed anything to spice things up a bit. For that reason, and also because of the erotic videos Kevin bought for them to watch together, she was more than agreeable to most of the things he suggested they do.

One night, after several rehearsals with Janine as Donna, Trace said it was time for Kevin to pay his penance. The next morning Trace used the soap and aftershave Kevin provided for him and he shaved off his mustache. He was careful not to smoke or to drink his usual tumbler of Gentleman Jack Whiskey before dinner. Instead, he grabbed a beer as Kevin would have.

It was a Friday night, and as that was customarily Donna and Kevin's night to go out to dinner together, Donna didn't think it at all unusual that Kevin was waiting in the living room for her when she arrived home from teaching. That he had a bath tub filled with bubbles for her and champagne already poured, sitting on the closed toilet seat, was a little odd, but she was game. He'd been very attentive lately and she loved it.

She went to their bedroom and removed her clothes, then walked into the bathroom and gingerly felt the temperature of the water. This was going to feel so good. She'd really had a hard day at school. Kevin handed her the champagne glass after she had settled herself into the water and then sat down on the toilet lid.

He nervously rubbed his hands together and asked about her day. As she elaborated at length he kept refilling her glass. When her skin was all rosy and pink and she had finished three glasses of the champagne, he gently pulled her to her feet and toweled her off.

"I'm, going to ravish you in an all new way tonight. I want to tie you up on the bed and have you squirm as I kiss and lick you all over."

"Umm," she said, "sounds nice."

He walked her into the bedroom and she saw that he had lit a few candles and draped a few scarves around the posts on the brass headboard and foot board. "Just lie down, right in the center here," he coached as she slid over the crisp sheets.

Then he took first one hand and then the other and gently stroked them to the fingertips before attaching the scarves to her wrists and the bedposts. Then he took each foot in its turn and kissed all the toes before tying her ankles to the posts at the foot of the bed. He stood up and looked at her, spread eagled with anticipation in her sparkling eyes. He leaned over to kiss her gently on the lips and then tweaked both her nipples bringing them instantly erect.

He opened his nightstand drawer and took out a black cloth. "Now, for the 'piece de resistance'," he said as he gestured with exaggerated finesse.

When she saw what appeared to be a sleeping mask and a blindfold, she became instantly tense. "No, don't do that, I don't want that," she said.

"Oh, we must have this. My fantasy requires this. C'mon it won't be so bad."

With that he put the black sleeping mask against her eyes, securing the mask to her face with the elastic string around her head. Then he took a dark brown kerchief and tied that over the mask, just to be sure she couldn't see anything. It would be a disaster if she was able to see even the slightest shadow, since there was such a pronounced difference in size between Kevin and Trace.

"Please, Kevin, I don't like this, you're scaring me," she cried.

"Shh, it's okay. You'll get used to it. Try to get into this. Imagine you're a beautiful slave girl and you've been tied up and blindfolded because the King wants you and no one can know of it. Not even you, because you're married to his brother." With that he leaned down and kissed her thoroughly, gently at first and then roughly. Then he moved down to her throat and licked her from there down to her navel. "Give me a minute while I look at you and undress myself," he said.

Trace came around the corner from the living room and silently walked into the bedroom, stopping at the foot of the bed. He was completely naked and it wasn't hard to see that the sight that greeted him pleased him very much. He was rampart hard, sticking straight out and pulsing while his eyes roved over Donna's breasts and belly, finally resting on the dark triangle between her legs.

Somehow Donna had a sense of something and she started to squirm, pulling on her scarves trying to get loose. "Kev, I don't want to do this tonight. Let's just do it regular, all right?"

Kevin moved over to the bed and stroked her hair and her forehead while Trace continued to get his fill of her. He motioned for Kevin to get up from the bed and then he leaned down over her face and brought his lips to hers. He gently rubbed his lips over them, enjoying the feel of her and coaxing her lips wide apart with his. When their tongues touched he had to disguise his moan as a gasping sound.

When he took her whole bottom lip into his mouth she gasped. This was certainly new. He didn't give her a chance to dwell on it though as he slid his tongue into her inner cavity and laved the roof of her mouth. Then he ran his tongue down her throat directly to her nipple, licked it and then bit it.

"Ow! That hurt!" she cried. Trace lifted his hand up in the air as a gesture to Kevin to say one of the things they had rehearsed.

"Shut up bitch! You're just a slave. It's going to get a whole lot worse before it gets any better." With that Trace cupped both of her breasts in his hands and squeezed them firmly then bent down and suckled on the nipples. When she started moaning from the pleasure of it he stopped and taking her nipples firmly between his thumbs and forefingers he pinched them and pulled them hard.

When Donna screamed Kevin took a step toward her but Trace's penetrating glare cut him off. When Trace started chewing on her nipples, she cried and begged him to stop. "Kevin! Stop it! Stop it! I can't stand it."

Trace motioned with his hand again and Kevin said, "You'll take it bitch! This is what I want to do to you and I'm going to do exactly as I please. I own you and don't you forget it! Just lie there and take it. Take it like a good little slave!"

Kevin was becoming distressed with Trace's treatment of Donna, but he didn't know what to do about it. He couldn't cross Trace on this. He knew he'd kill him if he did. The weird thing was that he was sort of enjoying the attention Trace was paying to his wife. He was also immensely proud of how good she looked lying there with all her nakedness displayed. He was almost delighted that Trace could find such great pleasure in his woman.

He didn't mind sharing her really. He just minded him hurting her. Just then Trace took both of his thumbs and gouged them hard into the middle of her nipples depressing them in a good two inches. Donna screamed out in pain but Trace was oblivious to her screams. He kept pressing his thumbs down and rubbing them in wide circles, pressing her nipples and breasts almost flat. When she sobbed Kevin's name over and over again begging him to please stop, Kevin made to go to her. Trace shot him a fierce look that stopped him in his tracks.

Trace deserted her nipples to move on down to her stomach. He grabbed his penis in his hand and with gyrating motions of his hips he rammed it into her stomach, moving all around, careful not to put too much weight on her or to touch his chest to hers as Kevin was nearly hairless with no muscles and Trace was covered with hair and bulging muscles.

He took his hand away from himself and put his palm up against her fleshy mound, cupping her, and at the same time inserting his middle finger between her nether lips and thrusting it into her repeatedly. When she started to moan he looked to Kevin with a pleasantly surprised expression. Since both of his hands were occupied, one in her and the other supporting him, he gestured with his eyebrows for Kevin to say something. "Yeah, I know you want me, you want me deep inside, don't you?"

She moaned again and said, "Yes, Yes, You own me, I'll do whatever you say. Take me any way you want me. Just take me!"

With that Trace removed his finger from inside her and shimmied down between her legs. The second he put his mouth where his finger had just been she arched off the bed, striving to meet his lips and tongue. He tongued her thoroughly, laving her up and down, around and around, and ended by concentrating on the ultra sensitive area near the top of her slit.

When he started gently sucking on her clitoris she buckled and spasmed, flooding his mouth with her wetness. He quickly straddled her and with his lips still coated with her essence he kissed her thoroughly, slavering her with the wetness of her own orgasm.

He then rose above her, looking down at the picture she made, a captive, blindfolded Donna, who had no idea who was rising above her ready to penetrate her soft flesh. He gave a groan signifying his immense pleasure and then positioned himself at her opening. He looked to Kevin and gave a slight nod.

Kevin leaned down toward her ear and whispered, "You are now mine!" and with that Trace plowed into her, causing her to sink into the mattress. He thrust in and out of her making the headboard creak with the force of his exertions. He had been so ready for her for so long that he doubted he would last more than a few more penetrations, so he pulled partway out to allow himself to gain his control.

He hadn't counted on her following him back up from his thrusts and so she held onto him for one extra second more than he had counted on, the walls of her vagina beckoning him back. It was the undoing of him. He gave one final thrust, sending the headboard into the wall and then he exploded inside her, releasing his hot pulsing stream deep into her.

God, how he wished he could collapse on top of her or at least beside her. But he knew the jig was done and she would be expecting Kevin to untie her and remove her blindfold so they could bask in their sated glory, each telling the other how wonderful they were. Trace pushed himself off the bed with his arms and gingerly lowered his feet to the floor. He motioned for Kevin to undo her and then he walked naked from their bedroom, through their living room, through their sliding patio door and then through his patio door.

Janine was waiting there in a chair in their darkened living room. "So, how'd it go?" she asked.

He grouchily mumbled something that sounded like, "shaddup", and just walked down the hallway toward the bedroom, dripping his excellent jism from the tip of his penis onto the carpet. He felt empty in more ways than one. Now what was he going to look forward to? The hunt was over.

Chapter 34

Reston, VA

After Trace left the bedroom Kevin sat on the bed while he removed the scarves and blindfold from Donna. When she was untied she put her arms around his neck and laid her head on his shoulder. They just sat in silence for several minutes just holding each other.

When Donna lifted her head to look into Kevin's face she was surprised to see tears in his eyes, ready to overflow and cascade down his cheeks. She was amazed at the dichotomy of him, so rough one minute and so gentle and caring the next.

She wiped one tiny rivulet away and lightly kissed his chin, saying "Well, that was really something! Have you been reading Trace's Penthouses or something? You've become quite kinky lately."

"Yeah," he mumbled, "a real sex machine. I'm sorry I hurt you. I guess I got too carried away with my passion." Abruptly changing the subject, he got up and started to dress as he said, "Where do you want to go for dinner? I'm starving."

"Yeah, I'm not surprised. I'm kinda hungry too," she replied. "How about Outback? I could go for a big juicy steak."

"Okay, I'll wait for you in the living room."

As she started selecting clothes from her closet, she called out to him, "What do you think about inviting Janine and Trace?"

The thought sickened him. "No, let's just go by ourselves. We'll see them tomorrow night."

While Donna was dressing she ran her hands over her breasts and thoughtfully considered how tender they were. And, her pelvic bones actually felt bruised. She marveled at how Kevin could be so timid and gentle one minute and brutal and aggressive the next. She was a little surprised that he had the capacity to hurt her as he had by biting so hard on her nipples and then jamming his thumbs down so hard into them.

She had never felt pain quite like that. It was physically hurtful and at the same time mentally debasing. She would have to talk to him about that. As she pulled on her skirt and slipped into her shoes she looked over at the bed, devoid of covers and top sheet with the scarves still draped around the posts. In the middle was a large moist spot where Kevin had climaxed into her.

She walked over and removed each scarf and then dropped them into her nightstand drawer. She wondered how he would like being her slave for a change. With that thought on her mind and a smile on her lips she joined him in the living room where he was distractedly flipping through the TV channels with the remote.

It was two weeks later when Donna was folding laundry in Janine and Trace's laundry room that she got the shock of her life. Her dryer had gone on the fritz that Saturday morning, and since Janine was getting her hair done, she decided to use Janine's dryer instead of waiting until Monday when hers would be fixed.

Trace and Kevin had just come back from an archery tournament and were in the kitchen getting some beer. Donna was just about to call out to them when she heard Trace say to Kevin, "You gotta find a way. I gotta have her again. I'm almost obsessed with it!"

"Trace, I can't. I just can't! We were goddamn lucky before. I won't risk it. Besides, we're even, that was the deal, "tit for tit", remember?"

"Yeah, well you're still enjoyin' my wife's tits and I've got the pictures to prove it!"

What the hell were they talking about? Donna's heart started racing as she was absorbing the words and their implications. Kevin was arranging sex for Trace? Kevin was enjoying Janine's breasts while Trace was taking pictures of them?

Just as she was about to leave the laundry alcove off of the kitchen hallway and confront them, she heard Trace say, "Here comes Janine now," as he spied her car turning into the driveway from the kitchen window. "Wait'll you hear what I did to her this time. You know last week I made her work all day at the diner with nipple clips on. I even went in and pulled her into the ladies' room around 2 o'clock to make sure she still had 'em on. What a hoot! This morning I put walnuts over her nipples and pushed 'em in deep and then duck taped 'em on real tight. She cried for awhile because it hurt so bad. I think this might be worse than the clips. I told her she had to go around all day that way and that she'd better not touch 'em or they'll stay on for a week! I told her it was her punishment for not being able to suck us both off last night."

Just then Janine came into the kitchen through the garage door. "Hi, guys," she said as she put her purse on the counter.

"C'mere," Trace said and turned her around to face Kevin, "show Kevin your titties, now." With that he pulled her loose sweatshirt way up to her neck. Janine turned red, embarrassed and humiliated as they both stared at her bound breasts, concave in the center where a walnut was crushed into each nipple.

At that moment Donna chose to make her presence known and opened the laundry room door that had been ajar. When she saw Janine, she gasped and covered her mouth with her hand. As soon as she saw the depressions in the center of her breasts she was reminded of two weeks ago when her own nipples had been painfully pressed in by Kevin's thumbs.

Realization came to her then as she stared at them in shock and they all stared back at her in shock. That hadn't been Kevin after all! The man that had *had her* was Trace! With a sickening lurch of her stomach she ran to the bathroom and vomited up her breakfast.

As she knelt there heaving and holding onto the toilet seat, Kevin came up behind her and put his hands on her shoulders. She abruptly stood up and pushed against his chest, sending him into the towel rack. "You bastard! You gave me to him! You bathed me and trussed me up and then you let him look at me and touch me and fuck me! How could you do that? I'm your wife!" she sobbed heartbrokenly.

When he reached out to her again she slapped at his hands and shouted, "Don't you ever touch me, ever! You hear me! Ever!"

"Jesus, Donna. I'm so sorry. Please believe me. I had no choice. He was going to kill me if I didn't let him have you!"

"Then you should've let him kill you, instead you let him kill me!"

"We thought if you had a good time we could get you used to the idea of the four of us 'swinging' together. It's done all the time now."

"Not with me it's not! And you knew that! Don't tell me you didn't know that I abhor Trace!" The thoughts came back to her then of the things that had been done to her by him and she was brought low to her knees again, gripping the cold porcelain basin. The coldness seeped into her fingers and traveled the pathways to her heart and there the coldness turned to ice and froze her heart solid.

She stayed in Janine and Trace's bathroom for the better part of an hour, listening to their pleas and explanations through the door. But she just couldn't absorb it all. She had gone numb. The realization that Kevin and Janine had been having an affair together and that Trace not only condoned but encouraged it with his presence and suggestions was bad enough. But the ultimate betrayal of her as a sacrifice to atone to Trace for Kevin's use of his wife was more than she could ever get over.

She knew that from this moment on, she would never have a peaceful night's sleep again, that she'd always be afraid to close her eyes. She would be plagued with the despicable images of Trace abusing her breasts and taking his pleasure in her body. Whatever feelings she had ever had for Kevin had been destroyed forever. She would never be able to forgive him or to trust him. So that afternoon she packed a suitcase, oblivious to all their begging pleas, first from Kevin and then from Janine.

Trace knew better than to show his putrid face, if she'd had a gun she would have shot him.

She put her suitcase in the trunk of her car and drove off. She had lost her husband and best friend in one quick revelation that she wasn't even supposed to hear. What if she hadn't found out? Would they have done it to her again? The thought nauseated her and she had to pull over to the side of the road to wait for the queasiness to subside.

"Where to go from here?" she asked herself. She checked herself into a hotel and ordered a bottle of vodka sent up. She took it with her to the bathroom and drank almost half of it while she scrubbed herself in the bathtub until her skin was almost raw. When she looked down at her nipples she remembered the pain Trace had administered to them, imagining his delight at her suffering. Hatred burned deep within her and she started to cry. Loud, wrenching sobs echoed back and forth off the tile and she slipped her whole body under the water, wishing she was strong enough to end this anguish right now by not coming up. But she was not.

The next day she hired an attorney. Without going into too much detail she briefly described what had happened to her to cause her to seek his counsel. The man was a well-known divorce lawyer who at the age of sixty had heard quite a few tales, but this one would've made his hair turn white if it hadn't already been so.

As she detailed some of her demands, he added others, convinced that this woman shouldn't have to suffer anymore, especially financially. By the time separation papers were served to Kevin, the attorney had arranged to have a moving van remove practically all the contents of their townhouse and all the contents of their bank accounts. They were demanding the immediate sale of the townhouse with three quarters of the profit to go to her and an alimony payment that would keep Kevin at the poverty level for a long time.

Donna took a few days of personal leave to set up housekeeping in a high-rise apartment building that had a very efficient doorman. Kevin was bound to find out where she was sooner or later and she did not want to see him, ever again. She wasn't worried about him coming to the school to see her since the security at most of the local high schools was better than the security at Lorton Prison.

Her attorney had expressed some desire to see criminal charges brought forward and, although she would have loved seeing Trace go to jail, she knew she'd never be able to go through all this in a public courtroom. And even if charges could be brought against Kevin, if he was in jail, he wouldn't be able to pay her the alimony she desperately wanted to punish him with. However, the threat of her pressing charges for their criminal behavior was enough to keep them all away from her, which was exactly what she wanted. She just wanted to be left alone to try to get some semblance of normalcy back into her life.

Two months later she found out she was pregnant. She'd gone to her doctor for a routine checkup which had included blood tests done at a lab a few days before her appointment. When her doctor told her the news her first reaction was that it wasn't possible. Kevin had had a vasectomy a few years after they were married when they'd decided that they didn't want to have any children.

Then she remembered with a jolt. She wrapped her arms around her midsection, squeezing and squeezing as if she could push out the unwanted child. With everything she'd had to deal with lately, why did this have to happen? Why did Trace's seed have to find her egg? It wasn't fair! It was only one time!

She sure hadn't sanctioned that and she wouldn't accept this either. But she knew she couldn't just get rid of it. She'd been raised Catholic, and even though she didn't go to mass every week, she still went often enough to consider herself a practicing one. No, she just wasn't the type of person who could have an abortion, regardless of the circumstances. Even though she felt pretty sure that the church would believe this baby to have been conceived during a rape and would approve of it, she knew she couldn't kill it.

Oh, what was she going to do? She did not want to have a baby. She'd grown up in a family that had twelve children. She was the oldest and because of that she'd felt like the last four had been hers personally. She couldn't remember her mother feeding or changing any of them after Charlene, the sixth one.

She always felt that the reason she did so well in school was because it was not home. No matter how hard school was it was ever so much easier than being at home. She excelled beyond her parents' expectations and had earned a full scholarship for college. From the first day she left home to become a teacher she knew that she'd had enough of raising children. Now she only wanted to teach them.

As she drove home from the doctor's office she cried softly about her predicament. She cursed Kevin for letting this happen, Trace for actually impregnating her, and Janine for seducing her husband in the first place. Hadn't they even given this the slightest bit of consideration when they were planning their debauchery? Leave it to two rutting males to forget all about birth control. It did surprise her a little that it hadn't occurred to Janine, who had obviously been in on all this. Why was she, the innocent in all this, the only one being punished? With that thought she quickly turned her vehicle around and went to see her attorney.

This new development made her attorney see dollar signs exploding in air. Trace was a highly successful airplane pilot and salesman. He made a lot of money selling high ticket used jets to corporate types. He also spent a lot of money on all his sportsman-type hobbies. Not any more. His child support payments would make it worth her while to carry this child to term and then hire a nanny to take care of it. It would be worth it to know that Trace would have to sell his prized bows, rifles and skis because of one ill-placed ejaculation. His selfish, rutting urges were going to cost him over a third of a million dollars, payable in monthly increments of $1600 spread out over the next eighteen years.

Six and a half months later Donna gave birth to a baby girl. She named her Melanie after the nurse that stayed with her throughout her labor. Before she left the hospital she had already hired a nanny, determined to have minimal contact with her daughter. The hospital staff tried to encourage her to nurse but she kept thinking that she didn't want Trace's daughter sucking on her there as he had so she made the nurses feed her with a bottle.

She knew she shouldn't be thinking this way but she really couldn't help it. She didn't want this baby, his baby. As soon as the baby was born her attorney notified Trace that it was time to begin paying support. It had been established long ago that there would be absolutely no contact between Trace and Donna and that if he violated that agreement then she would press criminal charges against him. So everything was handled by her attorney, and when Trace insisted on a paternity test before he would agree to pay any support, her attorney arranged to have the test done using his power of attorney as Melanie's guardian. When the tests confirmed that Trace was the father, he made an attempt to establish visitation rights. The attorney said he could see the child if he wanted, after he got out of jail, if that's what he wanted. The message was well received and the subject of visitation rights never came up again. Donna had never even known about the paternity test or its outcome.

Over the next few years the child became very attached to her nanny since her momma was hardly ever around her. Donna made the important decisions regarding her care, but spent very little time with her. When Melanie came to her in the evenings after her bath she would read her a story while she sat on her lap.

One day Melanie looked up at Donna and with her freshly-scrubbed, angelic face resting on a pudgy hand propped on her knee, she asked, "Why don't you like me, Mommy?" It was then that Donna realized that Melanie was her child not Trace's, and she didn't deserve the steely coldness that Donna had been giving her.

She decided to seek professional help. She had to get rid of this anger or her child would be suffering right along with her. When her attorney recommended Dr.Sandler, she took his advice and made an appointment. Her attorney had also arranged for Trace to pay for the counseling, citing her reasons for needing it in the first place.

Donna's anger was so deep it was hard to get her to let go of any of it. David tried many different things, but once he knew the whole story and the complexities of it, he knew that there would only be one way to get rid of it. That would be to wipe the slate clean; to make her forget what had happened or to recreate the events in a different way. He couldn't attempt any of these therapies without her consent and there was certainly no guarantee that he could even pull it off, even with it. If he told her too much he was dooming himself to failure and if he altered her memories without her knowledge he was being very unethical. He didn't know what to about the dilemma.

His idea was to use relaxation imagery hypnosis to filter out the memories that she didn't really want to have. This was very possible and he, in fact, had done it several times with good success. The difficulty here would be that a child had been conceived, how would he erase that? He would need to invent a new, more pleasurable way that she had been conceived so that Donna would have the best chance of loving her and being a good mother to her.

Chapter 35

Fairfax, VA

What would happen if he could reconstruct the conception with a man she found desirable? Could he create a whole romance in her mind? A chance meeting with a handsome stranger followed by a torrid affair and then the tragic demise of her lover, leaving her anguished but pregnant with their cherished love child?

If he could do all this, would it work? Would it be somehow better to simply focus on erasing the bad rather than creating good? And what were his obligations as far as approval of the procedure from her? If he told her what he was going to do one way or the other he stood a good chance of it not even working.

He went to his reference books and pored over them for several hours, not even coming close to a situation like this. In the end he opted for a trumped up romance, not because he thought it more ethical, for it probably was not. But because he didn't know how she'd handle the loose end of how the conception had occurred if her mind was a total blank on the subject.

He was familiar with the legal aspects that had already been resolved with Trace, from both her recounting of the story and from what Philip Garnesworth, her attorney, had explained to him regarding the payment of his psychiatry fees. Child support was deposited automatically into her account on the 15th of every month from the county child services department who collected it directly from the father on the first. Counseling fees were billed to the attorney who forwarded it to the father for payment. Unless there was a glitch, there was no reason for her to have any further contact at all with Trace to confuse the issue of paternity.

He sat at his desk for hours mapping out a plausible scenario for her romance and finally decided on a chance meeting with a prolonged seduction, figuring that she would never have been the type for a one-night stand. Hypnosis would not allow him to invent anything that she wouldn't ultimately do in real life. Would she have an affair, even if she were in love?

She sure was bitter over Kevin's infidelity. Maybe she wouldn't. Donna and Jenny were similar in temperament and in their conservative ideals. Maybe he could talk to Jenny this weekend. He could find out if she would succumb to a physical mating if she really and truly fell madly in love while married to another man.

A thought occurred to him then. If his memory served him well, which it almost always did, Donna was only a few weeks pregnant when she had left Kevin. Maybe there could be a one-night stand kind of thing, if he could persuade her that she had sought solace in a stranger's arms nearly right away.

He would talk to Jenny. It would be a good time to probe her for a few fantasy ideas that he could use for Donna now and then later, for her. He hoped. Usually he was anxious to leave work to go play. Now that he was going to go play, he was cheerfully turning it into work. Who could ask for a more interesting occupation?

Chapter 36

Herndon, VA

Jenny woke up early the next morning and started packing for the beach. Her mother had gathered some beach toys for the kids and packed the lunch she had prepared for them. She had insisted yesterday that she be allowed to make their lunch, so Jenny had called David to tell him to cancel the Sutton Gourmet basket. The pile she was amassing by the back door was beginning to make her think that they were planning on going for a week instead of for just one day. Good thing she had taken a van off of the front line to use for the weekend.

By the time David arrived she had both kids dressed and fed and she was ready, except for trying to find some batteries for the portable radio. She finally just emptied two flashlights of their batteries and off they went. They were leaving by 8:00 so they could get to the beach by 9:30, well before the Sunday beltway traffic and so they could park close to an area near the water to make it easier to go back and forth to the van all day instead of unloading all their stuff. After the kids were settled in their car seats Jenny took out a Thermos and poured some coffee for David and herself. They both took it black, one of the many things that Jenny was just starting to notice they had in common.

The drive was very pleasant. It was one of the few times she could just sit back, relax, and enjoy the signs of summer changing the scenery all around the beltway. Everything green and flowers were blooming in front of the houses she could see set back from the road. At least where she could see some houses, there were only a few areas that didn't have those enormous noise-reduction walls.

The sun was glinting off the gold statue atop the Mormon temple. It was so bright it hurt to look right at it. It was going to be a beautiful June day, and apparently a lot of Washingtonians thought so too, as there were convertibles everywhere with one or two riders lifting their faces up to the sun. One day, she thought, I think I'd like to have a convertible of my own.

They exited the Beltway at route 4 in Maryland, also known as Pennsylvania Avenue Extended. Leaving the city behind, they headed for the Southern Shore and St. Mary's County. About forty minutes later they were at Breezy Point, a quaint little marina and beach just a few miles north of Solomon's Island. Jenny had been here many times over the years, but David had never ventured here before.

Pulling into the parking space Jenny pointed out, he took a look around and knew why this had not been on his list of things to do and see around Washington. He saw a rundown concession stand next to a cinder block building that housed the restrooms. Beyond that was a small marina with various boats anchored here and there. A quick perusal assured him that there were none here that he would ever consider owning.

Directly in front of the van, about thirty feet away, were picnic tables and beyond that, the waters of the Chesapeake Bay. There were about twenty picnic tables scattered among the shade trees. Behind them was a playground with a slide, monkey bars and two gigantic steel swing sets with swings made from straps of rubber.

The tables were quickly being commandeered by families from all different ethnic groups and blankets and chairs were being positioned all around them marking off their respective territories. Children were running around everywhere in various stages of dress. Some were still in pajamas, some all dressed up in summer dresses and some in their bathing suits already down by the water. And it smelled god awful. What a day this was going to be!

When Jenny stepped out of the van she took a deep breath and smiled as she looked around. There was a salty-fishy tang to the air that was reminiscent of an old-time Atlantic beach shore. As she turned her head she took in the familiar sights. She noted the quaint little concession stand with the best crab cake sandwiches she'd ever had, the tile-lined restrooms that she used to linger in on hot summer afternoons, their coolness a respite from the scorching sun. The marina was way off at a distance, filled with the activity of people coming and going, anxious to enjoy their day on the water. She lingered over her favorite part, the people and the memories they brought to her mind.

People came from all over to this little hidden strip of paradise. She could hardly wait until the late afternoon when all the delicious smells of Asian cooking and the aroma of Soul food would blend with those of Mexican spicy tortillas frying at all the table side grills. When the smells would waft over to her beach chair, she would sniff long and deep trying to decipher one from another, until she just had to go put her marinated steaks on just to compete with them.

The playground was just as she remembered it, filled with the sounds of children playing with abandon. A toddler with just a diaper on was sitting in a blow up baby pool splashing with glee down by the water's edge while his older brother, still in his pajamas, was eating cereal from a small Fruit Loops box watching over him. There were people already in the water playing with a beach ball. It was going to be a grand day!

Quickly she staked out their table by putting a basket on it and then returned to help David with the kids. She and David took turns unloading the things they needed and watching the kids. A few minutes later the adults ate their breakfast of cinnamon rolls, orange juice and coffee relaxing in beach chairs while they watched Rusty and Paisley build who-knows-what in the sand.

"How in the world did you ever find this place?" David asked her.

"My aunt and uncle live pretty close to here in Huntington, MD. When we used to bring my brother here to spend a few weeks every summer with them, we'd all meet here and have a huge family picnic. I've been coming every year since then. I usually try to come on the 4th of July. They have the most marvelous little parade! The local children have their little handmade costumes and they have four or five cute little majorettes. One or two always end up dropping their batons and then have to run after them. A boy scout troop of seven or so lead the parade carrying this huge American flag that looks like it was really there at Fort McHenry when it was getting shelled. And then, of course, they have the traditional convertible covered with streamers carrying 'Miss Liberty'. It's small town America of forty years ago. I just love it here. My grandparents used to go to a beach just north of here called Chesapeake Beach to play the slot machines years ago when they were legal here in Maryland. I remember they had an amusement park there, but that shut down when the gamblers stopped coming."

"There are some nice sailboats out on the bay," he commented as his eyes skimmed the horizon. "Do you sail?" he asked.

"No, I have been deep-sea fishing though. Every couple of years a bunch of us from work charter a boat and go out to catch fish. We usually catch so much that one of the guys who lives in D.C. ends up giving it to a youth shelter, after we all clean them of course," she said with a shiver and a small laugh.

"Do you sail?" she asked.

"Used to. Don't have the time anymore. I still own part of a sailboat with three other doctors. It's docked in Annapolis. I haven't been out in it for over two years now though. Sure is a good deal for the other three!"

"Well, maybe one day you can teach me how to sail, one day when we don't have the children with us!" she said as she jumped up to get Paisley who was crying because sand had gotten in her eyes. Jenny took her to the ladies' room and cleaned her off, removing her own over clothes before carrying her back outside. Dropping her clothes on the blanket, she walked her right out into the water.

Paisley loved the water. She had no fear and was quite eager to be put down so she could be on her own. When Rusty was born she and her mother had been overly careful not to get any water in his eyes when he was being bathed. They used washcloths to carefully wipe off his face and now it seemed he was somewhat afraid of the water. He certainly wouldn't put his face in it.

They had learned not to be so protective when Paisley came on the scene. The first time Jenny gave Paisley a bath she put her whole head under the water and held it for a few seconds. Now look at her, she'd rather swim under the water than be on top of it. She laughed when Jenny dunked her. Jenny and Paisley played together in the water with her inflatable toys until Rusty decided he wasn't getting much attention and wanted to join them. David decided to join them also.

As he stood up and pulled his shirt over his head Jenny had her first look at his chest. It was quite impressive to say the least. He had a very muscular build with broad shoulders and a slightly tapering waistline, but the most spectacular part was the hair. He was covered with it, a brown so deep that it looked black. She was instantly reminded of Sean Connery's chest in that James Bond movie, the one with Ursula Andress. She could never keep the titles straight.

The coverage was so complete that she could hardly make out his nipples, but she could see where it started thinning out as it disappeared into his bathing suit just below his navel. She was sure she had been staring because when her eyes met his face he cocked his head, raised his eyebrow and gave her a huge smile before he grabbed up Rusty and charged into the water towards them.

They had the best time playing with the rafts they brought. It was hard trying to get on top of them without going over the other side and then once you were up, everybody tried to push you off. The kids were in their inner tubes watching the antics of the adults and everybody laughed hilariously each time someone was unseated and dunked into the water.

When they finally wore themselves out they plopped down on the sand at the water's edge. It was the first time David had seen Jenny in a bathing suit also, and now that she was out of the water and not carrying Paisley in front of her, he could see that she filled out her one piece suit very nicely.

Her modest neckline only allowed for the slightest peek at her cleavage unless she was turned on her side as she was now, facing him. He could see the rounded swell of the tops of her breasts and the dark line created by them pressing together. He didn't have to gauge where her nipples were because their distension was clearly outlined through the fabric.

He felt his pulse race and a warm feeling came over his groin as blood surged to his center. It throbbed to create a rather hard projection that was not exactly welcome at this time. He rolled onto his stomach, burying it in the sand so to speak. His eyes followed the curve of her waist past her hips to her thighs and down her legs to her toes. If he could have changed anything about her it would have been her hips, just a touch more to grab onto would be nice, but slender was good, too.

He was wondering just how long he was going to have to maintain this position when Rusty jumped on his back yelling, "I'll hold him, you bury him!" to Paisley. With that he rolled over and they proceeded to try to bury him in the sand. They really weren't making much headway until Jenny brought the buckets and shovels over and lent her assistance.

When he was completely covered from his neck down, they patted the wet sand down all around him. When Jenny patted his inner thigh on one leg it was the undoing of him again, and the sand cracked all around his groin area. He wondered just how long he could stand this torture of wanting her without having her.

Jenny took Paisley to the ladies' room to shower some of the sand off and David took Rusty. Then they all spread out the tablecloth and unpacked the lunch basket her mom had provided. Jenny's mom had made some sandwiches and there was fresh fruit and cheese along with a cooler that had fruit juices and sodas in it.

Jenny eyed the concession stand and debated about getting a crab cake sandwich but decided not to this time, her mother had sent so much food. While the kids napped under an umbrella, Jenny applied a liberal amount of sunscreen to them and began to slather herself. It was getting really hot so she went back to the van for her hat and then moved her chair under a tree.

"Do you mind if I join you?" David asked as he dragged his chair over to hers.

"Of course, not! Why would you even ask?" she replied.

"Oh, I just thought you might want some introspective time alone. The kids can be all-consumming at times."

She laughed, "Yeah, I know, but it's really nice to talk to an adult every once in awhile."

"What else do you miss about being with adults?" he asked in a low sultry voice.

She turned to face him and asked "What do you mean?"

"You know what I mean. Do you miss the intimacy? Do you miss sex?" Her eyes went wide as she registered her shock at his question. "Well?" he prodded.

She cleared her throat and said in a soft voice, "Well, yeah, I guess I do. A little."

"What do you miss most, the companionship or the intimacy, excuse me, let me clarify, the sex?" he asked.

She thought for a moment before she answered. "Well, I'm not really sure, the companionship I guess. The sex at the end wasn't really all that great, at least not so that I'd miss it."

His eyes bored into hers as he said silkily, "It can be great if you're with the right person." He took a big swig of his soda and turned back to face her again. "I want you to think about something for me. Think about it for a few minutes and then tell me honestly what you think, okay?"

"You're not going to psychoanalyze me or anything are you?" she looked at him hesitantly.

"No, no, nothing like that."

She looked skeptical but said, "Okay, shoot."

"If you could dream up your own romance, set it up on any terms, any place with anyone, how would you do it? What's your ultimate fantasy for falling in love? No. No questions. Just go take a walk over by the marina and think about it."

She raised her eyebrows in a questioning look, but he merely waved her off indicating the direction of the marina. She slowly stood, wrinkled her nose at him and walked off, turning back once to check on the kids. He watched her walk away, enjoying her little wiggle in her wet cut-off jean shorts that she had thrown on over her bathing suit. She was a nice little package.

After she made the loop around the marina and came back to their picnic site, she took a root beer out of the cooler and plopped down into her chair. "Okay, tell me why you want to know first." That was all she said.

He got up, adjusted the angle of the umbrella, and came back. He lied to her, "I'm trying to get an idea for a book I want to write but I need some help on the romantic part. Pretend you're my female character and you're married. What would make you be unfaithful? As part of the plot I need her character to be unfaithful, but it has to be believable. I need your help with this. I don't have anybody else to ask."

She looked at him with a doubtful expression and then shrugged, "Okay, how long have I been married, and are we happy, any children?"

"You've been married ten years, you're not happy, you're not unhappy. No children."

"Then I guess I would have to be head over heels ga ga with someone to cheat on my husband. It would have to be a situation that just came up. Nothing planned, purely spontaneous, because if I thought about it, I'd talk myself out of it."

"Okay," he said leading her on, "What kind of guy would it have to be?"

She closed her eyes, put her head back so her neck rested on the top of the chair and raised her face to the sun. Dreamily she said, "I walk into a room and there he is, exuding maleness, his penetrating eyes never leaving mine. No, no, back up, how about this? I walk into a country and western lounge, he's singing a beautiful love ballad, our eyes meet and then it's as if he's singing it directly to me. He never takes his eyes off of me. When he's finished singing that song he starts singing George

Strait's "I Just Want to Dance With You" and then he walks over to where I'm sitting, reaches his hand out to me and asks if he can have this dance. How's that for a beginning?"

"Not bad. Not bad at all." He reached out to take her hand and gently squeezed it. She timidly looked over in his direction and smiled. Just then Paisley woke up with a loud wail. She had rolled over in her sleep and landed in the sand. Her mouth was crusted with sand inside and out.

"So much for fantasizing!" Jenny said as she jumped up to take care of her, gently coaxing her to drink water and then to spit it out. It took her awhile to get the hang of it and then she thought it was so much fun she didn't want to stop, even though the sand was all rinsed out.

David and Jenny played gin until Jenny's nose twitched in the air and she recognized the delicious aroma of Beef Teriyaki sizzling in a wok on a grill somewhere just behind them. The cooking festival had begun! She scampered over to the cooler in the van and took out the steaks she had been marinating in a burgundy wine sauce for two days. David helped her light their grill, which was little more than a Hibatchi attached to a long black pipe stuck into a cement footing buried in the sand. After the coals were almost white with heat and the flame was all but extinguished they put the steaks on to cook. It did Jenny's heart good to see people's heads turning at the other tables looking for the origin of the delicious smell wafting over to them.

Dinner was of course, excellent, although nothing ever tastes as good as it smells when the smells have kept you salivating for twenty minutes. They feasted on steak, baked potatoes, a cold green bean salad and her mom's home-made applesauce as they watched the sun starting to set, turning the sky different shades of mauve, lavender and purple. It had been a marvelous day. After leisurely enjoying a chocolate mousse for dessert they started packing up for the drive home.

Jenny was thinking about all the things she had to do when she got home. The kids would each need a bath, and so would she. She needed to go over her accounts and pay some bills and she desperately needed to do some laundry. It was piling up in the laundry room making it hard to even open the door to get in. Having one day off a week was really the pits. And here she'd spent it actually having some fun. The traffic on the beltway was heavy but everything was steadily moving along. It would be almost completely dark when they pulled into her driveway. It was too late to watch a movie, she hoped David had forgotten that they'd planned to.

David was thinking that it would really be nice if he didn't have to go home after he dropped Jenny and the kids off. It would be wonderful if this was his home and they were his family. He had enjoyed his daughter immensely. He thought of her in his mind that way because in his mind that's the way it was. She was his daughter. Every day he saw more and more of himself in her and he just idolized her all the more for it. He would spend his evening thinking about Jenny, wanting her in his arms, lying beside him in their king-sized bed talking about their future together.

By the time they arrived at Jenny's house, they were all pretty tired and cranky. The day in the sun had taken the best out of all of them. It was all they could do to unload the van and the sleepy kids before David had to get into his car and drive home. He was even too tired to try to maneuver a way to kiss her. He called goodbye to her from the bottom of the stairs while she was running the bath water for Paisley and stripping her down.

She called back to him, " Thanks for taking us today, we had a really good time! Make sure you don't nod off on your way home, you look pretty tired!"

"Okay, I'll be just fine, you get some sleep and I'll call you tomorrow!" he called back.

As he drove home he thought about a lot of things, Jenny, Paisley, Jenny's fantasy guy and whether that could also be Donna's fantasy guy, and his bills. He needed to find a way to get more money. The bequest from Benton Riveria was almost gone. Pretty soon he'd be in dire straits again. God he wished

Linda would fall off a bridge or something. Her alimony payments were breaking him.

Chapter 37

Fairfax, VA

The next morning David answered a call from his bank letting him know that his credit card was over the limit and requesting him to refrain from using it until it was paid down below the credit limit. He banged on his desk and swore, something he rarely did. Good God, he had to find a way to get more money! He fervently wished that there was another Benton Riveria on his deathbed bequeathing him another monetary gift of appreciation for his services.

He had a lot of rich clients, maybe some day there would be. With that, his mind ran through the possible prospects of each patient, categorizing them in his mind as to their level of inheritance and the likelihood that they would leave any of it to him. He realized that many would if the thought ever occurred to them to do so.

And then it came to him. He could control their thoughts to quite a large degree. They all trusted and relied on him to reshape their thoughts in one way or another. How hard would it be to persuade them to include him in their wills? Benton Riveria had done it as a benefactor. He had believed in David's work. Most likely they would all leave something to some kind of charity or religious affiliation. Could he convince them to make the "David L. Sandler Foundation" their charitable institution?

His mind was racing at the possibilities. Of course he could! A few subliminal suggestions here and there in everyday conversations, maybe a sentence or two on their bills and finally a few well-placed suggestions during relaxation sessions should do the trick. Oh, this was not good. He couldn't believe he was actually contemplating doing something like this. He put it out of his mind and started working on Donna's case.

But all day long the thoughts kept coming back to him. The more he pondered this scheme, the more convinced he was that it would work. And why shouldn't it work? His foundation was worthy. He deserved a share of his patients' estates as much as any other charitable cause they might have. More, in fact, because his was personal. He helped them all to overcome serious problems when others hadn't been able to do a thing for them. Indeed, they owed him a part of themselves when they passed. After all, they wouldn't be contributing to his income anymore since they wouldn't be seeing him again. It only seemed fair that they compensate him for all he had done for them. And, it wasn't stealing if they acted on his suggestions. They were, in fact, only suggestions.

A quote from an old psychology textbook, "Hypnosis:The Power of Attention," came to mind, "hypnosis leads to changes in brain activity that separate it from all other states of awareness. It can create a pleasant state of focused awareness with a high rate of suggestibility." It was this precept that allowed him his great success. Now his success would be even greater.

He picked up his rolodex and scanned the cards, trying to pick out the perfect patient to try his theory out on. It wouldn't hurt to try. If it worked, he could always refuse the money from the estate. Katherine Cheney. Perfect. Absolutely perfect. She was one of his oldest patients, both in age and in treatment time with him. She was 83 and she was totally committed to him and to his treatments. He had cured her of migraines that she had suffered with for over thirty years. Heck, she might have already included him in her will for all he knew! His excitement was growing and he couldn't wait to try out his new idea.

When Katherine Cheney came in for her session a few days later, he commented to her that she looked a little tired, though she looked exactly the same as she always did. She was uncommonly tall for a woman born over eighty years ago, she was, in fact, pretty tall by today's standards too. She would have been considered willowy in her earlier days but now she walked with a marked brittleness to her stride and, of course, her cane thumping along beside her indicated her fragility as well.

She had snow white hair that looked as soft as rolled cotton from a box and her cornflower blue eyes complimented the fairness of her complexion. She over rouged her cheeks and she was constantly lining her lips fuller than they really were. This gave her a slightly theatrical look. She showed stately elegance, always dressed in a dark suit with a white frilly blouse secured at the throat with an heirloom cameo.

You would have to look really hard to notice that the right heel of her expensive Aigner low pumps was over an inch higher than that of her left. She had scoliosis, an abnormal curvature of her spine, that had gone far too many years without diagnosis, and rather than walk with a gait, she chose to modify her shoes to camouflage it. She was an extremely proud woman and even at 83 she was meticulous about her appearance.

Even though she hadn't felt tired in the least, it did affect her that David thought she looked tired. They took their usual positions in his office, she reclining on an exceptionally comfortable leather chaise with her shoes on the floor beside her and he in an easy chair flanked by two small tables. Katherine had been using the self-hypnosis techniques that David taught her along with his counseled relaxation sessions for years, so it was never hard to get her into a trance-like state.

With her eyes closed and her hands together on her abdomen, she started her breathing rituals. She focused on a gently sloping hill in the summertime on the farm she had been raised on. She pictured herself as she used to be, a little pig-tailed girl of eight or nine, lying in the sweet smelling clover, feeling the June sunshine washing over her face.

Even though her eyes were closed, in her trance they were open, staring at the blue sky above and all the wispy clouds drifting slowly around. She was lying with her feet toward the top of the small rise and her head buried in clover at the bottom. She liked it this way. It gave her a floating away feeling in her limbs. The blue was magnificent, as light as old washed out denim, and the soft white wispy clouds were inviting her to jump onto them. From the perspective in her mind she was above them looking down, ready to jump from one cloud to the other and on to the next and then the next

After watching her regular breathing for a few minutes David judged where she was in her focused state. Softly he whispered, "Katherine, do you ever think about what it would be like to die? Do you ever wonder about heaven? Is it like living on the farm again, being cherished and taken care of and being Daddy's adorable little girl all over again? Is it sweet like that? Will there be someone to read you stories and to play with you in the orchards? While you're imagining your beautiful hillside strewn with clover and morning glory flowers, try to picture this as your idea of heaven. Are you ready to leave this world to go there? It should be very easy for you to get things ready so you can go there. Make sure you haven't forgotten to do anything here that will keep you from enjoying yourself there."

Dr. Sandler continued on, "Are all your papers in order? Does your family know of all your wishes? Have you started giving away all your very special mementos to those who are worthy to take care of them for you? Have you remembered to thank everyone properly by including them in your will? This is the time to show them how much you have appreciated them, what they've meant to you and all they've done for you over the years. Don't forget all your faithful servants, your driver and your housekeeper, your cook and your gardener. They've been with you for a long, long time. And your doctors, don't forget to thank your doctors for all they do for you to keep you living such a healthy, happy and long life. Isn't it wonderful that you've been pain-free for so, so long. That wouldn't have happened by itself, you know. You needed help to do that. Dr. Sandler has been so very helpful to you. Don't you think he deserves a very special reward? You could contribute to his practice. He would really appreciate knowing how much you care and how much you want to help others with similar problems. Are you getting ready to go back home? You want to make sure you go with everything done. Don't put anything off. You don't know when your family will be calling you home to be with them again and you don't want to leave anything undone. Take care of everything soon so you can feel good about yourself and be prepared for the trip home. It could be soon. You could be home again, real soon."

He stopped speaking and studied her intensely. Her breathing was the same and she had just the faintest touch of a smile at the corners of her lips. He left her alone to her thoughts. When she roused herself a few minutes later, she still seemed a little lost in thought. "You did very well today," he said. "You seemed to have a lot of purpose in your focus and very good concentration." He handed her a four-leaf clover saying, "I found this on the floor by your shoes."

She took it gingerly from him, holding it between her thumb and forefinger, mindful not to touch the leaves. As she stared at it in total amazement, a huge smile came upon her face and tears filled her blue eyes. "I was really there," she whispered. "I was really home."

She slowly got up, slipped her feet into her shoes and picked up her pocketbook from his desk, all the while not taking her eyes off of the four-leaf clover.

"See you next week," he said as he walked her to the door.

"Don't be so sure," she said with a smile. Then she was at the elevator door. Her driver stood there waiting to push the button for her.

Chapter 38

Fairfax, VA

The next day as Dr. Sandler worked at his desk on a speech he was scheduled to deliver at a conference the following week, he was continually interrupted by his thoughts of his session with Katherine Cheney. How would he know for sure that she would act on his suggestion? Even after she did, if she did, he would have no way of knowing until he received the proceeds after the probate of her will. And then again, when would she die? She could live to be 110 for all he knew.

He would have to hedge his bets, and not count on her to do the right thing, which was to change her will and then promptly die. He would need back ups, maybe several. As he reached for his rolodex a thought was nagging at him, telling him that this wasn't very kosher of him. This wasn't something a psychiatrist of his caliber should be tinkering with. He ignored that thought.

It was becoming a challenging game to him. If he could sway one patient to include him in their will, he would win. Now, who would be the next player? He thumbed through the cards, mentally discarding anyone who wasn't likely to die any time soon and also those who weren't truly capable of achieving a high degree of relaxation in therapy with him. When he was finished going from A to Z, he had five names in front of him. Jessica Tyler, Shawn Vanscoy, Betsy Drayton, Leroy Dressler, and Nancy Meridan.

The only one of the five that had a really good likelihood of dying this year was Nancy Meridan. She was in the last stages of terminal ovarian cancer. It had been determined that she probably had less than three months to live. She was dealing with the pain through a self-hypnosis program that Dr. Sandler had prescribed. He used to see her three times a week when she was still getting around, now he actually made a few house calls at her family's request.

Nancy was a widow in her late fifties, but since she was a devoted Christian Scientist, she had never had the routine pap smear that would have allowed her to live probably well into her eighties. When she became so sick from the lack of medical attention that she collapsed while shopping, she was rushed to the hospital in an ambulance, totally unconscious.

It had taken the whole afternoon to track down anyone in her family and by then all the tests had been done. Of course, any further treatment was canceled as soon as she regained consciousness and she checked herself out and went home. Her spiritualist recommended hypnotherapy to deal with the pain while she fervently prayed for a full understanding of the divine principles of Jesus's teachings and the ultimate healing that would come from it.

Jessica, Shawn and Leroy were on a path of self-destruction and unless they made a quick turn around, they could be leaving the planet soon also. Betsy, bless her heart, was so obese and so out of shape that no one would be surprised if her body shut down on her tomorrow. Nancy looked like the best candidate for now, and she certainly had a big chunk of change to designate to him in her will, if she hadn't already promised it all to her church.

Of course, wills could be changed and he was confident he could coerce, er... convince her into doing just that. David reached for the phone and dialed her number. He spoke with her daughter who was extremely pleased that he had taken the time to call and inquire about her mother, and "Yes, it would be wonderful if he could drop by this afternoon to see her."

A few hours later he was sitting in a chair beside Nancy's bed in her bedroom. The house was a magnificent manor in Great Falls. Parts of it had already been taken over by her Church, as it had already been decided that the house and grounds were to go to the Church on her passing. She had encouraged them to set up their offices in the unused bedrooms as the lease on their old office building had expired and wasn't being offered to them for renewal.

Her whole family were devoted practitioners of the faith and they had also moved in to help with the renovations needed and to be near her to take care of her. It was a pretty busy and noisy household for an invalid to be dying in, but he supposed she didn't feel that way or she wouldn't have had them there.

It had given him a good excuse to close the door to ensure their privacy. "Nancy," he called out to her very softly. "Nancy, it's Dr. Sandler, I've come to check up on you. How's your focusing going?"

"Oh, Dr. Sandler, how good it is to see you!" she breathed. Her skin was ashen and her hair looked so very dry and brittle. Her hands on top of the sheets looked like they were made of wrinkled parchment and he was almost afraid that if he touched them they'd crackle. He looked into her dull eyes. She had changed a lot in just a few days, it was good he came now he thought.

"Are you managing the pain?" he asked, "or is it managing you?"

"A little of both," she said with a raspy whisper. She had apparently succumbed to the idea that the healing miracle wasn't going to happen for her. God wanted her home, and she was okay with that. "I can't seem to get into it as easily as I could before, my focus must be off."

"Well let me help you, that's what I'm here for." He adjusted her hospital bed so she was reclining in a comfortable position and then he pulled out a little bottle of almond oil from his jacket pocket. He removed his jacket and draped it over a chair.

David lifted the sheet from the bottom of the bed and raised it to just below her knees and then he removed a sock from one foot. He stood at the foot of the bed and poured some almond oil into his palm and rubbed it between his hands to warm it. He then lifted her right foot from the heel and started to gently massage it.

As a fledgling intern in the psychiatric ward at Georgetown Medical Center, he had learned from one of the best in the field of hypnotherapy to utilize whatever sense he could to maximize relaxation: Taste, smell, sound, sight, but most especially touch. Dentists used it all the time, so did acupuncturists and reflexologists. There had been many times he'd relied on touch when nothing else seemed to work.

Years ago, when Nancy and her husband had lived on a farm in Texas, they spent their evenings in prayer together and then, because there was no television, they would occasionally rub each others feet using a little lard in their hands to moisturize them and to help their hands from getting chapped at the same time. It was pure heaven. After a long hard day on the farm there was nothing better than having a foot rub. If Nancy could have been honest with herself, she would have said that she missed those foot rubs more than anything else she missed about her husband.

The searching out of information like this from a patient was what Dr. Sandler was so very good at. He asked so many questions and really listened to all the answers. At times, he felt that he probably knew more about his patients than anyone else in their whole lives had. When he discovered Nancy's little key to total relaxation, she had become his patient for life, short as it was to be.

After they had signed over oil rights to their farm and became instant millionaires, their lives changed dramatically. They moved to a mansion, raised three children, worked hard managing their money, and remained devoted to their beliefs. They became too busy with the social whirl and business world to even talk to each other much, much less indulge in the foot rubs. She'd always missed that. She hadn't had one since they packed up and left the farmhouse in Texas twenty-five years ago. Not until Dr. Sandler came into her life did anyone care enough to ask her what would make her sublimely happy.

As he gently massaged her heel and moved slowly up to caress her arch she moaned ever so softly, almost in a sexual way. He paid special attention to her instep and then her toes. She really liked that. Each toe received its own protracted attention. She had nice feet. She'd paid to have a manicure each week ever since she'd had her first session with Dr. Sandler. This was something new to her too, with all the money she had, she could have been enjoying this all along if it had ever occurred to her that she could have easily paid someone to do it for her.

He carefully placed her right foot back on the bed and raised her left one by the heel. "Nancy, concentrate on the sensations, feel the pressure of my thumbs as they massage your instep going in circles, little ones and then bigger ones and then joining with the other to knead the ball of your foot. Imagine you're on that horsehair couch covered with the chenille throw to keep it from being so scratchy. You're wearing a cool summer dress and you've hiked it up past your knees enjoying the gentle breeze from the fan on the coffee table. You've untied the belt at your waist, where it's been cinched in all day, and your sore feet are being lovingly stroked and prodded. Your toes are being pulled ever so gently, one by one, first the baby one and then the area in between, then the next one and the area in between. There is no more pain, only pleasure. The pain is leaving as the pleasure is entering. No more pain, just pleasure. Only pleasure. Pleasure one person has brought you, your friend and your doctor. Hasn't he been so good to you? You know he has. Has anyone cared for you as he does?"

"Does anyone give you the immense pleasure that he does? Wouldn't it be nice to show him your delight in him? Pretty soon you're going to go to a place where you can always feel like this. There will always be someone with strong hands to caress your feet like this. Before you go be sure to take the time to show how much you appreciate the one who gives you such great pleasure. Reward him for his dedication to you. He would like to know you haven't forgotten him and what he's meant to you. A codicil in your will would be a good way to communicate to him, long after you've gone, that you still remember his hands and his gentleness with you." He moved up to caress and knead her calf and she let out the most delightful groan.

He felt very powerful right now, knowing that he was controlling her thoughts through his manipulations of her body. "Be a benefactor to his foundation and ensure that your message gets to him. He needs to know that he's made a difference in your life." He put her left foot down and then grabbed a foot in each hand as they rested on the bed. He massaged the tops of them and then stroked her feet up past her ankles turning his hands as he inched up her legs deeply kneading her calves with his thumbs. When he got to her knees he rubbed the backs of them with his fingertips and that was their signal to suspend.

She slowly opened her eyes and smiled up at him. He replaced the bed cover and walked to the head of the bed. She took his hand and touched his cheek and said, "Thank you so very much for your loving ways, you are one of the kindest people I know." With that she closed her eyes and drifted off to sleep. A wonderful sleep such as she hadn't known in months. Later that day, after she awoke, she called her attorney and asked him to come by the following morning.

Chapter 39

Tyson's Corner, VA

On his way back to his office Dr. Sandler stopped by Jenny's work to visit her, but first he used the men's room at the dealership to wash his hands. As a doctor he was less squeamish about soiling his hands than most people. He had learned early in medical school that you could wash anything off as long as it didn't go in. However, he was still fastidiously clean or he just wasn't comfortable.

Jenny was nowhere to be seen, but he knew she was scheduled to be working now because he had memorized her schedule as he did every week when she posted it on the door of her refrigerator. Assuming she was on the lot somewhere or out on a test drive, he went to the showroom and asked the receptionist to take a message for him. That's when he was informed that Jenny had had an emergency call from home and had checked out for the day.

His heart leapt to his throat and he instantly thought of Paisley. Questioning the receptionist did no good. She had no idea what the emergency was and neither did anyone else standing around. He quickly went into Jenny's office and dialed her number. There was no answer. His palms were starting to get sweaty and he could feel his pulse throbbing in his ears. He didn't have Jenny's mother's number with him but it was programmed into his car phone so he ran out to his car and punched in the code.

Again, no answer. He drove to Jenny's mother's house, stopping at the Emergency Access Center that was close to her home. He left his car at the curb as he ran inside and looked around for Jenny, her mother or her father. He didn't see them so he hopped back into his car and drove like a maniac the rest of the way to Jenny's parents' house, screeching to a halt as he pulled in front of their house. It didn't look like anyone was home, and after ringing the bell several times, it was confirmed.

He felt like a madman. Where could they be? He noticed the next door neighbor sitting on the ground weeding around a flower bed. He called over to her, "Any idea where everybody went?"

"Yeah," she called back. "Rusty got hit in the head with a swing and they took him to his doctor to get a few stitches. It wasn't too bad. Didn't bleed too awful much."

He felt the air whoosh out of his chest and he sat on the front stoop trying to gather himself back together. This father stuff wasn't all good. He was shocked at how scared he had been. Now that he knew everything was all right he started to get angry. What would he have to do to get *into* this family? To count in such a way that he would be called if it were Paisley who was hurt. If not for the neighbor it might have been several hours before he found out what had happened.

He didn't like this. He had a right to know right away if his daughter was hurt. Marriage to Jenny was the answer. Then he'd be connected to Paisley just as any father would be.

When Jenny and her parents and the kids arrived home an hour later in their separate cars, they all had the remnants of ice cream cones in their hands or on their clothes. Rusty was sporting a bandage just above his eyebrow and the area around his eye was puffing up and discoloring. He ran to David to show him his battle wound. Paisley was in her car seat having thoroughly enjoyed her ice cream as evidenced by her face and hands and hair.

Jenny was a little surprised to see him there and gave him a questioning look.

"What are you doing here? Something wrong?"

"Yeah, you might say that," he mumbled. He explained what had happened and Jenny was very touched that he had been so concerned about Rusty. She hadn't understood that he was only there because of Paisley.

Since it was late afternoon and he had no other reason to go back to the office, he asked Jenny if she'd like to go out to dinner. She knew that there was no way her parents would let her take Rusty home that night. They would want to be the ones to care for him since he was "hurt", and Rusty would want to be there to milk it for all it was worth. She accepted with the provision that Paisley could come with them.

Her mother overheard and said, "Go out to dinner and come back for her later. She needs a bath and a nap now anyway."

So David and Jenny got into their separate cars and drove to her house. When they got there, Jenny got into his Trams Am and they continued on to dinner from there. This, Jenny thought, is definitely a date.

They went to a little restaurant called Sylvans in the shopping center where Jenny did most of her grocery shopping. It was a small cafe specializing in Italian and Greek dishes. When they had been seated at a table and handed menus, David grabbed her hand. "I was beside myself with worry today! When I stopped by the dealership and they told me you left because of an emergency, I thought something might have happened to Paisley. Or to Rusty," he hastily added as an afterthought. "And then when I couldn't find anything out, I was so frustrated."

Jenny was genuinely touched by his free-flowing emotions. He really cared about her kids. It warmed her to know this, this was truly an amazing man. Most of the men she had dated could've cared less about her kids.

"I'm sorry, David. When I got the call from my Mom, I didn't really think of anything except getting to the doctor's office."

"Well maybe in the future you'll give a care for my heart," he said. Then added, "Maybe I should get you a cell phone. Then you'll always be able to get in touch with me should you need me."

"Oh, I don't think that's necessary!" she said as she squeezed his hand before removing hers. "It wasn't really that big a deal. Kids get hurt like that all the time."

180

Without thinking he replied, " Well, I want to know when mine gets hurt!"

As Jenny raised an eyebrow he realized what he'd said and he covered by saying, "You know what I mean. Paisley and Rusty are special to me. I think of them as the kids that are going to be mine when we marry some day."

"David, I wish you wouldn't keep saying that. It makes me feel pressured. We aren't even a couple. This is actually our first real date!"

He smiled at the uncertainty in her eyes and winked at her. Then he said, "Well, talk about pressure! This had better be a date to remember!" He turned to the waiter who was just approaching their table and ordered a bottle of champagne, knowing full well her weakness for it.

They both ordered the chicken Parmesan with spaghetti on the side and shared a huge antipasto salad. Jenny was thoroughly enjoying herself, listening to David regale her with stories of his medical school days. As her glass emptied, he refilled it. When Jenny excused herself to go to the ladies' room he used his cell phone to call her mother to let her know that they would soon be on their way to pick up Paisley.

As he had expected, he was told that she had just fallen asleep and wouldn't it be better to just leave her there with them tonight? He agreed and had already paid the check when Jenny arrived back at their table, somewhat flushed in the face. He led her out of the restaurant and eased her into the Trans Am, marveling at how she could still keep her propriety regarding her short skirt while getting into that low-slung seat. Must be some kind of instinct, he mused, figuring she probably did that maneuver several times a day with customers without the benefit of being a little pixilated. Assured that he would probably be seeing quite a bit more than her shapely legs tonight, he closed her door and went around to his.

When Jenny reminded him that they needed to pick up Paisley, he told her of his phone call to her mother. A little miffed that he took it upon himself to intervene, she just nodded.

How much champagne had she had to drink? She couldn't even remember if they'd had dessert or not. Not that it mattered, she was quite full and more than content to just go home and get ready for bed. However, David had other ideas. When she tried to say good night at the door, he simply ignored her and led her up the stairs to her room. "David, what in the world are you doing?"

"This," he said as he reached for her and brought his lips down hard over her mouth. He wasn't at all gentle as he moved his lips over hers trying to maneuver hers to open for him. When she gasped for air he slid his tongue into the opening, the pointed tip stroking and chasing hers around the moist recess. She pushed against his chest and managed to disengage his mouth from hers but it settled on her cheek and then slid to her ear. The wet, slimy sensation of having his tongue licking her ear nauseated her and with all her might she shoved against him and ran for her bathroom. She had just managed to get behind the closed door when her stomach lurched and she spun around just in time to get the lid up before all was lost.

Twenty minutes later when she finally emerged from the bathroom, she found that David had left, leaving her a short note. "Sorry you're not feeling well, and doubly sorry that it was all my fault. Can we not let this be our first date? Call you in the morning. Love David."

Chapter 40

Fairfax, VA

Several weeks later David was in his office dictating patient notes when his receptionist walked in and placed an envelope in front of him. Her only comment before retreating and closing the door was, "I think Mrs. Cheney has overpaid her account."

David turned off his recorder and lying it aside reached for the envelope. Inside was a cover letter folded around a check. The check was payable to him in the amount of $19,733.40. It was issued from the offices of an attorney located in Washington, D.C. He scanned the cover letter. The estate of Katherine Cheney was dispersing funds per her request and because he had been a benevolent servant to her she had settled these funds on him.

Well, this was surely good news, in a way. He was sorry about Katherine's passing, he hadn't even known of it. He was sure he'd seen her less than a month ago. "Benevolent servant?" What did that mean? And what an odd amount. It was a bit curious but he didn't care, he could sure use the money. Better yet was the knowledge that he had caused this, he had manipulated her will to his. His blood surged and he felt invincible. This had almost been too easy.

He picked up the phone and dialed the number on the letterhead. He had to check out one thing. The date she had amended her will. He had to make sure this was his doing, not something she had done months ago. Not everyone was like Benton Riveria, but you never knew.

He was connected to the secretary of one of the attorneys listed down the side of the letterhead and, as luck would have it, she was familiar with this particular testate case. He started the conversation with feigned shock at Mrs. Cheney's benevolence, "I just can't believe she did this. I am totally in shock. What a sweet dear woman. Did she specify her intentions for the use of these funds?" knowing that the payee was simply Dr. David Sandler, and that there were no specified stipulations for endorsement, he just wanted to get her talking.

"No, Dr. Sandler, she did not. Her desire was to reward those persons who had served her well," she said crisply.

"Served her well?" he queried. That was unusual phrasing.

"Yes, you were listed in conjunction with her driver, her cook, her gardener and her housekeeper." He detected a slight attitude of superiority in her voice. "In fact, you all split the proceeds from one of her life insurance policies. She changed the beneficiaries just a few days before she died. That is why you have the proceeds so quickly. Benefits from life insurance policies aren't usually held up in testate and $98,667 divided by 5 was your share."

David was a bit offended by this news, but took it graciously. "Well, thank you for clearing this up for me. It's awfully nice to know that she appreciated my services." He emphasized the word services and then hung up.

After cradling the phone he retrieved the tapes of Katherine Cheney's recorded patient file and fast forwarded to her last appointment. There it was, clear as could be; "Don't forget all your faithful servants, your driver and your housekeeper, your cook and your gardener..." And only a paltry twenty grand. He obviously was getting through, he just needed to choose his words a bit more carefully in the future. He then destroyed the tape by pulling the ribbon out and tossed it into the trash can beside his desk.

He decided then that it probably wasn't a good idea to keep tapes of these sessions, so he destroyed all of his audio files, except Liesel's. He thought he just might want to listen to hers one more time before he destroyed them. He loved listening to her sultry voice and of course her story could be quite erotic from a man's perspective.

Chapter 41

Fairfax, VA

After weeks of research and planning Dr. Sandler was ready to alter Donna Bristol's memories of the night she left her husband. The technique he decided to use to induce her hypnotic state was one he'd never tried before so he had some trepidations, but all in all he was very excited about what he might be able to accomplish for her if it worked.

Without telling her exactly what he would be attempting, he described the state of focused concentration he would put her in. She would be more relaxed than she'd ever been in her life. He would use the method she herself used all the time, soaking in hot water. She already understood its soothing effects on her. She'd always retreated to a warm bath to ease her mind. Now the only detail to work out was where she would be comfortable doing this.

He made several suggestions; including his place, her place, or a hotel suite. It was important that she choose the location because if she felt out of place or threatened in any way, they would accomplish nothing. He even broached the idea of a chaperone being present, but she waved off that idea. She trusted him and had for several years.

She never once doubted his professional integrity and that was something that made him very proud. After discussing all the possibilities together, she decided that her own bath tub was familiar and conducive to what Dr. Sandler had in mind. They arranged to meet there Friday after work. Melanie and her nanny would have dinner out and attend a show so there would be no one to disturb them.

Even though Donna wasn't exactly sure what to expect she was excited because David was excited and he had assured her that she would be a new woman. She would be rid of her anxiety problems and her inner turmoils and she would be able to become the mother she wanted to be for Melanie. She would no longer look at her and remember the night of her conception. Only Dr. Sandler knew that wasn't exactly true. She would remember the night of Melanie's conception. She would just remember it very differently. She would remember it very fondly.

Friday evening at six o'clock, Donna opened the door of her high rise luxury apartment to her therapist. She had already prepared the room as instructed. When Dr. Sandler entered her bathroom he was pleased to see that she had even moved a boudoir chair next to the tub for him to sit in. She had filled the tub to full capacity with hot water and bubbles and had attached a terry cloth covered pillow with suction cups to the tub for her to recline against.

Candles were lit throughout the spacious tub alcove. The tiles covering the walls in the rather large bathroom had designs painted on them here and there, reminiscent of ivy climbing the walls. There were a couple of Boston Ferns enjoying the misty humidity hanging from the ceiling in the corners.

Also as instructed, Donna had prepared herself. She was wearing the heaviest Terry Cloth robe she had and her hair was piled on her head wrapped with a thin hot towel. She'd had exactly two glasses of wine as prescribed. There was a stack of large bath towels on a stand. They were ready.

David removed his tie and suit coat and rolled the sleeves of his white shirt up to his elbows. He took Donna's hand and led her over to the tub. "I want you to step in and see if the temperature is all right. If it's not we'll adjust it. And remember what I said. The robe stays on to weigh you down and to keep you from being self-conscious about being in your bathing suit underneath."

He assisted her in getting into the tub. "How's the temperature?" he asked.

"I could stand it a trifle hotter," she said and he reached over and turned on the hot water tap.

"Did you remember to unplug your phones?" he asked.

"Yes," she said, "I think I remembered everything you said." After a minute she said, "Okay, that's hot enough."

He turned off the tap and took her elbow to help her lower herself down into the tub. When she was all settled in with the robe plastered down against her he took a bath towel and placed it over her. It floated on the water until it settled down against her body. The bubbles were just about dissipated and because of the water displacement caused by her body, some sudsy water sloshed over the side.

She relaxed her turban-wrapped head against the bath pillow and closed her eyes. A marvelous low sigh escaped from her lips. David took a seat in the chair and took a small notebook out of his breast pocket.

For the first few minutes he instructed her to close her eyes and to do some deep breathing, bringing in huge chest fulls of air and exhaling them ever so slowly. Then he began a recounting of the car ride she had taken from her house in Reston on the night she left Kevin.

"Your suitcase is packed. It's in the trunk and you're driving and crying, unsure exactly which way to go. There's no one you can go to. You left behind the only people you care about. But now you don't care about them. You only care about you. What is it you want? You have a sense of freedom, although you're not really enjoying it yet, but you will. You're free to do and go as you please. Where do you want to go? What do you want to do?"

"You pass by an ABC store and you think maybe this would be a good time to get drunk. Why not? Who's to know? It's Saturday night, party night. You feel like having a party, if only a pity party. You turn down the access road and back track to the liquor store. You go in and buy a bottle of vodka. You don't have anything to mix it with so you buy a good bottle. The kind with lemon flavoring. The young clerk gives you a big smile and you are bolstered by the fact that he's coming on to you. You smile brightly for him and then practically bounce back to your car. On to the party!"

"So, where's this party gonna be? Can't just sit in your car and drink, you might get into trouble that way. And you don't want any trouble. You decide to go to a hotel. A nice one. You deserve the best. You see the lights at the top of the Sheraton building and remember the times you ate in the restaurant there. Well, you think, now might be a good time to check out the rooms. You park in the parking lot and carry your suitcase to the front desk and check in."

"On the way to your room you pass by the lounge and hear some great county music. It's dark inside and you really can't see much of anything except that there are some people dancing on the dance floor and they look like they're having a swell time. You go to the elevator and when the door closes you press your floor."

"You wish you had let the bellman carry your suitcase. At least you'd know where the ice machine was. Now you go the wrong way down the hall before you realize the numbers are going up instead of down, but when you turn around to go the other way you find the ice machine. Letting yourself into the room you put the suitcase on the stand, your purse on the dresser and the bottle of vodka on the bathroom counter. You go get some ice."

"You come back to the room and lock yourself in and then you start a bath. A nice warm bath. While the water's running you fix yourself a drink in the little tumbler glass you find on the counter. It's embossed with an "S" in a circle. You rub your thumb over it. How did they know you were *Sexy*?"

By the time you get out of the tub, your skin is pink and your face is glowing. You stumble trying to put your underwear on. Maybe you should have eaten something this afternoon. Your stomach growls in agreement. Room service or restaurant? you ask yourself. You know, that country lounge looked friendly and maybe a few bar appetizers would suit for now."

"You dress in tight jeans and a country shirt from your line dancing days. You didn't bring any boots but your loafers will do. You blow dry your hair so it fans all around your face, little curls accentuating your rosy cheeks. A dab of lipstick on your pouty lips and you grab your room key and charge card and put them in your pocket."

"On the way out the door you take a look around and spot your latest drink by the sink, you grab it and close the door behind you. On the elevator going down to the lobby you finish your drink while you preen in front of the mirrored doors. You leave the glass on the floor in a corner of the elevator. This is not like you but you don't stop to think much about it. You really don't want to think about much of anything tonight, you just want to wallow."

"As soon as the elevator opens up you hear the familiar strains of 'I've Got Friends in Lonely Places' and you sashay over to the opening of the lounge. You lean against the wall there for a moment or two trying to adjust your eyes to the dim light inside. You step inside and there, standing on the threshold, your eyes are drawn to the only lit place in the room, center stage."

"It's then that your eyes connect. He sees you at exactly the same time you see him. He's singing and strumming on a guitar. And now he's smiling just for you. He is as handsome as sin. And the particular sin that comes to mind startles you. It is not like you to size up a strange man like this, but you are intrigued by him."

"Even though he's half sitting, half leaning against a stool, you can tell that he's quite tall. His long legs covered in denim are supporting him, one booted foot hooked on a rung and the other firmly planted on the floor. He's wearing a red brushed flannel shirt open at the collar revealing burnished bronzed skin with tawny golden hair to match the hair gently waving around his face, sticking out from under his cowboy hat."

"The planes of his face are chiseled and tanned giving a harsh appearance until you notice his eyes. They are sparkling blue eyes twinkling with firelight as they reflect the light coming off of the small strobe spinning above the dance floor. They crinkle at the corners each time he sings a word that moves his lips into a smile and it softens the whole look of his face."

"He has an aura about him that is friendly and confident and you just know that everything he does is outrageous, wild and spontaneous. He is the one everybody wants to be with at a party. He is the one who can tell a joke and cause everyone to roar hilariously at the punch line. You don't know how you know all this, you just do."

"Your heart flutters a little as you realize he's not taking those eyes off of you. You smile back, rather timidly and then a waitress approaches and ushers you to a small cocktail table one row back from the stage. She asks your preference and you wisely decide food before another drink so you order a coke and some potato skins. She brings your coke and a big bowl of popcorn."

"As you watch the man on stage you feel like you're the only one in the room. He appears to be singing directly to you. His voice is clear with a husky, honeyed maleness in it that makes it seem like he's doing a lot more than just singing the words. It's like he's caressing them before they pass over his sensuous full lips. When the potato skins come you become self-conscious about eating them in front of him."

"When he starts singing George Strait's 'I Just Want to Dance With You,' with his eyes locked onto yours, you begin to tingle and a slight shiver escalates up your spine. When he walks over to your table and extends his hand in invitation you rise as if in a trance and walk right into his arms. He finishes singing the song as he dances with you on the dance floor.

'I caught you lookin' at me
When I looked at you
Yes I did
Ain't that true?
You won't be embarrassed by the things I do
I Just want to dance with you' "

"Since you stepped into his embrace you haven't missed a step even though the woodsy pine scent of him is making you light headed. His big hand on the small of your back is reassuring you and gently guiding you at the same time. He looks down at you and you look up at him and it's one incredible sensation after another. You are not even aware that your body is dancing on autopilot while the rest of you is sending reinforcements everywhere to combat the flushing, tingling, swooning feelings you are experiencing."

"When he playfully inserts his leg between your thighs and rubs it gently against your crotch, you use every bit of will power not to push back against him. Things are moving way too fast for you and as the song winds down you move away, look up into his eyes and murmur a soft "Thank you." He sees you back to your table where a cocktail waitress is delivering another bowl of popcorn, and you order a vodka tonic to calm your nerves."

"For the next half hour you watch him and his band as they perform one country hit after another. It appears that he's really playing the guitar he has strapped around his neck for some of the songs and not just using it as a prop. There is another man, much older and somewhat grizzled-looking, playing another guitar off to the side and every once in awhile he looks over at you and flashes a toothless smile."

"When you smile back he blushes up to the tops of his ears. The drummer in the back has a long ponytail and a sparse goatee. He looks very young and it appears that he is very serious about his music, never once looking up until each song has ended and then focusing solely on the singer to get his cues for the next song to be played."

"The last song they play is, 'I Tip My Hat to the Keeper of the Stars.' You sip on your third vodka tonic as you listen to the words and you know that he is singing them directly to you. Every inflection in his voice being duplicated in his eyes.

'It was no accident, me finding you.

Someone had a hand in it long before we ever knew.

Now I can't believe you're in my life.

Heaven's smilin' down on me as I look at you tonight.

I tip my hat to the keeper of the stars.

He sure knew what he was doin' when he joined these two hearts.

I hold everything when I hold you in my arms.

I've got all I'll ever need, thanks to the keeper of the stars.'

The message is quite clear, something has happened between the two of you, something stronger than just lust."

"After the last song he thanks the members of his band as he calls them by name and says that they'll be back the following night. As the crowd disperses and the band steps off stage he walks right over to you. He puts out his hand and introduces himself, 'Hi, I'm Marty Logan. Mind if I join you?' "

"You shake his hand enjoying the feel of having his warmth envelope you. You feel his touch all the way to your knees. 'Please,' you say and he settles into a chair right next to you. He hasn't relinquished your hand and you don't object as he places it between both of his on the table."

"You tell him that your name is Donna. He asks you where you're from and when you tell him he raises his eyebrow in question, but he doesn't ask. You tell him you're changing your life tonight and the two of you talk and drink and laugh until the lounge is practically empty and the wait staff is putting the chairs on top of the tables."

"He says he's not ready to give you up for the night and gives you a choice between his room or yours. You don't say anything, you just push your chair out and stand. He puts his arm around your waist and leads you to the elevators. When you get in he asks which floor and you tell him. He pushes the button and the doors close. As soon as the doors are closed he turns you to face him and gathers you into his arms. He leans down to kiss you and just before his lips meet yours you close your eyelids shutting off one sense to allow the others to more fully savor this first kiss."

"When his lips meet yours you marvel at how soft they are as they brush over yours, contouring themselves to the shape of his. You hear his low moan. His reaction causes you to part your lips slightly and he takes advantage of the opportunity to insert his tongue between your parted lips. This is such a heady feeling you can't help but lean into him. All at once you both are licking and sucking and crisscrossing your tongues together."

"You reach your arms around his neck and lift up onto your toes to get closer to him and he threads his fingers through your hair pulling your face closer to his. You both end the kiss at the same time and pull back to look into each others eyes. Instantly you both press your lips back to the others, frantically moving your lips back and forth trying to gain entry, trying to quench some deep burning passion spreading like something molten all along your nerve endings."

"When you hear the ding of the elevator bell you both pull apart and face forward prepared to pretend to anyone on the other side that there was nothing going on between the two of you just moments ago. When the elevator doors open he puts his arm around your shoulder and walks down the hall with you to your room. You fish the plastic key card out of your jeans pocket and he takes it from your hand and opens the door. Then he flicks on the wall switch beside the door illuminating the hallway of the room."

"He steps inside and closes the door securely behind him, never taking his eyes off of you. As soon as the echo of the door closing stops, you both realize that you are in your own quiet corner of the world and you turn to reach for the other, desperate to feel those feelings once again. When your lips meet this time your passions cannot be denied. You are frenzied as you try to get enough of each other. Tongues delving deep, tracing and probing, lips nibbling and caressing, trying to meet each other in one of life's most intimate dances."

"He reaches behind you and turns off the glaring hall light leaving just the wall sconce over the king-sized bed to softly illuminate the room. Never taking his lips from yours he reaches down and puts his arms around your legs and lifts you up into his arms. He walks with you in his arms like he's holding a rare treasure and you feel like he could carry you like this forever and be quite content with the slight weight of you in his arms."

"As you're poised over the edge of the bed he reluctantly lays you down causing the separation of your lips and an immediate feeling of deprivation. He anxiously removes his boots and settles himself along the length of you, careful not to crush you. He gathers you back into his arms and fits every inch of his length against the corresponding length of you."

"You hear his groan as he experiences the softness of you coming up against the hardness of him. You moan too, as you feel the heat and hardness of his manhood probing against your hip. His lips are kissing your neck and throat and then you feel the warm breath of him against your ear and it sends shivers up and down your spine. You long for his lips to find their way back to your mouth but they are moving in the other direction."

"When his hands leave your shoulders and caress your buttocks, kneading them firmly and at the same time pulling you closer to him, you move with him feeling his engorged shaft searching out a place to be pleasured by. You put your hand between your two bodies wanting to feel him, needing to be reassured of his immense need for you because suddenly you have an overwhelming desire to be his."

"As soon as your hand touches the swollen mass that is him he groans and covers your hand with his. As you both exert pressure going up and down his groin he says your name, 'Donna, oh, Donna, God you feel so damned good.' He removes your hand and rolls you onto your back. He takes both of your hands in his and raises them up over your head, securing them together with just one of his. With the other hand he starts to unbutton your shirt."

"You squirm because you really don't like having your hands caught up like that. But as soon as he opens your shirt and kisses the flesh swelling above your bra, you forget all about your hands. There's a fire raging in your veins and it's moving to the very core of you. With one hand he unsnaps the front closure and pulls the lacy bra away from your breasts. You hear him inhale appreciatively. That and the cool air causes your nipples to tighten and all at once there is a yearning for his lips to enclose around them that is so compelling you can't stand it. Reading your mind, he complies as he puts his lips around first one rosy peak and then the other gently sucking and nibbling on them."

"You are going out of your mind with passion and you arch up against him telling him with your body that you need him. He releases your hands and raises himself off of you, with one leg on the floor and the other kneeling on the bed, he reaches for his belt and undoes it. Then he pulls his shirt out of his jeans and quickly unbuttons it. His smoldering eyes are fastened on you as he throws it to the floor."

"His broad chest is covered with curly golden brown hair, almost every inch of it until it reaches his navel where it whorls around his navel before it disappears into his jeans. Then he zips down his jeans and removes them. He's wearing nothing underneath and his throbbing penis is jutting straight out, quivering up and down with his desire for you. You take your hand and wrap it around his shaft pulling him back towards you. His groan is so deep in his throat it almost sounds painful."

"He undoes your belt and zipper and eases your jeans off your hips and down your legs, letting them fall off the end of the bed. He reaches his hand down and cups your mound over your lacy underwear. It is driving you crazy to have that barrier there, keeping his hand from making contact with your bare flesh. It's driving him crazy too, and with one quick motion, he hooks a finger under the waistband and pulls them down past your knees to your ankles and over your feet where they fall gently to the floor to land on top of your jeans. He lays down on you, gently gyrating his penis against your inner thighs. You feel like you're going to die if he doesn't enter you soon."

"While one hand is hefting and squeezing a breast the other is kneading a buttock, pulling you closer. When that hand moves around front and a lone finger strokes your feminine flesh you arch your body so that his finger enters you. As he delves into your moistness with one finger, he whispers breathily into your ear, 'You are so ready for me, as I am for you. I can barely control all the sensations you are causing in me. Forgive me, if I can't take my time.' "

"With that he positions himself above you and his penis finds its niche nestling in the velvet lips opening to him. With one forward movement of his hips he gains entry, with another he is buried deeply within you. As he gasps and clenches his teeth together you sigh and lift up to meet his thrusts."

"The pleasure is just too exquisite and just when he doesn't think he'll have enough control to satisfy you, you surprise him by wrapping your legs around his hips and pulling him in close, your fingers digging into his buttocks. Suddenly you buck up against him and he feels you spasm. Your slippery shaft pulsates and grips him tightly."

"He moans your name and lets his body explode into you, his penis jettisoning his sperm into your vagina like a hydraulic pump, retreating and plunging again with each release. As you both tumble through space on your way back to earth and to each other you realize that it has never been this good. Never. You smile as you realize you've just had your first one-night stand. He smiles as he realizes he's just had his last."

David looks over at Donna's face to see how she's doing and sees a tender smile touch the corners of her lips. Quickly he takes a sip of water and continues on.

"Together you lay side-by-side stroking each others backs as you try to catch your breath. He pulls you close for a kiss and then turns you in his arms so that his thighs are rubbing against your bottom. As you snuggle against each other he murmurs that he'd like to have a repeat performance in the morning. He kisses the back of your neck and the next thing you hear is his slow even breathing."

"When you awake the next morning you both open your eyes at the same time and smile brightly at each other. You make love two more times before calling room service for breakfast. After breakfast you go to his room to shower together and start all over again. By late afternoon you both dress for dinner. He dresses in the clothes he will be wearing for his last show there and you put on your favorite black sheath that you don't even remember packing."

"He tells you that you are beautiful and helps you put on your necklace. Your eyes meet in the mirror and you see the appreciation in his eyes. Over dinner you discuss your plans to meet the following weekend. He assures you that he has plans to see you often, probably more often than you will want to see him. You are very happy to hear this for you believe that you are beginning to fall for him."

"During the week Marty is a flight instructor and also teaches parachuting in a little suburban airport outside of Indianapolis. Tomorrow he is scheduled to fly his band home. They've been on the road for three weeks and are anxious to get home. Marty promises you that this is not just a groupie thing between the two of you. He says he can't explain it but he feels like you belong to him now. A gift from heaven that he doesn't deserve."

"When it's time to go into the lounge for his show he arranges a table right up front for you. You watch the show like a love-sick teenager. One of the songs he sings gives you goose bumps as he looks directly at you. 'Touch Me, Turn Me On and Burn Me Down.' His last song of the night he dedicates to you, Michael Martin Murphey's 'I'm Gonna Miss You Girl'. Tears trickle down your face and he catches them with his fingers as he sings directly to you."

"When the applause dies down he leans down and kisses you and tells you to wait for him while he helps the band pack up. Afterward you go for a walk around the hotel, looking up at the stars and marveling at the circumstances that brought you together. Since his flight out is very early and you have to teach the next day you both decide it's best to say goodbye tonight. He walks you to your door and kisses you deeply."

"The kisses are drugging and pretty soon you decide it would be better to be in the room doing what you're doing than out in the corridor. It's two in the morning before you open the door again and really say goodbye. He says he thinks he's in love with you. You ask him when he'll know for sure and he replies, 'As soon as I get back to my lonely room'."

"You wake up early the next morning but he's already checked out and gone. As you pack up and dress for school you start dreading all the things you have to do today. You wish you could just spend the day thinking of him. Somehow you manage to get everything done despite thinking about him all day anyway."

"The week drags by as you try to teach, set up a new apartment and pine for Marty's return. When Friday rolls around you are glad to find a few minutes just to relax and watch some television while you do your nails."

"As the 7:00 news program starts you settle into a corner of the couch and begin removing the old polish. You're really not paying too much attention until you hear the word 'Indianapolis', then you look up to see the charred remains of a plane. The newscaster is talking about a group of parachutists. Your heart feels like an anvil is sitting on it, the blood trying to lift it up with each pump."

"There is a survivor and she is being interviewed. She's a young college student on break. This was her first jump. Her friends had persuaded her to join them on their weekly outing. She was all ready to go and Mr. Logan was reassuring her and checking her chute when the plane suddenly shifted and began a downward spiral. He had pushed her out the door just as the turbulence of the plane slammed him and all the others towards the front of the plane. Luckily, on the way down she had fallen clear of it and after her chute opened, she watched horrified as the plane nose dived into the ground. They listed the names of all the victims, the pilot and the instructor's names were last. The instructor had been Marty Logan."

"You cried nonstop for days. You called in sick for work and you just about stopped eating. After two weeks you finally stepped back into your life and moved through it like a zombie, unconsciously blocking out the painful memories. Six weeks later when you discovered you were pregnant, you felt comforted that you had something of Marty to keep you going. You cherished that little life growing inside you and you vowed that you would be a good mother to Marty's baby."

"When you told your lawyer that you were pregnant you didn't bother to correct his assumption that it was Trace's. He deserved to pay for what he had done to you and you decided to keep Marty out of it. Nobody needed to know about your very special weekend with him."

"The day she was born you saw Marty's face reflected off of the mirror in the delivery room. He was smiling at you and it seemed that he was trying to thank you for his beautiful baby girl. The minute you looked at her you saw that she had Marty's sparkling blue eyes and his tawny gold hair. The night you and Marty made her lies hidden deep inside you because you couldn't deal with the pain of losing him. When he left you, he didn't want to go, so he left you with a part of him to treasure always."

David looked over at Donna's face. There were tears squeezing past her closed eyelids, spilling out at the corners and streaming down her face. He stood up and leaned down to caress her cheek and then pushed the lever for the tub letting the water drain out. He walked out of the bathroom to give her a few moments to compose herself.

When Donna came out into the living room she was dressed in a comfortable lounging pajama outfit. David walked over to her and handed her a small tumbler half-filled with brandy. She said thank you and gingerly took it out of his hands. It was then that she noticed the embossed "S" cut into the front of it. She leisurely stroked her thumb over it, a smile turning up the corners of her lips.

David was observing her closely trying to make out her feelings. "Do you feel all right?" He asked tentatively.

"Yes", she sighed, "just a little melancholy settling in." After a moment or two she looked over at him and said, "You're really good at what you do. You've made me remember something I had really hidden away. But now that some time has passed I think I can deal with the memories. Thank you for giving Marty back to me."

David got up and walked over to her, "I hope you always feel that way, please don't ever let me see that now you're drowning in grief." With that he bent down, kissed her on the cheek and walked to the door.

Just as he got there it opened and Melanie and her nanny came into the room. Melanie was so excited she nearly knocked him over in her haste to get to her mother. "Mommy, Mommy, we saw "Annie" and it was so terrific! Can you and I go see it again?"

Donna leapt up and opened her arms to the running little girl. As soon as she was in her arms she hugged her and lifted her up and kissed her cheeks. "Of course we can!"

Donna looked over at David and said "Good night Dr. Sandler and thank you for all you've given me."

She set Melanie on the floor and took her hand as she led her to the kitchen, "How about some milk and cookies before it's bedtime?"

Chapter 42

Fairfax, VA

As David drove home from Donna's apartment two thoughts were foremost in his mind. The first was that he had done an absolutely amazing job creating a part of Donna's life that she was now *remembering*, something that had actually never happened. And the second, was that two weeks of reading and researching erotica had made him horny as hell. He and Jenny had seen each other only a few times since the episode of their "first date" but as he was very anxious to experience his own orgasm instead of relating fantasy ones, he decided to call her and see if he couldn't push her a little farther along.

When he dialed her number she answered on the second ring, a good indication that she was trying to get to the phone before it woke Paisley. "Hello", she breathed.

"Hi, am I calling at a bad time?"

"No," she replied. "I just got Paisley down and was on my way into the kitchen, how are you?"

"I am missing you, that's how I am. If you're not busy can I come over?"

She quipped, "I'm not sure the laundry will understand being stood up again, but I'll risk it. What do you have in mind?"

David made his voice sound huskier than usual and said, "I want to neck on the couch, any problems with that?"

There was silence on the other end for a moment as Jenny remembered the kisses they had shared so far. Maybe she hadn't given them a fair chance. After all, she'd had an awful lot to drink the night of their date. After a long moment of indecision Jenny answered, "Does this mean I shouldn't have had that garlic chicken for dinner?"

"No problem," he retorted, "I'll stop at the grocery store and grab a garlic bulb to chew on. How 'bout I show up all smelly and ripe in about a half hour?"

"Okay." she said.

The moment she hung up the receiver she dashed up the stairs to take a quick shower and fix her hair and makeup. Getting out of the shower she went to her walk-in closet and leafed through her clothes. What exactly does one wear for making out purposes? Something easy to get out of or not so easy to be taken out of? Something soft and enticing or something not so alluring. Whatever she wore would speak volumes to him about her attitude for this little sofa romp. And what exactly was her attitude, anyway? She was so undecided about this relationship, but she was also very lonely and desired the companionship only a man could provide.

Strangely enough she was excited about the prospect of testing their pheromone compatibility without the benefit of alcohol to tip the scales. After their last fiasco she was genuinely surprised he was willing to attempt another liaison so soon. What a turn off she must have been. Tonight she would know for sure if he had the "kiss connection". She chose a pair of tight fitting jeans and a soft crop-topped sweater.

She had just finished applying a light coat of mascara and a light pink shade of lipstick when she heard his car in the driveway. She knew he wouldn't ring the bell but she hadn't unlocked the front door for him so she ran down the steps still brushing her hair.

It surprised her to see him juggling three garlic bulbs when she opened the door. "Is this enough to cover your offensive odors?" he queried.

"Well, I really didn't have any garlic, so I hope it won't be necessary, you didn't already eat any did you?" She frowned and then laughed when he purposely let them all fall to the ground and grimaced as if he had.

He stepped inside and closed the door, locking it behind his back and pulled her into his arms for a quick kiss. "What do you think?"

For a moment she thought he'd read her mind and was asking about the kiss, when he'd actually been asking about the garlic.

"About what?" she stammered.

He took her hand as he turned out the porch and foyer lights and walked with her through the kitchen to the family room. "Which couch has the better success rate, the one here or the one in the living room?" he asked.

"Well actually, neither has ever been successful," she said, "they're both new since my divorce."

"Ah, then let's try this one," he said as he led her over to the sectional sofa in the family room. He sat down and pulled her into his lap. "Jenny, you are so beautiful that sometimes I can hardly believe that no one has snatched you up to be their bride," he said as he gazed into her green eyes.

"I'm just very particular," she said, "I insist that all my dates fall in love with my children first. So far, you're the only one to pass the test."

He softly replied, "I do love your children, but I cannot say that I loved them first."

He looked at her lips and lowered her head to his. His lips feathered hers lightly just barely touching them before he increased the pressure and hungrily devoured them, savoring her sweet little pink mouth. Her lipstick tasted of strawberries and her tongue tasted of sweet tea. He grasped her head with both hands, luxuriating in the feel of her long silky hair wrapped around his fingers.

His mouth moved over her face kissing her cheeks and temples and then her eyelids and nose. As his thumb outlined the outer edge of her ear his mouth moved to join it, gently sucking on her earlobe and then breathing her name in a gasping hot breath into it. His lips inched their way down the column of her throat stopping at the base to press his lips to the soft vee he found there. When his lips rejoined hers they were almost rough with passion.

Jenny was submitting herself to his attentions but she really wasn't enjoying this as much as she knew she should be. Her thoughts were jumbled in her head about why she wasn't responding to him. One thought crossed her mind that maybe if she became a bit more involved instead of being so passive she would feel something. So as his kisses deepened she accepted his thrusting tongue and ran hers around the inner rim of his lips.

The jolt he experienced from her sudden spontaneity caused a leap in his groin area and he knew that she had to feel his stiffness against her bottom as she sat there on his lap. One hand moved around her to support her back as the other dropped to her shoulder and then to her breast, massaging it lightly through her sweater.

When she didn't make a move to stop him he put his hand under her sweater and cupped her breast through the lacy material of her bra. His low moan vibrated against the corner of her mouth as he pulled the material away from the nipple so he could pluck at it. When his thumb and finger tugged lightly on her nipple it budded to a hard peak instantly and Jenny, feeling her own jolt of electricity jumped from the pleasant sensation.

The combination of her involuntary reaction repositioning her on his erection and his hands exploring the curves of her breasts was enough to almost send him over the edge. His desire to have her was overwhelming him, he couldn't think of anything except taking her now on this sofa.

Jenny's thoughts were in a turmoil, some of what he was doing to her felt good. Lord, it had been ages since anyone had touched her breasts and they tingled with the heaviness of her arousal. But the kisses, they just weren't hitting on anything. Her lips were numb to his ministrations and now she was beginning to feel uncomfortable in his arms. She really didn't want to go any further with this but his hands were already fumbling with the button on her jeans.

She moved to cover his hand with hers but he'd already sensed that she was timid about the area he was moving towards and instead put his hands on the hem of her sweater and quickly pulled it up to her shoulders and then over her head. Her bra had already been worked off of her breasts and shoulders and hung down around her waist.

As he sat back to admire her he raised one hand to heft the fullness of one round perfectly formed breast. He sighed and said, "You have the most beautiful breasts I've ever seen. They are in fact, quite perfect."

He then bent to put the tip to his lips. He licked and suckled her unable to get enough of the taste of her. He did the same with the other and then he gently moved her off his lap and laid her down on the sofa, intent on holding one full ripe breast in each hand as he licked between them.

If there had ever been one erotic region capable of overriding all the others it was her breasts. To be touched and fondled there was the epitome to her and even though she knew that she didn't want to make love with David, she didn't want him to stop caressing her there, at least not yet, this was heavenly.

David's passions were beginning to control him. He had to have some release. The swelling against his zipper was straining to be freed. As his lips continued to pull against her nipples his hands found her zipper and pulled it down. The jeans were so tight that he didn't bother trying to take them down, he just reached his hand into the opening and worked it down into her underwear, his fingers brushing up against her soft furry mound.

Suddenly she tried to sit up, both hands grasping at his. With his hand firmly gripping her, he used his torso to keep her down. He wasn't about to stop now, he'd come so close. He worked his hand lower, he was constricted by the tight jeans but he managed to get a finger positioned at her labial opening and began to stroke her there.

Jenny was in a panic, she did not want his hand there. The weight of his upper body had one arm pinned so with the other she tried to pull his hand out of her pants. It just dove deeper and then she felt his finger penetrate to the opening of her vagina and enter her. "Oh, no!" she thought, "now what have I done?"

She knew that by not stopping him sooner she had lead him on and now he wasn't at all interested in curtailing his ardor. He wouldn't stop until he had satiated himself inside her. She was scared. She moved against his finger trying to pull away. He took it as an invitation to probe further and thrust his finger all the way into her. She was a little dry, not the warm welcoming stickiness that he had been expecting. He was more than ready but apparently she was not. He shifted himself so he could remove her pants.

Jenny was unsure what to do but when David shifted a little and her other hand was freed, she pushed against his chest saying, "David, I'm not sure..." before she could finish her sentence he had covered her mouth with his. He was not going to listen to any objections, he had sensed her backing away and he wasn't going to have any of it. He moved his lips over hers until she was forced to grant his tongue entry. He would keep his lips on hers as long as it took to claim her. With his hands he jerked on the waistband of her jeans, arduously inching them down until they were past her hips.

In a fit of desperation, Jenny tried to turn her head but his lips followed and captured hers again as soon as she'd gasped a breath. Her hands pushed against him, but his single mindedness would not let him acknowledge her denial. When her hand found its way between their bodies she felt the incredible hardness of him and knew that he would not curb himself. He was too far gone and it was her fault as well as his. She made a decision then that she felt she had to, to protect her body from his unwanted penetration. Borne out of her belief that life was full of sacrifices and compromises, in her mind she negotiated a way out, her body would be spared the assault she really did not think she could bear. She would work on the self-esteem problems later.

She wrapped her fingers around the bulge in his pants and was rewarded by the sound of a mournful groan from him. She moved her hands to his waistband and undid his belt. He didn't know what had caused her change of heart but he wasn't about to question it. He removed his hand from her pants and helped

206

Jenny undo the button and zipper on his pants. He stepped to the floor just long enough to drop his pants and remove his briefs. It was a relief to have his engorged member freed and he quickly turned to get back to Jenny and to the removal of her clothes. He was surprised to find her in a sitting position, her eyes at the same level as his penis. The sight of her naked breasts caused his erection to stiffen even more and he groaned with the surge of it.

Before David could reposition himself back on the sofa with her, Jenny wrapped her fingers around his penis and started moving her hand up and down on it. David placed his hands on her shoulders and allowed her to caress him for a few minutes, but he knew it would only be a few minutes before he would loose control and he was not going to loose this opportunity to claim her as his in favor of ejaculating all over her breasts. Although that idea had quite a bit of appeal, too.

He reached out and squeezed both breasts and then pulled on her nipples. She moaned and he reached his hand down and uncoiled her fingers from him. By his actions Jenny realized that he was not going to settle for a hand job and immediately took him into her mouth. His gasp of delight was the only sound in the room, save the ticking of the mantle clock.

Jenny pulled him towards her by putting her hands on his buttocks. She allowed him to fill her mouth and to hit the back of her throat as he repeatedly thrust into her and pulled back out. She hadn't done this since she'd been with R.J., but it wasn't something you ever forgot how to do, she just didn't remember how big these things were. She used all the tricks R.J. had taught her trying to get him to climax as soon as possible. When she reached down with one hand and lightly stroked his swaying balls while sucking on the head of his penis she knew she'd been successful in hurrying him along.

He suddenly lurched into her and he held her head against him as he pulsed several times, each time squirting a load of sperm to the back of her throat. She eased off of him careful to suck the tip so it wouldn't drip onto the carpet. Then, with her mouth full, she hurriedly ran to the kitchen sink and spit, rinsing her mouth several times. On the way back she took a swig of her tea that had been left on the counter. Even though it was now cold it tasted a lot better than the watery saltwater pudding that had just been there. Mentally she reminded herself to give the sink a good scrubbing tomorrow.

David was sitting on the sofa, his arms resting along the back, his shirt still on as well as his socks, his flaccid penis curled into the hairs that were his lap. He looked up at her and grinned, "Well, needless to say, you surprised the hell out of me! Where did you learn how to do that?"

Jenny reached down to retrieve her sweater and pulled it on. "It was something R.J. insisted he was entitled to while I was pregnant and recuperating. He was very specific in his coaching."

He reached up to her hand and pulled her down beside him. "I owe R.J. a very big thank you. You are incredible." He leaned over and kissed her on the temple. Just then Jenny heard a sound coming through the baby monitor that was over by the lamp. The extension was in Paisley's room.

She jumped up to go see what was wrong while David reached for his clothes to put himself back together. When Jenny reached Paisley's room, she was sitting up in bed looking at her. Jenny picked her up but could not maintain eye contact with her, she didn't want her to see the shame that was in her eyes. Jenny whispered, "Oh baby girl, I hope you never have to make these decisions in your life. You would be ashamed of me if you knew what I just did. I'm ashamed of me."

A small tear trickled down her face and Paisley reached up to touch it. Jenny took her downstairs and she and David played with her and fed her some juice until she was ready to go back to sleep again. Jenny's full concentration was on Paisley, as she couldn't quite bring herself to meet David's eyes.

When it was time for everyone to go to bed and for David to go home she and Paisley walked him to the door. As they stood in the foyer David hugged Paisley and then gave Jenny a long sensual kiss and a pat on her bottom. Jenny watched him walk to his car, bemoaning the fact that she now knew that he wasn't the one for her and that she'd done a very stupid thing tonight.

After putting Paisley back in her crib Jenny went back downstairs to turn off all the lights and to get some Scotch to swill around her mouth. When she walked past the reflection of herself in the hall mirror she saw a woman she didn't know. Upstairs in her bathroom she took a long shower and then got ready for bed. She finished brushing her teeth and looked at herself in the mirror over the sink. Her thoughts were all degrading ones.

She had betrayed herself by doing something despicable because it was coerced, not done out of love. She felt flushed and hot inside and then noticed a rash around her neck going down to her chest. Good God, was she allergic to David's semen? Or was this just a bad case of nerves? She hoped it would be gone by morning. She hoped this feeling would also be gone by morning.

She was so angry with herself because she knew better. She knew better than to lead a man on, especially when she had no desire to let him continue to his end. And now look what she'd done. She'd established a sexual relationship with David when she didn't want one. His kiss and pat on the bottom as he was leaving was a sure indication that he expected things to go on from here.

The next time they were together he would expect that they would be going to bed not watching videos or playing chess. He'd come right on in, grab her for another unfeeling kiss and whisk her upstairs for her to lay beneath him while he shoved himself into her over and over again.

Why had she been so stupid? Now she had cost herself one of the best friends she had. She felt dirty even though she'd just showered. Her behavior had been dishonorable to all women. She felt like she'd been a whore tonight only there was no money on her nightstand. She wondered how many women over the years had compromised themselves as she had tonight. It was little comfort to her to know that probably hundreds of thousands had back in the times that maiden heads were a defining point in a woman's life.

She tried to imagine how differently she would have felt if she'd just let him take her the traditional way and of course, she felt a little bit better. And of course, she wasn't pregnant. Damn! She could have avoided everything if she had just remembered to use that excuse to end everything! Although with her luck he'd probably been prepared with a few condoms. Oh My God! She could have AIDS from what she'd done tonight! She put her face in her hands and started crying. How could I have been so stupid? She walked over to the nightstand and downed the scotch, shivered and crawled into bed.

Chapter 43

Fairfax, VA

David couldn't remember a time when he had enjoyed driving his Trans Am as much as he did tonight. As he drove home from Jenny's he enjoyed the absence of traffic and he found himself taking the long way so he could enjoy the car's superb handling on the winding country roads. It had been an almost perfect day. He was still elated over Donna Bristol's session and he was absolutely euphoric after his lovemaking with Jenny.

Well, it wasn't exactly lovemaking, but it certainly had been quite wonderful. And for the second time his semen had become a part of her. She was truly amazing, who would have thought she was so skilled in the art of oral sex? Somehow it had never even occurred to him that she would do that kind of thing.

This was truly a bonus he hadn't counted on. He was more than anxious now to make her his permanently. He wanted to be Jenny's husband, the recipient of all the sexual prowess he had just discovered in her and he also wanted to be Paisley's father in name and actuality. With the advent of tonight's consummation, so to speak, he was much further along in his quest for both. Now he just had to get the financial aspects of his life in line.

He wanted to give Jenny and Paisley all the things they deserved. He wanted Paisley to have all the advantages he'd never had. He wanted her to have a house in the country with stables for the horses she would learn to ride. He wanted her to go to the best private schools in Northern Virginia and he wanted her to go to any college she chose, not one the state would mandate for her as they had for him. He wanted to be there for all her special accomplishments, being supportive and proud, something he had never enjoyed no matter what he had achieved.

He wanted Jenny and Paisley to be the family he had never had. He would try to develop a better relationship with Rusty as he was part of the package in the whole family deal. Maybe later he and Jenny could even have another child together, conceived in the more conventional manner this time.

Driving on the moonlit country roads he eased the car around the turns as he recalled the last hour spent with Jenny. If this was a sampling of the connubial bliss he had to look forward to he would be a happy husband indeed. Although they hadn't technically made love together he felt sure that would happen the next time they were together. After all, a woman who went down on a man certainly wouldn't be squeamish with any other aspects of sex. It would be his turn to grant her some of the pleasure she had given him.

He wondered if she was multi-orgasmic as he pulled into the parking garage of his apartment building. He was deliriously happy that he was going to be finding that out real soon. A thought crossed his mind. Maybe she hadn't been as sexually inactive these past few years as he had been led to believe. Or maybe she was capable of self-pleasuring. All of a sudden he had some questions he hadn't had before and he was bothered by them. More than ever he was determined to stake his claim to her and her body before somebody else came along.

Upon entering the elevator he remembered that he hadn't collected his mail for a few days, so he went to the lobby and opened his mailbox. There was quite a bundle waiting for him and he browsed through it as he made his way to his apartment. Dumping it all on the desk in his study he removed his jacket and sat down. After sorting through it he piled the bills one on top of the other. There was almost $25,000 on just three credit card bills.

Each month he was getting more and more in debt. Soon it would be difficult to make the minimum payments on everything. What had turned out to be an almost perfect day was quickly deteriorating into a nightmare. What was he going to do about making more money? He could do a few lectures but that would require travel expenses and time away from Jenny. He could write another book, but that would take the better part of two years and again, time away from Jenny.

So far he had *suggested* contributions from eight patients but so far none were cooperating by dying. Since reading the obituaries had become a part of his morning routine he had to assume than none of his patients had succumbed, but of course none of them were on death's door either. The check for $19,733.40 from Mrs. Cheney's estate had been the last monies to go into his coffers. He needed more money and he needed it sooner than they were providing it.

He began to think about what he could do to speed things up a bit. He went to the kitchen and filled a brandy snifter with some Grand Marnier and took it with him to his bedroom. The Master suite. And what was he the Master of? Where was his mistress? He stared at the large empty bed. He ached to feel the warm body of Jenny lying naked beside him on this bed. Soon. He would have her here soon.

The next morning as he was eating his bagel and sipping his coffee he read the Saturday Washington Post. After checking out the Sports section he turned to the Style section to out check the obituaries. As he turned the page he was surprised when he recognized a woman's photograph. The picture was of a younger version of one of his patients.

Nancy Meridan had finally gone to join her maker! He almost couldn't believe his good fortune! What wonderful timing this was. He scanned the article to see if he could glean a few details about her death. She had died on Thursday and there was a request from the family for donations to the American Cancer Society in lieu of flowers. That was a little odd.

He would have thought she would have preferred the Christian Science Church to be designated to receive memorial funds. The viewing was yesterday and the service was today at St. Catherine's of Sienna in Great Falls. That was very odd. St. Catherine's was a Catholic Church. He had attended a few weddings there over the years so he was absolutely positive about that. Nancy had been a Christian Scientist for many years.

He decided to go to the service and see what was up. After all, he had a stake in the disposition of her finances, if all went as planned.

He sat in the back of the church acknowledging Nancy's children with a slight nod of his head. During the very long service the Christian Science Church was never mentioned by anyone who came up to eulogize her. He thought he recognized a few church members from his visits to the house at the cemetery an hour later, but he couldn't be sure. But whoever they were, the family wasn't recognizing them at all.

Later at Nancy's house, he noticed things had been rearranged downstairs to resemble a traditional parlor and dining room instead of the meeting rooms and offices he had seen when he was there before. He had an uneasy feeling about all this and approached Nancy's daughter, Carol to offer his condolences.

"I was so very sorry to read about your mother's passing in this morning's newspaper. She was one of my favorite patients."

Carol wiped at her eyes with a tissue and took his hand in hers, "Thank you so much for coming on such short notice, even though it's been expected for quite sometime we're all still in a state of shock."

"Speaking of shock," he said, "I was surprised it was to be a Catholic service. Wasn't she a pretty devote Christian Scientist?"

Carol's face became stern and her lips tightened, "Oh, them. We just kind of humored her the last few years as those leaches grabbed onto her, waiting for her to die and leave all her money to them. If it hadn't been for them, she'd still be alive you know."

He was stunned by her vehemence. "I thought the whole family were believers and had been for years."

Carol leaned in conspiratorially, "Nah, we just pretended to be for Mama's sake. It made her happy, that was all that mattered."

David blinked in confusion. "I guess that makes her donation of this house to them hard for you to deal with."

"Oh, no!" she whispered. "They're not getting anything! My brothers and sisters and I are contesting everything! If they ever do end up with anything it'll be at least five years down the road and it won't be much. We're going to fight them until there's no money left to do it with! They killed our Mama, just as sure as if they'd put a gun to her. She wasn't even sixty years old yet. They don't deserve anything!"

David fought to hold back his anger, "Well, surely she left money to other people and her family, what about them?"

"Oh, all that was taken care of last year. All our money was put in trusts and gifted over to us. We'll be fine while the lawyers duke it out over the rest. We really don't care about the money, we just don't want them to have it."

David bit his tongue. These niggardly people were going to keep him from getting his part of her will and there wasn't a damned thing he could do about it. Hell, he didn't even have the satisfaction of even knowing if it had been changed for him!

On the off chance that she would see his name mentioned in it whenever it was read, he didn't want her to remember him badly so he feigned commiseration and wished them well and left. It was with a very sad countenance that he walked to his car and drove home. After changing his clothes he picked up the phone and called Jenny at work. She was with a customer and unavailable to come to the phone, so he left a message. He walked by his study on the way out the door and his eyes fell on the neatly stacked pile of bills. His insides wrenched with the realization that if he didn't do something soon, all would be lost.

Chapter 44

Washington.D.C.

Betsy Drayton was getting ready for her appointment with Dr. David, as she called him. She always looked forward to her sessions with him, he was so handsome and he was such a gentleman. She had met him a year and a half ago when she was referred to him by her endocrinologist. She had been in and out of so many doctor's offices in the last five years that she had been practically ready to give up on the idea of ever losing any weight. Then she met Dr. David. He was her savior, of sorts.

She was obese by anyone's definition of the word, in fact most of her medical charts that she had stolen a glance or two at had the words "grossly obese" in the first sentence or two. She had been 320 lbs. when she had first started seeing Dr. David and now she was under 250 with hopes of being under 200 by Christmas time.

It was absolutely amazing to her that he had been able to accomplish what endless dieting, liposuction and stomach stapling had not and in such a short period of time. Remarkable too, was the fact that she was not hungry all the time and her compulsive eating was a thing of the past, and almost effortlessly on her part. The man was a magician.

Six years ago Betsy had won 16 million dollars in the Maryland State Lottery. She had been 26 at the time, struggling to finish college at the University of Maryland while working part time as a cashier for Giant Food. As she rang up her customers' purchases she took note of the new items that appealed to her and when her shift ended she grabbed a cart and went looking for them. Then she went home to watch TV or to study with her new arsenal of test foods. Her back was just beginning to give her real fits of intensive pain from all the standing when she discovered she had the winning lottery ticket, so she took a year off from everything. Except eating.

She had no real friends either at work or at school and her dysfunctional family was back in Nebraska, oblivious to her new-found fortune. Both her parents had beaten her until the state stepped in and took her away at the age of six. She'd been in a different foster home almost every three months until she was sixteen, when she ran away to be on her own. She ended up in College Park, Maryland at the University of Maryland because she'd overheard some teenagers say that's where they wanted to go after high school.

She was fat and ugly, at least that's what all the kids at school used to say, but she was smart. While working as a bagger she got her GED and then enrolled in college, starting out just taking classes part-time. She found a room to rent on campus and was able to take a bus to and from work and school. When she turned eighteen she was promoted to cashier and added a few more classes until she was going to school full-time, working part-time and eating all the time.

After her one-year sabbatical she took stock of herself and didn't like what she saw. She now had the money to do practically anything she could imagine, but everything she imagined involved a prettier, slimmer Betsy. She had dreams of being on a cruise ship being escorted around the deck arm-in-arm by a handsome man. She dreamed about skiing down the slopes of a Swiss mountain and later relaxing in the lodge being entertained by a handsome man. She dreamed about riding horses in Montana and sitting by a campfire at night next to a handsome man.

She could do all these things, but where to get the handsome man? She knew that handsome men wanted beautiful women, not fat, ugly, rich ones. So she decided to use her money to become the best woman she could be.

She spent months at expensive body spas, which did improve her skin and she lost a little weight, but only temporarily. Over the next few years she had her teeth done. She had her nose fixed. She had her hair done. She had liposuction, her stomach stapled, her blood changed. She tried numerous diets and fads, bought every new work out tape, took aerobic and yoga classes, and anything else she read about, that she thought would work, she tried. So far no handsome man had ever looked at her twice. But now there was hope. Things were really happening now.

The hypnotherapy Dr. David was using was curbing her appetite and making her actually enjoy exercise. She worked herself up to walking five miles a day. She could probably walk ten, but she found that after five the constant rubbing of her thighs together caused painful chaffing, but even that was getting better all the time.

As soon as she reached her target weight of 150 pounds she was going to book passage on a cruise ship and find that handsome man she had been dreaming about. She might not be beautiful by then, but at least she'd be pretty, slim and very rich. There had to be a handsome man somewhere who would appreciate those attributes.

She strapped her fanny pack around her waist and walked down ten flights of stairs before getting the elevator to go down the remaining floors to the lobby of her apartment building on Wisconsin Avenue in Northwest Washington, D.C. When she walked through the revolving doors the doorman signaled her driver to pull up for her. He drove her to Fairfax, letting her off to walk the last five miles to Dr. Sandler's office.

By the time Betsy arrived at his office she was usually pretty winded and very tired. After drinking some water and eating a piece of fruit she would settle onto one of the sofas as the chaise was a bit too delicate for her cumbersome form. She had hopes of one day being able to use one airline seat instead of two, not needing a seat belt extension and reclining on Dr. David's chaise.

As far as she was concerned that day was in the foreseeable future due to these sessions. While she would rest and float in and out of drowsiness David would structure a daydream for her. He would take her to her favorite places with his soft droning voice. Today he mentally rowed her out to the middle of a beautiful Vermont lake, somewhere north of Rutland.

He was deliberately slow in his descriptions of everything and painstakingly real in his detail of the scene. So there she was in the middle of this serene lake on a warm summer's day. Exhausted as she was from the efforts of rowing, she was sleepy and totally relaxed. He was effluent in his praise of her, repeating over and over how very proud he was of her.

He spoke of a cabin not far away where a man on a high deck was focusing in on her through his binoculars. "He watches you every day. He thinks that you are beautiful and he can't wait for the day to come when he will be allowed to meet you. For now he's satisfied with gazing at you from afar but soon that won't be enough for him. He will have to walk out to his pier, untie his kayak and paddle out to where you are. You must get ready for him. You must be the best you can be for him."

As he tells her that she loves salad, that she can't get enough of it, he moves over to the fanny pack that she threw on the opposite sofa. As he carefully unzips it he tells her, "You love carrots and broccoli and cauliflower."

He takes out her prescription bottle and opens it. "Twinkies, ice cream and cookies are not for you. They make you gag with their sweetness." He takes a pill from his jacket pocket and adds it to hers and replaces the cap.

"Chips and bread and pasta turn sour in your mouth. You mustn't swallow them, they turn rancid inside you."

He replaces the bottle and zips up her fanny pack. "You see a sudden glint caused by the sun reflecting off of his binoculars. You raise your hand to shield your eyes and make out his form. He is so tall and so muscular looking. You wave and then turn your boat around to head back to your dock. Maybe by tomorrow you'll be ready."

He lets her rest for awhile longer, knowing that these sessions are exhausting for her. Her emotions get so worked up and her heart gets to racing like a catamaran on the ocean. When she opens her eyes, he is sitting at his desk making some notes.

He looks up and smiles at her. He always makes sure he smiles at her with a hungry look in his eyes. It's important that she think he finds her desirable. Otherwise she'll never believe anybody else will.

As Betsy prepares to leave he looks down at her chart and asks her how her allergies are affecting her this season. Betsy is allergic to many things. It's the reason she's always had so much trouble with her skin. Most things just cause her discomfort in the form of rashes or hives, like tuna, eggs or shellfish. But some things are deadly to her, like penicillin, bee stings or nuts.

She jiggles her fanny pack to indicate the contents inside and says, "As long as I have my medicine everything's fine. Thank God I live in this century. I would have died awfully young had I lived in the last one!"

"See you next week," he said as he watched her attach her fanny pack to her hips. He wondered where she had been able to find one with such long straps. Inside it was her medication to control her allergies along with one identical capsule that had been emptied and refilled with ground up peanuts.

Chapter 45

Fairfax, VA

It was lunchtime, and while David waited for the deli across the street to deliver his lunch, he called Jenny at work. He hadn't spoken to her since Sunday night. He had wanted to see her Saturday night after she got off from work. It ended up that she had a late delivery and didn't get home until close to ten. She had called to tell him that she was just too tired to do anything but go to sleep.

On Sunday evening she had already planned to have dinner at her parent's house with her brother and sister. Monday she was working late again and Tuesday a group of her friends were getting together from work to go to the movies.

He was beginning to wonder when he would ever see her again.

She was actually trying to avoid him without being too obvious. She needed some time to sort out her feelings. She didn't love David, but she liked him a lot. He was practically her best friend and she didn't know how to deal with all this without losing that friendship.

If she had any sense she'd forget about her emotions and this damned chemistry thing and snatch him up. He was a good catch, such a gentleman, and so nice. He was handsome in a Gordon McRae kind of way and smart, heck he rivaled her in jeopardy responses and was quite the chess challenger. He loved the kids and they just adored him. And he was a doctor! What more was she looking for? Just the spark that made it all work, that's all. Just an itsy bitsy tiny spark.

When she finally picked up the line, he breathed a long sigh, "Well, it's so nice to hear your voice again, I was beginning to forget what you sounded like."

"I'm sorry David, it's just been very hectic around here. This is our busy season, you know."

221

"Yes, I know." he replied.

"Any chance you'll be free tonight?" he asked.

"I had to switch with one of the guys. I've got to work tonight and tomorrow night, but I'm off Friday night."

He didn't like this one bit but he didn't say anything except, "Friday night it is. What do you want to do?"

Normally Jenny would just turn it back around to him but she already had a hunch she knew what he wanted to do. So instead she said, "I can get some tickets to Wolftrap if you want. I think John Denver's playing."

He thought for a minute and then said, "It sounds like you're having a rough week. Maybe it would be better if we just stayed home and had some pizza and watched a movie." She knew it! Great. Now what?

"Okay. That'll be fine," she said with little enthusiasm.

He said "I'll call you Friday to see what time, meanwhile try to get some rest, you sound tired."

"David, we need to talk..." she started.

"We'll talk on Friday. I've got someone at the office door." She turned the phone in her hand and looked at it as if she'd never seen one before. He'd hung up on her!

After lunch David met with Jessica Tyler. She hadn't been arrested lately and none of her exploits had been featured in the style section so he didn't know what she'd been up to this week. But he was sure it wasn't good. He was having a real hard time trying to help her and he didn't know if it was because he couldn't find the right technique or if it was because she truly didn't want his help.

He had cured her of the shoplifting, but now she was drinking. He had raised her self esteem and convinced her she wasn't the ugliest woman on the planet after her husband had dumped her for a ditzy socialite and now she was granting her favors to any man who winked at her. Her depression was the key here and he was more than a little curious to see how she was responding to the medication he had prescribed for her.

When she came into his office he noticed right away that her condescending attitude was back as she sneered at his receptionist for not buzzing her through right away. That was a good sign. She was back to thinking she was better than anyone else instead of believing she was pond scum. In his line of work it wasn't as important to escalate his patient to a decent level of humanity as it was to return them to the person that they were before they had the need for therapy. In Jessica's case that meant that if he could get her back to being vain, conceited, arrogant and selfish then he was a success.

"That woman is so annoying!" she grumbled as she pranced into his office and plopped herself down on one of the large overstuffed couches.

He knew if he told her that less than an hour ago there was a fat sweaty woman laying there that she would jump up and scream as if it were covered with spiders. A smile twitched at the corners of his lips. "Come, come Jessica. What did she do to you this time?"

"She keeps asking me what my name is. Lord, doesn't that woman ever read the newspaper?"

"You're just famous to the gentry, not the everyday working schmoo. And how are you feeling today? You look incredibly breathtaking, if you don't mind my saying so."

She flashed him a big smile and made an exaggerated gesture of crossing one leg over the other, letting the heel of her stiletto pump slip off of her foot. She gently flexed her ankle up and down causing the shoe to dangle from her toes enticingly.

"What's your week been like? Good?" he asked. She proceeded to catalog her conquests while he watched her eyes trying to discern the truth.

"Yessss," she hissed at him and then excitedly told him about this new drink she had discovered at one of the local bars. Something called a Fuzzy Navel: Peach Schnapps, Orange Juice and lots of vodka. When he drolly replied that he was reassured that she was at least getting her vitamin C, she laughed hysterically.

Try as he might he couldn't get a glimmer of an idea for relaxing her so he opted for a more traditional approach. "Jessica, can you find something in this room that pleases you that you can focus on for a few minutes?"

She got up and walked around, looking at the pictures on the wall, the clock on his desk, an oriental lamp on an end table. She stopped in front of a big flower arrangement on the coffee table in front of the other sofa.

Her hesitation caused him to ask, "Do you like flowers?"

"No, not really," she replied, "not unless somebody's sending me some and then I never know what to do with them. But my mother liked flowers. She was always working in the gardens."

"Would you like to talk to me about your mother?"

She turned and looked him right in the eyes, almost defiantly and then dropped her eyes to the carpet and said, "Yes, I think I would."

That was the beginning of his breakthrough with her. They talked for the next two hours. If he'd had a scheduled appointment after hers, he would have been tempted to still continue on with her. This was that important. He had discovered a little girl still looking for her Mommy, who used to put buttercups under her chin to see if she liked butter.

Gwendolyn Tyler died in a car crash when Jessica was eight years old and as life hadn't been fair then, why should it be fair now? Jessica was punishing herself because her mother had left her. A nagging thought kept occurring to David. Was Jessica just a little too anxious to go find Mommy again?

Nothing in this life was making her happy. Maybe she thought joining her life with her mother's would be better. At least he had some background now for their next session. He was finally getting somewhere with her now and his professional pride soared. Again he'd found the key. Everyone had a key.

Chapter 46

Herndon, VA

Friday evening came too soon for Jenny and not soon enough for David. Every night when David went to bed he envisioned Jenny there beside him gently stroking his chest and murmuring sexy things to him. He also pictured Paisley joining them in the mornings all rumpled and sleepy-eyed looking for a warm body to snuggle up to.

Jenny had given much thought to what she was going to say to David tonight and she dreaded the whole idea of it. She knew they couldn't go back to where they'd been but she couldn't go forward, either. Why couldn't she fall in love with him? Then things would be perfect.

They ordered a pizza and when it arrived they took it and some wine and soda to the park just around the corner. The kids each ate one piece before the temptation of the slide and the jungle gym got the better of them. While Jenny kept her eye on the kids she noticed the other families clustered around.

Since it was the start of the weekend practically every child was attended by both a mother and a father. They all looked so happy to be spending time together. One particular husband who was still in his business suit when he arrived at the park, spotted his wife and daughter and headed over towards them. When the wife saw him coming she apparently said something to the little girl on the swing because she turned quickly, glowed with a great big smile and jumped off the swing to run to him. He scooped her up in one arm and nuzzled her neck never missing a step in his quest towards his wife. When he reached her he greeted her with a peck on the lips and whispered something in her ear that caused her to laugh musically. Then he rubbed her slightly rounded belly and gave it a pat.

David, watching Jenny, and seeing her wistful expression said, "It can be like that for us, if you'll let it." Jenny, awakened from her reverie, turned to look at him.

"Marry me Jenny. Let me come home to you and our children every night." Jenny just smiled. God, he made it all sound so simple.

"You know that I'm in love with you, I would do anything for you Jenny. You and the kids are my whole world."

Oh, no! she thought, when had it gone so far?

"David, I can't, I'm not in love with you." There she'd said it. She scanned his face for his reaction.

He smiled and tenderly touched her hand, "I know I've had a head start on you, but you'll catch up. You'll come to love me, you'll see."

Just then Jenny saw Paisley from the corner of her eye, getting ready to walk right into the path of an empty swing that a little boy had just jumped out of. She jumped up to get to her but David had already grabbed her and pulled her out of harm's way. Well, just maybe she could fall in love with this superman, given enough time. She took Paisley from David. She was crying now because he had scared her when he grabbed her so suddenly. She rocked her in her arms and smiled at David.

David carried Paisley back to the house on his shoulders and Jenny helped Rusty walk his bike back. He had scraped his knee falling off the jungle gym and said it hurt to bend it. They both worked to get the kids bathed and ready for bed and then David read them a story while Jenny cleaned the bathroom. When they were both down for the night Jenny went to the kitchen and got a glass of water and made a big deal out of taking three Tylenol.

"You can't have a headache, we're not even married yet," David said as he smiled at her.

"I don't have a headache. I have cramps."

"Oh," he said. After a moment of silence he asked, "Are the cramps very bad?"

"No," she answered "not terribly. The back ache I get is actually more bothersome. But I'm pretty stoic, I've never used it as an excuse to slow down any."

He took her by the hand and led her over to the sofa. "Lie down," he said simply.

Great, she thought, he would be the type who wouldn't care about the timeliness of a woman's cycle, although that seemed extremely out of character for him. He was usually very fastidious about staying clean. To top it all off, now he'd also find out she was lying to him. Her period was still a week and a half away. Before she could formulate a way in her mind to ease into a conversation about their physical relationship, he gently pushed her down and flipped her over onto her stomach. Then he straddled her hips with his thighs and began massaging her lower back. His fingers were strong and capable.

He massaged her through her shirt for awhile and then pulled it out of her jeans and raised it up to her shoulders. He undid the back clasp on her bra and moved it out of the way. He was then free to massage her whole back, which he did as expertly as if he was a Swedish masseur. It felt wonderful. How could you not love the man? His attentions to her back and shoulders were causing her to relax and sink into the sofa as if she was reclining on a soft spongy cloud. Before she knew it she was barely conscious, drifting on a puffy marshmallow raft.

David hadn't meant to put her into a hypnotic state, it had just happened. But he knew the minute she had succumbed to it though, as her muscles lost some their tense definition. While he gently kneaded them between his hands, her breathing became very regular and shallow. Normally he would have just let her fall into a deep slumber. She certainly could use the rest. But he saw this as an opportunity to try to secure her feelings for him.

Softly, he leaned over and whispered into her ear, testing her state of relaxation as well as suggesting an emotion to her. "Love me, Jenny. I need you to love me. You know you already do, just let it happen. Let us both have what we've always wanted. We can be a loving couple raising happy kids together. You know

I'm devoted to you and the kids and I know I can make you very happy, if you'll just let me. You love me Jenny. You already know you do. Admit it to yourself. You find me very desirable and it's time you let down your guard and let your body love me as well as your mind. It's meant to be, you and me. I am the man you've been waiting for. Stop resisting it. Let yourself fall deeply in love with me."

He sat back up and drew soft circles all around her back and shoulders, crooning softly about how much she loved him, how much she needed him and how much she was attracted to him. Then he moved off of her and pulled her shirt down to cover her. He also covered her with the Afghan Jenny always kept on the arm of the sofa. He kissed her softly on the cheek and then let himself out using the front door, pushing in the button on the door knob to lock it as he closed it behind him.

When Jenny awoke several hours later she was confused about why she was asleep on her sofa in the family room instead of on her bed. Then she remembered David had been rubbing her back for her. Sweet, wonderful David. She must have fallen asleep. With his incredible massage technique she didn't wonder why. She looked up at the clock on the mantle. Two thirty in the morning. She supposed he had left and gone home.

She felt a strange twinge of remorse, a kind of an empty feeling. Was she missing him? She got up to go upstairs to her room and felt her bra loose under her shirt. Gosh, she hoped she hadn't slept through a frontal massage! The thought caused a feeling of sexual anticipation between her thighs. Was her body warming up to him after all?

She locked the deadbolt on the front door, noting that the bottom lock was already pushed in and went up to check on the kids. After assuring herself that they were fine she walked to her room removing her clothes as she went. She slipped between the covers naked. Something she rarely did. As she closed her eyes and felt the heaviness of her head on the pillow she also felt her body reaching out for something or someone. It would be nice to have someone hold her close at night.

Chapter 47

Fairfax, VA

Shawn Vanscoy was Dr. Sandler's least favorite patient. He was a spoiled arrogant brat as far as Dr. Sandler was concerned. His father was a well-known Hollywood actor, who would have disowned him years ago, except for the negative publicity it would have caused. So for the last four years his father had gritted his teeth while he paid for Shawn's rent, car payment and drug treatment programs.

After failing at several drug rehab centers Shawn had been referred to Dr. David Sandler by one of his father's producers. Having him see a hypnotherapist was going to be Shawn's father's last bid for getting his son straightened out. After that he couldn't care less what the press said about him. He'd show them the receipts for all the bills he paid for Shawn, which lately seemed to also include the support of his latest partner, Jeremy.

Shawn was slowly killing his body. One look at him and it was evident that he lived the life of a druggie. His eyes were listless and sunken into the sockets. His skin was pasty white except where it was black and blue and faded yellow from the stick marks on his arms and neck. Rarely did he put together a completely coherent sentence and even more rarely were the times that he combed his hair.

As he came striding into David's office with his "man's bag" tossed over his shoulder he nearly tripped as his foot caught on the leg of the coffee table on his way to the sofa. "Whoa!" he yelped as he recovered enough to fall onto the sofa. With a loud *thwack* his body hit the leather and bounced once before he was able to gain a sitting position. He looked over at Dr. Sandler sitting behind his desk with a cocky smile as if his entrance had been part of his grand plan.

"Yo, Doc! What's shakin'?" he asked.

"Shawn, you are definitely a sight of sore eyes," he said smiling at his own twist on the play of words. "What have you been doing to yourself?" David asked him.

Shawn just replied, "Anything I can get my hands on. You got any good stuff I can get carry-out like?"

"Shawn, I've told you before, I can't give you anything. You have to go to the clinic and get methadone injections. It will help you a lot if you can just get over there and do it."

Shawn put his feet up on the coffee table and David glared at him until he put them down on the floor again. "I don't understand why I just can't inject myself, I have been injecting myself for years. I want to do the treatment but I don't want to go to the clinic. Everybody recognizes me there and I don't like it." Well, he had a point, his face was very familiar due to the tabloids.

"If I can arrange a way, how would I know that you're not selling it on the street or trading it for something else?" Dr. Sandler asked.

"You don't, unless we do it here. But you gotta know that this is my last way out. Dad's not paying when the lease is up again. He canceled all his charge accounts in my name. If I'm not clean by your say so in four months, Jeremy and I will be living on the street. So what have you got to loose, except a patient?" Shawn said matter-of-factly.

What indeed? Thought David. It wouldn't actually bother him any if he did loose this one. After most of his sessions with Shawn he found himself regretting that he had even taken this referral. He hadn't accomplished a single thing in his treatment with him. Still, if Shawn was going to kill himself, he should at least be able to profit from it somehow. An idea came to him and he didn't even think it all the way through before he acted on it.

"I'll tell you what," David said, "I'll give you your Methadone treatments to take home when you come here each week. But I want something in return."

"Yeah, what's that?" Shawn asked.

"I want you to name me the beneficiary on your life insurance policy." He tried to say it in a joking way by adding, "Because if I let you do it yourself, some life insurance company is going to be paying up real soon."

"Oh, yeah, we'll see about that! You got yourself a deal!" Shawn said enthusiastically.

He stood up and reached his hand over the desk. David met his eyes then looked at his outstretched hand. He took it in his and shook it briefly. Shawn continued, "You get me the Meth and I'll come pick it up. I'll take care of that insurance thing and get you a copy of it. But New York Life won't be paying off, I'm going to do it this time. I swear it. Jeremy and I are going to have a good long life together, you'll see."

"Okay," Dr.Sandler said, "you've talked me into it." Hoping that Shawn really saw it as being that way. "You've got to agree to one more thing though."

"What's that?" Shawn said, in a way that suggested he knew the deal was too good to be true. He knew there'd be a catch.

"You can't tell anyone. Not even Jeremy. What I'm doing isn't exactly legal or ethical you know. I'm not supposed to be providing you with drugs. Not even methadone. It's only supposed to be dispensed at a clinic where you can be monitored."

"Yeah, I know. No problem. No one'll know. Scout's honor," and he put up three fingers with the other two joined beneath.

The following week when Shawn showed up for his session he still stumbled against the coffee table, but twisting on his way down to the sofa he managed to toss an envelope onto David's desk. David picked it up and looked at the return address. New York Life Insurance Company, New York, N.Y. He took out the single piece of paper and saw his name listed as the new beneficiary to Shawn's $350,000 life insurance policy. Oh, this had been too easy.

"You know I was just kidding about this," he said to Shawn as he put the letter back in the envelope and handed it back to him.

"Yeah, well I wanted you to know I was serious about this," Shawn said. "Just keep it. No one else knows about it anyway. One day I'll die and if you're still around keeping me straight, you can buy yourself a Lamborghini."

"Okay, maybe I'll just do that," David opened his top desk drawer and put it inside then he took out a small box of pre-filled syringes and handed them over to Shawn.

After being assured that Shawn knew more about how to use them than he did, he sat back and watched as Shawn took them out of the box and put them into his shoulder bag. "So," he joked with Shawn, "you ever had a yen to try skydiving or bungie jumping?"

Shawn turned and smirked at him, "No, I like whittlin' and playing the piccolo! You'll be an old man before you get to drive that car, that I promise you!"

They had the best session they'd ever had and then Shawn went home to start his treatments, despite Dr. Sandler's belief otherwise.

Chapter 48

Fairfax, VA

Liesel... His favorite. She was beautiful and spunky. She reminded him of Jenny a little, except where she was tall, Jenny was petite. She was brunette, Jenny was blonde. Exactly what was it about her that reminded him of Jenny, anyway? He couldn't put his finger on it. Must be just the way they lived their lives. Unpretentious, naive and gullible as hell.

Liesel was really coming along well in their sessions. At first she had terrific problems dealing with her feelings of guilt. Guilt dealing with the fact that she wasn't prosecuting and incredible, wracking guilt over getting pleasure from some of the revolting things Jake had done to her. Her body had betrayed her and she was having a hard time coming to terms with that. And she was even having nightmares about other women becoming Jake's victims and other ones where he recaptured her. Dr. Sandler didn't feel that he had been instrumental in Liesel's overcoming any of her doubts or anxieties, unless just talking about them had eased them until they didn't seem to bother her as much any more. There was really not much more that therapy could do for her, but he was a little reluctant to end it with her. She was the high point in his day. Another Wednesday patient. He saved Wednesday for all his special patients, the ones that really challenged him.

When Liesel came in she was bouncy and all smiles. As she placed her handbag on the coffee table and gracefully settled herself onto the couch she smiled at him. "Wait til I tell you what's been going on. You won't believe it!"

He smiled over at her and said, "Okay, the floor is yours. Dazzle me!"

"Well," she started, "you know that Daniel, the man who rescued me, comes to visit every month or so, right?" When he nodded she continued, "Well, he fills me in on what's going on with the men at the mill and what they're doing to Jake. They keep chiding him about "Anna" and giving him a hard time like he's nuts or something. So Daniel sneaks into his cabin every once in awhile and leaves something there that had special relevance to him about me. Things that were mine, like pieces of the shredded jeans I wore when I was there, my shoes, my socks, my camera bag and such."

"Daniel thinks Jake is going out of his mind now, because no one believes him. They all keep telling him that he's crazy, and then he comes home to find something that wasn't there when he left that morning. He thinks "Anna" is haunting him!" she chuckled as she shook her head.

This retribution was doing wonders for her. He had to hand it to Daniel, he knew her well. A spark of jealousy flared for a moment but then he remembered that he had Jenny. Daniel could have Liesel. Apparently he already did.

"Daniel sounds like a wonderful man," he said.

She dreamily replied, "Yes, he is."

"How often is Daniel visiting these days?" he asked.

"He tries to get here at least once a month. The flight is so long that it takes up almost all his time off just for the travel part of the trip. We talk every night though and you wouldn't believe the cards that we send back and forth. I get at least four a week."

"And how are things going physically for the two of you?" he asked.

She sat back against the sofa and rested her head on the cushion, she closed her eyes and a smile crossed her lips as she replied. "Quite nicely, actually. I know you have been very concerned about how I would adjust to the physical part of a relationship after what happened to me, but it's really going a lot better than I would have imagined possible. Daniel is very gentle and extremely patient with me. Even though we haven't done much more than some pretty heavy petting, it's really not because of me. He wants the moment to be perfect and he says that once he gets me into his bed he's not letting me leave for at least a week. He's planning a trip for us at the end of next month.

He won't tell me where yet. He just told me to shop for a new bathing suit."

"Are the nightmares still a problem?" he asked when she stopped reminiscing about Daniel.

"I only have them every once in awhile now and they're not as bad as they were. I think just knowing that Daniel is keeping an eye on Jake and making sure he doesn't victimize anyone else has eased my mind a little."

"Still happy with your decision not to press charges?" he asked.

"No, I'm not happy about it. I'll never be happy about it. But, I can't put my parents through it and I think Daniel would sooner kill Jake before he would let me be in the same room with him, even if it was only a courtroom. He knows what it would do to me. I just want to forget about it the best way I can, which is to go on with my life as if it never even happened."

"Isn't that a bit hard to do, given Daniel's prominence in your life now?" he queried.

She looked at the ceiling and replied, "Sometimes. It's hard not to remember the way we met. Especially since he keeps telling everybody that it was love at first sight! God! I hope nobody ever finds out what he really means when he says that!"

"Have you ever thought about asking him not to say that since it bothers you?" David asked her.

She softly replied, "I'm sure he doesn't mean any harm by it. It's just a private joke between us. Only it's not so funny sometimes."

David nodded his head in agreement, "Well, you should tell him that. What else is making it hard for you forget?"

"Oh, lots of little things come up on a day-to-day basis. Things that you wouldn't even look at twice, now make me stop what I'm doing and just stare."

"What kind of things?" he asked.

She closed her eyes and thought about the things that had upset her lately. "Like a picture of a rustic cabin in a magazine, a Styrofoam food container, my camera. That's a biggie. My camera. I reach for it at least thirty times a day and each time I'm reminded of when he..." She stopped. He knew the whole story, she didn't have to continue.

She liked talking to him. He made it easy. Nothing seemed to shock or provoke him. He was sympathetic but not morose and he always knew just what to do to relieve her guilty conscious. He had completely arrested the problems she had dealing with the shame and humiliation. They were in the box.

"Do you want to put those things in the box?" he asked simply.

"Can we?" she asked. "What happens if I need them and they're in the box?"

"Nothing. Just because they're in the box doesn't mean they're inaccessible to you. It just means your bad feelings about them are in the box. Your camera will still have all the good memories attached to it and you'll be able to eat from a fast food container just as you did before. Only now you just won't cringe with loathing. Go to your place in front of the box. I'll meet you there," he said.

Her place. That was how she had dealt with all this. Going to her place. She removed her shoes and tucked her feet up under her and then she slumped back into the deep cushions of the couch. She closed her eyes and breathed deeply.

Chapter 49

Fairfax, VA

Dr. Sandler discovered Liesel's phenomenal ability to visualize during one of their earlier sessions when she was relating her ordeal to him. He happened to ask her how she managed to spend all that time alone, confined as she was, without any distractions for hours on end. For a lot of active people that would have been almost as harrowing as what Jake had put her through.

She told him that she had played so many games of scrabble that she'd probably never play it ever again and that twice she had played golf with her father. When he hadn't understood what she meant he asked her to elaborate for him. She explained that she was able to visualize the scrabble board with all its pink and blue squares for extra points, as well as all the words as they were played in turn.

She was actually able to keep track of the number of tiles played in each letter category in addition to the myriad arrangement of the words on the board, all in her head. The way she randomly selected letters to make words came from a progression of numbers she predetermined before the game. Each number correlating to a letter and each time she used a vowel she was allowed to replace it with the next vowel in the a-e-i-o-u sequence.

Of course she didn't have an opponent to compete with so she just kept trying to best her last score before the letters gave out or she couldn't make any more words with what she had. She always felt that this ability to visualize so strongly was why she did so well in the photography field.

Dr. Sandler was so amazed by this that he eventually brought in a scrabble board and had her play against him. He used the tiles and the board to keep track of their play and she just laid down on the sofa and visualized it all. She beat him, soundly;

partly because she knew a lot of off-the-wall words; partly because she was better at using the colored squares for her letters. The only mistake she made was that she counted 7 points for a "K" when it only called for 5. He was more than suitably impressed and he had a plan for her treatment.

He also asked her what she meant about playing golf with her Dad while she was held captive. She said that she got the idea of trying it from a book she had read a few years earlier about a P.O.W. who had trained his mind to play his home course so completely and so many times that when he finally went home and actually played it, he had his best round ever without having had a club in his hand for years.

So she decided to play the golf course she and her Dad had played together when they had vacationed in Hawaii on the island of Kauai. When he asked if she had beat her dad, she had laughed and said, "Oh, no! He's a much better golfer than I am." Which had struck him as hilarious. They both had a good laugh over that.

Because of her incredible ability to visualize, he chose that as the primary way to treat her. The idea had come to him when he had seen a small wooden box in a craft shop window. It was six inches long, two inches deep and two inches tall. It reminded him of a coffin because of where the brass hinges for the lid were and also because the wood was unfinished.

He took it in for one of their sessions and had her visualize it as a real coffin and then he had her recall every bad memory she had from her time on the mountain with Jake and then they assigned an emotion to it and she put it in the coffin. At the time he had only allowed two hours for this particular session. He hadn't counted on her memory being quite so prolific and the session ended up running over three hours. He was glad she had been his last appointment of the day.

After she was all finished she had a coffin filled with Anxiety, Dread, Fear, Humiliation, Shame, Panic, Depression, Sadness, Anger, Terror, Hate and Guilt. Lots of Guilt. That seemed to be one of her biggest problems initially. Then together they went to a local park and with a small garden trowel, they buried it in an out of the way place up against a stone fence.

With each succeeding session, whenever a forgotten memory came up, she would name it and then she would visualize the park, mentally dig up the coffin, open it and add the new emotion or feeling to it, then close it and rebury it. In this way she was able to get rid of the things she didn't want to keep around her but she could still recall what was buried there, just as people remember those who have departed and been buried. Dead and buried, unable to trouble them anymore or to cause them problems, but still be a part of their past life.

The graphic visualizing of all this worked well for her, putting her back in control. It absolutely floored David that she never brought up the same memory twice and there had to be a good couple hundred of them that she'd categorized and buried. The one problem that still nagged at her from time to time was the guilt. He reasoned that was probably due to the fact that she still had the ability to do something about it, and wasn't. He decided to help her do something about it. Something that would help him, too.

"Liesel, it's time to set this question of guilt aside and I think I've come up with a way. Basically you're bothered by the idea that other women or maybe even very young girls may be preyed upon by Jake sometime in the years to come. Do I have it right?" he asked.

She thought for a moment and replied, "Well, yes. And I think he needs help and he's not going to get it unless the courts intervene. And if he doesn't get help, he's just going to try it again. I just know it!"

"What if you could help those women and others just like them that have already suffered the same types of things, or will suffer them in the future. What if you could help forty or fifty women overcome these same things instead of just the one or two Jake *might* get to. Would you be interested in being their champion?"

"Of course, I would. I would be very interested. Tell me more," she replied.

"Well, just as you sent your problems away, never to be heard from again, you can send this problem away temporarily, to be dealt with at a later date. An assigned date in the future that you would know for sure that something was being done for the benefit of these abused women."

"Okay. Exactly what are you talking about? I'm not getting it," she said.

"Here's the deal. You figure out monetarily what a court of law would settle upon you if you followed some sort of civil lawsuit to its legal end. If Jake were wealthy and you sued him for damages, aside from the criminal charges. You take that money and donate it to a women's shelter or a treatment program set up to help women who have suffered at the hands of men like Jake. Voilá. You're off the hook. You've helped out the exact people you're so worried about."

"I must be really obtuse. I still don't get it. Where's the money?" she asked.

He replied with a question of his own, "First, how much should it be?"

She thought for a moment, "What I think or a court of law?"

"A court of law," he countered.

"Two hundred thousand," she stated.

"Fair enough. Now where's the money you ask? It's future money. You pledge $200,000 of your inheritance to a foundation or an association and then you live your life guilt-free for now, knowing that when you pass on that women with the same problems you're facing right now, will be taken care of then. You help out in a really big way, when it counts and when you can. Meanwhile, you're off the hook and guilt-free. All you have to do is amend your will now and be done with it."

She took a minute to absorb all this. Strange thing was, it was making some sort of sense. Her inheritance would probably be at least twenty million by the time she died, so $200,000 would hardly be missed. And missed by who, anyhow? So far there were no beneficiaries for her to even consider. She wondered if doing this would really salve her consciousness. Well, there was one way to find out and even if it didn't, she could always change it right back. What a novel idea he had. "How would this be set up?" she asked.

"Any way you want. I would recommend that you leave it in charge of somebody you trust who feels the same way you do and who understands the whole situation." If she bought this, he was going to do cartwheels. But she did seem to be going for it, he thought. "Maybe someone in the counseling profession that these women could go to. You could provide the fees for their recovery."

"You are a genius, Dr. Sandler! How is it that you are able to figure all this out so easily? I'll try it. What have I got to loose? After all it's only money on paper. I'll call my attorney and make the arrangements. You seem to know so much about all this, I wish I could just leave it to you for you to handle, but the likelihood is that I'll survive you, and then what?"

"Leave it to my Foundation. They'll take care of it after I'm gone. That's exactly what they do. They provide counseling for those who have a need but no money for treatment. The David L. Sandler Foundation will have trustees that will take care of everything for them."

"That's perfect!" she glanced down at her watch. "I've got to get going otherwise I'll miss Daniel's call. I'll take care of everything as soon as I can get in touch with my attorney in Washington, and thanks! You're the best! See you next week." She slid off the sofa and put her shoes on then grabbed her matching handbag and walked out of his office.

He watched her leave. She had a newfound spring in her step. She certainly was anxious to get home to get Daniel's call. Daniel was a very lucky man. Again, he felt that little pang of jealousy, but thinking of Jenny caused it to disappear as quickly as it had come. He and Jenny were going to have a wonderful life together. He shook his head as he rubbed his chin. Gullible. For such a smart woman, Liesel was quite gullible.

Chapter 50

In the Air—En Route to Dulles International Airport

Daniel sat in his seat looking out the window at the white clouds and blue sky. They were better than halfway there, heading to Washington, D.C. after departing from Portland. After talking to Liesel last night he was more than anxious to fold her into his arms and make love to her. She had sounded like a soft, sexy kitten on the phone, mercilessly teasing him with her banter.

She had been unusually bold this time suggesting that she turn his body into an ice cream sundae. Cover him from head to toe with chocolate syrup, cherries and marshmallow fluff that she could lick off. He had readily agreed to be submissive to this. In fact he had even offered to provide the "nuts".

During their long hours of talking it was not at all unusual for the conversation to turn to sex and for them both to say some pretty outrageous things, but when they got together, none of them ever happened. Liesel could be pretty bold on the phone, but she was extremely timid when he could actually get her into his arms.

He was pretty sure that the reason for this was that they really didn't have much of a chance to get warmed up to each other before he had to prepare to leave again. Three day weekends that included 15 hours worth of travel time were not enough for them to sustain this relationship. And he was not about to give up on it. He was in love with her, as he had never loved a woman before.

Sometimes he felt that his heart was outside of his body. It was so much more a part of her than it was a part of him. He had been very gentle and patient with her because of her experiences with Jake. They had talked about all that had happened and surprisingly, in great detail. Once he had even asked her what she would have done if Jake had raped her and she had discovered herself pregnant with his child. She told him that she would have loved the child, regardless of its parentage, saying, how could an innocent baby be held accountable for the sins of its parent? He was reminded of the awful thing his wife had done to their baby without his knowledge or consent. And here was Liesel, determined to keep the innocent life of a child fathered by a despicable monster like Jake. He was thankful for Jake's impotence, at least Liesel had been spared that misery.

He knew the areas that were likely to cause her some sort of stigma. He certainly knew that there would never be any nude posing for pictures in their relationship no matter how much she came to trust him, but that was something he never would have considered doing anyway. The oral sex on her would be very touch and go if they ever actually got to it and of course bondage of any sort was way out of the question!

All this was pretty moot though. They hadn't progressed past the petting stage yet despite all the patience and perseverance he could muster up. It was the time thing. He just knew it. No sooner were they laughing and playing and getting to know each other up close before it was time to fly off again. And that was the reason for this unscheduled trip.

On one of his trips east he had met her boss when they had attended a dinner party and dined together. Yesterday Daniel had called him and asked him if he could arrange some time off for her without him telling her about it. After answering a few rather pointed questions that had been directed at him, Daniel had his answer. Her boss could spare her for seven days starting tomorrow.

Daniel had to act fast. He made travel arrangements for himself, planned out the seven days and made all the necessary reservations. He called the mill and took a leave of absence and then on his way to the airport this morning he had stopped at Jake's cabin. Jake was already at work so he had plenty of time.

Remembering Liesel's exact words he walked down a dirt pathway to a small clearing and then he started looking.

It only took him about fifteen minutes to find it. Then Daniel went into the cabin and left something for Jake. He closed the door behind him and got back in his truck. There, in the cabin, in the middle of the mattress stuck through the dirty linens was a Phillips head screwdriver standing straight up.

He had driven his truck to the Portland airport where he arranged to leave it in long term parking and then boarded his flight to Washington. Now as he sat staring out the window, he was eager for this flight to end so he could surprise Liesel. He looked down at the heavy hardback book in his lap, Ken Follett's "The Pillars of the Earth." It was the same book he carried on all his trips to Dulles. He'd never even read the first page. He'd used it to hide the protrusion in his lap that was almost constantly there whenever he thought about Liesel. Which was almost all the time.

Chapter 51

McLean, VA

Liesel had just finished changing from her work clothes to a comfortable jogging outfit when she heard her apartment door bell ring. Who could that be? She never had any visitors, she hadn't been here long enough to make many friends other than those at work. Probably somebody selling something. She walked over to the door calling out "Who is it?" as she neared the door.

"Daniel," was the one-word answer she heard.

Daniel? Her heart started to race just hearing his name. Daniel couldn't be here. He was in Oregon. She looked through the peephole and saw only the lower half of a man's face. Those were certainly Daniel's lips and chiseled chin. She quickly stepped away from the door and began unlocking the series of locks. When she flung the door open he quickly gathered her up into his arms and spun her around, her feet a foot off the floor.

"Daniel," she whispered softly into his ear. He set her down and kissed her soundly. His hands cradling her head between them. When one wouldn't do, he bent down to take another, savoring the feel of her lips as he plucked at them with his.

"Surprise honey!" he said. And then he reached down to the floor and picked up a small white paper bag from Baskin Robbins. "I couldn't wait to be your ice cream sundae, so here I am. And...I remembered to bring the 'nuts' you said you liked so much." He added with a wolfish gleam in his eyes.

She smiled a shy smile and stood aside so he could come in. He bent down and kissed her cheek, already sensing her reticence. "I'll just put this in the freezer for later," he said. While he walked to the kitchen and put the ice cream and toppings away she closed and locked the door. When she joined him in the kitchen he turned and took both her hands in his.

"How would you like to go to a beautiful tropical island with me tomorrow?"

"Oh, Daniel. You know I'd love to, but I have to work. This is still a fairly new job and they won't give me any time off for at least six months yet."

"Don't be so sure about that. I'm so sure that they will, that I've got the tickets right here." He produced two airline packets from his jacket pocket.

"You're serious, aren't you?" she said with a stunned expression on her face.

"Babe, where you're concerned, I'm always serious. Go ahead, call your boss, you'll see." He handed her the phone receiver hanging on the wall beside him.

She smiled at him and said, "I can't believe this."

She dialed her boss at home. He picked up right away and when she identified herself she could almost hear the smile in his voice as he said, "Yessss? What's up?"

She hesitated for just an instant before she said, "Well, Daniel's here and he wants to take me on a trip. I told him I wouldn't be able to go with him but he said that I should call you. He already has the tickets so I know something's up. Has he spoken to you about this?"

Daniel leaned with his hip against the counter watching her expressions change as she spoke into the receiver. "Tomorrow! Seven days! Uhuh... Yeah... Okay. With pay? Yes. Thank You. Yes I will. Bye." She hung the phone back up on the wall.

"He said I could go. In fact, he said I had to go. I have to spend a day or two taking some pictures he wants for the magazine. Oh Daniel..." she exclaimed as she hugged him around his neck.

"Just exactly where are we going, Mr. Wonderful?" she asked as she turned to gaze up at him.

"St. Croix," he replied and watched as her face lit up.

How had he known that she'd always wanted to go there? Had she told him about the underwater National Park she'd always wanted to photograph or was this just a coincidence?

"St. Croix! Oh, Daniel!" She wrapped her arms tighter around his neck which required her to stand on her tip toes even as tall as she was. "I have always wanted to go there! I can't wait! When do we leave?" Daniel smiled and hugged her tightly to him.

"Let's sit down and I'll show you the itinerary. We don't have a lot of time though. Our flight leaves Dulles tomorrow morning at seven o'clock, so we've got to get you packed. And because we're leaving so early I didn't get a hotel room for me tonight. Is it okay if I stay here with you tonight?"

Liesel looked over at him, "How many rooms did you book for us in St. Croix?"

"One," was his one-word answer.

"Well, then I guess it doesn't matter, does it?"

He grabbed her hand, "Liesel, if it's a problem... If this isn't what you want..."

"No, No. Sooner or later we've got to face this. I think I'm ready."

"Good," he said and walked her over to the couch in the living room.

Her apartment was a one bedroom so there was no doubt where he'd be sleeping tonight and he had to bite his tongue to keep from expressing his extreme pleasure at the thought.

He showed her pictures of the hotel they would be staying at—The Buccaneer. They had a cottage right on the beach. He showed her pictures of the island and a list of all the things they could do. He had known that the underwater park would please her but he was a little surprised when she said something about taking advantage of the hotel's offer of a personal masseur, until he understood that he was to be the masseur.

He leaned over and kissed her deeply and was already enfolding her into his arms when she suddenly pushed hard against his chest. "Ohmygod! I've got to pack! What am I going to wear? Daniel! By keeping this a secret, I don't have anything to wear!" she moaned.

"Honey, the first time I saw you, you didn't have anything to wear either and you looked just fine to me." He deadpaned. He was not ready for the barrage of pillows that assailed him and was a little slow getting his hands up before one after the other they hit him in the face.

She ran into the bedroom and he wasn't far behind, grabbing her around the waist and picking her up in his arms. He walked with her to the bed and laid her down gently. Then he stretched himself down beside her and stroked her face with his fingertips. "I love you Liesel. You do know that don't you?" She nodded her head slightly, but did not reply in kind. It would take awhile, he knew that.

"Whatever you don't have, we'll buy there. But I don't think you're going to need much. A topless bathing suit and one evening gown should do it," he chided.

Her eyes opened wide and he said, "Just kidding. I'm not sharing these with anybody."

With that he cupped both breasts in his hands and squeezed them gently through the fabric of her sweat shirt. Then he hopped off the bed and said, "I'm going into the living room to watch the game. Call me if you need any help, okay? And let me know when you're ready to go to bed." As he said that last part he lifted his eyebrows up and down like Groucho Marx, causing her to laugh at his departure from the room.

Chapter 52

St. Croix, V.I.

They arrived in St. Croix late the next afternoon. Neither had slept much the night before, she excited about the trip, he excited and aroused lying next to her all night. She hadn't finished her packing until very late, partly because she had to run out to the camera shop at the mall to get film for her underwater camera and also by her office to pick up the assignment notes left by her boss, and partly because she was stalling. She wanted Daniel to make love to her, but not tonight. Not until they got to St. Croix. They slept the few hours before dawn snuggled in each other's embrace savoring the closeness and anticipating what tomorrow would bring.

They flew first class. Daniel pretty much had to, he was so big. But that wasn't the reason. He wanted everything to be perfect and he had spared no expense in arranging it to be so. He specified the most remote bungalow they had and he wanted fresh flowers and champagne delivered daily. The phone was not to ring for any reason. In fact he suggested that they unplug it and remove it entirely. If they needed to be contacted for any reason, a note could be slipped under the door. But since no one knew where they were going except Liesel's boss it was unlikely anyone would be trying to get in touch with them.

When they arrived on the island, a limousine from the hotel met them at the airport and whisked them away. They had champagne in the back seat and toasted to their time together. Liesel commented that this was to be her *sea duction*, and every time they toasted from that time on they both whispered, "sea duction" softly before sipping their drinks.

Arriving at the hotel, Daniel took care of the preliminaries while Liesel walked around outside admiring the view and mentally cropping shots in her mind. Two bellmen accompanied them to their room. Boy, for someone who didn't have anything to pack she sure had found plenty, Daniel thought as he turned to smile at her.

But in all fairness, most of it was her camera equipment and scuba gear. He'd never met anyone who had their own scuba gear. He could scuba dive a little but apparently he was nowhere near her league. It would be fun watching her. She was as excited as a little kid on her first trip to Disney World.

When they arrived at the door to their bungalow, one of the bellman opened the door and then both bellmen turned their backs on them and waited. It took Daniel a moment to understand. They thought they were newlyweds. What the heck. He picked Liesel up into his arms and carried her inside. They both stared into each other's eyes for a long moment and then Daniel set her down on the cool terrazzo tiles.

The room was bright and cheery. One king sized bed as he had specified was in the center. From the bed you could look out onto their terrace and beyond to the spectacular view of the ocean as it met the white sand. After tipping the bellmen, Daniel closed the door behind them and walked over to Liesel who was looking out the sliding glass door to the ocean.

He put both his hands on her shoulders and ran them up and down her bare arms. As he kissed the nape of her neck and nibbled on her ear lobe, he whispered, "Welcome to paradise. Just having you to myself for awhile makes this paradise for me."

She turned in his arms and put her head on his chest, wrapping her arms around his waist, feeling the hard muscles of his back. "Daniel," she softly whispered. "This is almost too good to be true."

Then the kid in her bubbled to the surface and she quickly said, "Let's put on our suits and go get in the ocean!" That wasn't exactly what he wanted to do right then, but then he did have seven days, they'd do what she wanted first.

"Okay. First we have to figure out which of these sixty-odd cases contain the bathing suits," he teased.

She whipped off her tank top and pulled down her shorts revealing a very nice body clad in a very skimpy bikini. She pulled open the glass door and ran out yelling behind her, "Last one in the water is a rotten egg!"

He watched her fanny jiggle enticingly as she ran down to the beach and right into the water. He shook his head. He felt like he had brought a little girl into the den of a wolf. A huge, hungry, sexually starved wolf. When it really counted, how was he ever going to be able to slow down and control himself? He found the suitcase containing his bathing suit and changed into it in the huge, lavishly appointed bathroom. Then he walked down to the beach to join her.

It was late afternoon and the sun was just beginning to go down. The beach was becoming empty as people left to get ready for dinner. Pretty soon they had it all to themselves. They swam out to the breakers together and then back, enjoying the feel of the water cascading over their bodies. Then they linked their hands and floated on the surface shielding their eyes from the sun as the current gently rotated them around and around. It was Liesel who decided that now she was hungry and maybe they should go back to the room. He agreed, even though he wasn't particularly hungry.

As they walked hand-in-hand through the water and through the sand back to their terrace they glanced at each other. It was Liesel's first time seeing Daniel with no shirt on and his massive chest reminded her of the body builders she'd seen on TV. Only his chest wasn't covered with shiny oil. His was covered with dark, thick, curling hair.

His long legs with their well-developed muscles had water running in rivulets down them causing the hair there to lay flat and straight against his tanned skin. And his arms matched the rest of him, hairy and rippling with muscles hewn from years of hard work and exercise. He was male incarnate and looking at his body was doing strange things to her insides.

Daniel glanced sideways at Liesel as they made their way to the patio doors and, although he had seen her unclothed before,

251

he hadn't been at liberty to stop and enjoy the view. He remembered her long legs vividly from the times that he had seen them. Hell, he'd had night sweats recalling them. Now as he casually eyed them up and down he felt a tightening in his groin that was a precursor of things to come as his eyes moved from her legs to her slim waist and then to her generous bosom.

The material of the bikini bra was thin and the outline of her nipples was clearly visible to him. He felt the flaccidness of him caused by the cold water leave him as waves of heat flushed through him. They were on the terrace now. What difference would it make if she knew that he desired her more than he could control? So instead of turning away from her, he grabbed her and brought her to him, crushing her against his lips, his chest and his erection.

His kisses were savage with their intensity. His tongue forced its way inside and plundered her sweet mouth. His hands held her face to his as he retreated and attacked again and again. When he heard her low moan of ecstasy and she answered his kisses with her own frenzied tongue searching out his, he reached down and lifted her into his arms. He carried her through the open doors and set her on her feet by the end of the bed.

Grabbing one of the towels he had placed on the bed earlier, he dried her off and removed her bikini top. When she was bare chested in front of him, he murmured, "Oh, how exquisite," and dropped the towel. He placed his hand under her breast, lifting the nipple to his lowering lips. When they met she felt the world start to slide away. She had never felt anything so wonderful as his lips kissing her there. When his tongue slid out to lick at the hardened peak, she thought she would die, the heat pulsing through her was so great.

His wet thigh slid between hers and she could feel his arousal meeting and pushing against her hip, straining against his suit. She put a hand on each of his hips and hooked a thumb from each under the elastic of his suit. She started working it down past his hips and then over his buttocks before pulling it loose around the front so she could ease it over his erection that was now rampart hard and sticking straight out, as it tried to find some cavity or crevice to ease itself against.

As his shaft touched her skin, he removed his mouth from her breast and groaned as he kissed his way back up her throat to her mouth. Taking her there was like claiming her as his. His lips branded her lips as his hand slid down her hip to her bikini bottom and he deftly eased it off her hips and down to her thighs.

His hand returned to find her woman's mound and without thought to the suddenness of his actions, he thrust one finger deeply inside her, relishing the feel of her moist, slick opening. Liesel thought her legs were going to give out on her. She couldn't understand how she was still standing with all these delicious sensations coursing through her. As soon as Daniel's finger had penetrated her she felt her body slump against his hand.

He had to be holding her up somehow. She couldn't feel her legs, only that part of her that his finger was moving in and out of. Daniel moved against her until the back of her calves touched the edge of the bed and then he gently pushed her down on top of it. Before following her down he grabbed the loose piece of fabric that was her suit from between her legs and pulled it off.

Then he stepped out of his trunks that had fallen to his ankles. He lay down on top of her, gyrating his hips against hers and feeling his chest rub up against hers. He looked down into her face and kissed her gently on the lips, and said, "If you mean to stop me, this is your last chance, although I'm not so sure I could stop now, even if you wanted me to."

"I don't want you to," she said softly and lifted her hips in welcome.

He didn't hesitate. He locked both arms on either side of her shoulders and raised his upper body off of her. Then he positioned his rod between her thighs, found the entrance and with one quick probe he thrust into her. "Ahh," was all he could say as the head of his penis found itself just touching the very tip of her womb.

He was too far in and he knew it. But God, it felt so damned good. Most men wanted an inch more to please a woman but he'd always felt that an inch less would have pleased most of his women better. He withdrew slightly when he found her moving back against the mattress and then pulled out more until she reached for him and urged him back.

He dipped his head to suckle on her nipples as he slowly eased himself back into her. When she moaned his name and moved her hands against his chest and stomach, he started an in and out rhythm that was as compelling as breathing. As he thrust repeatedly into her he bent his head to her throat. As he kissed and licked her there he whispered her name against her skin.

He caressed her buttocks and held tightly to them as he continued to plunge and retreat. Suddenly she arched up against him and he felt a trembling throughout her body. The realization that she was coming for him was too much for him to bear and he plunged once more into her and the full load from his heavy scrotum exploded deep inside her. His head fell down beside hers and he moaned her name over and over again.

When he was somewhat recovered, he rolled onto his side taking her with him, reluctant for any separation between them at all yet. Stroking her cheek and smoothing her hair away from her face he said, "Liesel, I have waited my whole pubescent and adult life for you and you are most definitely worth it. I love you, darling."

Liesel was still trying to find her way back from the odyssey she had just been taken on. As she opened her eyes she tried to focus on his as they swam in and out of her vision, she just smiled and said, "I'm still hungry, how 'bout you?"

He laughed heartily, pulling her closer to him. If he had anything to say about it, he was never going to let her go.

After a short nap they got up to dress for dinner. Liesel showered while Daniel unpacked his things and then Daniel showered while Liesel unpacked. Somehow neither one had gotten past the stage of putting on a hotel robe and before long, Liesel found Daniel taking hers off. After enjoying the pleasures of her body once again, he found the phone the hotel had unplugged and left on the top shelf of their closet. He found the phone jack to plug it into and called room service and ordered dinner. It had been a mistake to think they were going to leave this room tonight.

They had a lovely dinner of Steak Diane, new parslied potatoes and fresh asparagus followed by miniature Baked Alaskas before they found themselves in the huge bath tub licking champagne off of each other. Liesel looked over at Daniel on the other side of the tub, over the rim of her champagne glass, and gave him a little smile as she asked, "Is the area below the ear really your favorite place on a woman?"

Daniel laughed and said, "Hell no! But if I'd kissed you where I really wanted to he would've knocked me in the head while I was doing it!"

With that, he pulled her towards him and grabbed her by the crotch. "Do you think you're clean enough yet for me to kiss all my favorite places?" She raised her eyebrows as he pulled her up out of the tub with him.

At two in the morning when Liesel decided it was her turn to be on top, Daniel rolled her over and smacked her lightly on the bottom, "Go to bed woman! Tomorrow is another day! What vitamins are you taking and do you have any extra for me?"

Liesel laughed and ruffled her fingers through his hair. "I don't take any vitamins. But I do take Prozac."

Daniel almost asleep quickly rolled over and said, "What! What did you say?"

"I said I take Prozac. Dr. Sandler prescribed it for me. He says I need it to counter the depression I've been experiencing."

"Liesel, are you sure that's necessary? That's pretty dangerous stuff. How long have you been taking it?" he asked.

"Daniel, it's okay. He knows what he's doing. Remember it was your friend who recommended him to me."

"I know. I just don't like the idea of you taking an anti-depressant like that. Why don't you refrain from taking them while we're here and we'll see how it goes. Surely there can't be anything depressing about me." He leaned over and kissed her and plopped face down back onto the pillow.

"I don't know. He said it was pretty important that I keep taking them, even if I felt good," Liesel said.

"We'll talk some more in the morning. Get some sleep. I plan on an early morning invasion of that area between your legs and I want you awake to enjoy it." He made a mental note to find those pills in the morning and flush them down the toilet.

Liesel watched Daniel sleep. He looked like a tousled god. What a hunk he was she thought to herself. And the things he could do to her body. She'd never known it could be like this. Was it because she loved him? She suspected it was. She couldn't wait for what tomorrow would bring and then a thought occurred to her. She never would have met Daniel if it hadn't been for Jake.

So now she had a grateful feeling towards him. She wondered, is that supposed to go in the coffin, too? Dr. Sandler's trick for the removal of all her guilt had certainly been a winner. Ever since she had signed the new testament papers delivered by courier yesterday to her office, she hadn't had a twinge of guilt. Could he be wrong about the Prozac? She rolled over and went to sleep.

True to his word, the next morning she was awakened by the soft brush of Daniel's hair against her inner thighs. As he spread her legs wider to accommodate him, he noticed her body tense up. He remembered that Jake had done this to her and a feeling of intense hatred burned in him. When he got back, he was going to bash his head in if it was the last thing he did.

He tried to reassure her by kissing her gently on her thighs and stroking along her hips with his fingertips. When the tenseness eased, he lightly pressed kisses to her nether lips, lingering in all the special places experience had taught him about. Then as she opened up a little more for him, he used his tongue to explore every inch of her. She had a musky warm scent and it was driving him crazy. He couldn't seem to get enough of her taste or her smell.

Suddenly he was ravenous for her and he forced her to open all the way up for him. With each of his hands clutching a handful of her fleshy bottom he lifted her higher so that his mouth had complete access to all of her. He felt her begin to shudder and concentrated on that very sensitive area at the top of her slit. He licked and sucked and tongued her until she began to spasm uncontrollably, bathing his face with a new wave of her wetness and pulsing against his face. When the last vestige of her orgasm died off, he kissed her tenderly and then wiped his face teasingly in her furry thatch.

When she opened her eyes again, he was leaning over her with a great big smile on his lips. As he leaned down to kiss her on the lips, she quickly covered her mouth, mumbling that she hadn't brushed yet. He removed her hand and before he kissed her deeply, he whispered, "Neither have I."

Daniel went into the bathroom to comb his hair. On the counter he saw a little baggie with ten small white pills in it. He assumed they were the Prozac pills they had talked about last night and opened the zip lock seal. He dumped them into the toilet just as Liesel walked into the bathroom.

"What are you doing?" she asked in a loud surprised voice.

"Just getting rid of your Prozac pills for you. You don't need them," he said emphatically.

She reached over him to the counter and picked up another baggie with green pills in it. "These are my Prozac pills."

"Then what were these?" he asked, innocently.

"Those," she said rather blandly, "were my birth control pills."

Chapter 53

Fairfax, VA 1989

Dr. Sandler sat at his desk in his home study running his fingers through his hair and wondering what in the world he was doing. His eyes took in all the vials and pills scattered in front of him and his huge Physician's Desk Reference book open on his lap. He had no doubt that this was going to work. He just wished there was some other way.

If Linda would just die or even remarry, that would help a lot. Neither was likely and he knew that if he was to assist her death in any way, her family would come looking for him. It was no secret that their divorce had caused bitter feelings between them, and even if she died accidentally, everyone would suspect him. He would get caught if he took that avenue. This way was at least foolproof. There would never be a way to link him to these pills.

Whenever the pills were taken, his unsuspecting patients would be far from him, doing the normal things occurring in their lives. It would be totally random. Even he wouldn't know when or where their reactions would occur. It could be at home, at work, in a restaurant or in a movie theater. It would be whenever they remembered to take their pill and then it would have to be one of the few that he had doctored and intermingled with the rest.

The pharmacies would be the first place they'd look, then all those with access to the pills. He would never even be considered, even if he had been the prescribing doctor. A part of him was excited just to see how it would all play out.

As soon as he had arrived home from the office he had taken out his home rolodex patient file. After sorting through and taking out the ones belonging to patients he knew to be quite well-to-do and biddable through hypnosis, he scrambled them upside down with his hands on top of his desk blotter. Much like a five year old getting ready to make the "pond" for a game of Fish. He selected six cards. These were the *lottery winners*. The *death lottery*.

He had tried several times to pick his victims with impartiality but had been unsuccessful each time. He cared about them all in one way or another. He'd had his greatest career success to date with Donna, he was amused by Jessica and he often found himself fantasizing about Liesel. Heck, he even found Shawn to be an intriguing challenge. When he hit on the idea of a lottery, it had taken off the pressure of deciding who was going to die. Let fate pick the *winners* or *losers* as was the case.

As he scooped some pills into a brown vial, he thought about the patient that would be taking them. These pink and fuschia ones would be Henry's. Sinequan laced with Nardil and more drug in each, than would normally be in a single capsule. The large dosages by themselves would be lethal. The combination was insurance.

Ah, Henry. You'd probably like to be put out of your misery anyway. Henry Blocker had started out as a pro bono case. Two years ago his wife had been in a serious car accident. It left her in a vegetative coma with virtually no chance of ever awakening. Henry had been at work at the time and the hospital staff had only been able to locate her family who hadn't bothered to contact him and he had spent the entire night trying to find her.

Henry and his wife Sally had met through a special education program at the community college. They were both slightly retarded and had been virtually dateless until they had met each other. There was an immediate bonding between the two and they fell in love and married despite Sally's family's objections.

Their wedding night had been awkward for the two of them, but once they figured out how the game was played they became insatiable for each other. Sally would be waiting for Henry to get home from his job at Burger King and they would dash to the bedroom to make love before fixing dinner together. They were blissfully happy living a very simple life in a small apartment rented over a garage. Henry finally found the hospital that Sally had been taken to at 4:30 in the morning.

For three months Henry listened to the doctors as they tried to be realistic and at the same time offer some hope. Sally's family was constantly in attendance during the day when Henry was working and Henry spent the better part of each night by her bedside talking to her as if she was fully awake.

One night as he sat in the chair beside her bed holding her hand he became agitated. These doctors didn't know what they were doing. His Sally was right there, waiting for someone to find the way to wake her up and so far no one had. He thought that it was high time for him to take care of matters. He didn't see how Sally could possibly stay asleep if he could wake her up from the inside like he did when they made love. Surely those spasmodic explosions he had felt generating from deep inside her inner core would wake her. He just knew if he could get her to climax that she would come back to him.

It wasn't that late yet, so he moved over to the drape separating her side of the room from her roommate's, who was also comatose. Then he removed his pants and draped them over the chair. He gently drew the sheet down past her knees and pulled her nightgown up to her shoulders baring her from her calves to her neck.

The sight of her beautiful pale breasts displayed under the fluorescent light over her bed caused him to gasp with remembered pleasure. He slipped out of his shoes and climbed on top of her. Straddling her, he played with her breasts and sucked on her nipples until he was sure she had to be quite aroused and ready for him. He kissed her on the lips but she was totally unresponsive and had a funny taste so he abandoned that idea.

He used his fingers to stroke her and although she wasn't as wet as she usually got for him, he thought she was wet enough, given the fact that he had been dribbling all of his precome up against her opening. He positioned himself and gently eased himself inside. God, how good it felt. Before long he was thrusting and bucking trying to get a response out of her. She just lay there, eyes closed, lips partially open with her breasts jiggling up and down and back and forth with his movements.

Just then Sally's mother and sister pulled the drape back and screamed. Henry, just about ready to unload himself into Sally, cried out in anguish. The anguish of losing Sally, the anguish of a long needed physical release and the anguish of humiliation all ran into each other and escaped as a primitive keening that was heard throughout the ward.

Of course security had been called along with a battalion of doctors and nurses. No one knew what to do for sure. After all, she was his wife. Sally's mother ranted and raved about Henry being perverted and insisted that he would probably dig up Sally's coffin to have at her if someone didn't do something and arrest him.

Sally's doctor didn't think they could do that. Nor did he want to. It was apparent to him that Henry adored Sally and that he missed her tremendously. Henry was so upset he couldn't get any words out for his own defense other than saying over and over again, "I was trying to make her wake up. She likes to wake up this way."

It was finally decided that Henry should have some counseling. That seemed to appease Sally's mother and Henry didn't seem to care much about what happened to him at this point. So Sally's doctor had called his long-time sailing buddy, Dr. David Sandler, and asked him if he could see Henry as a favor to him.

Henry had been virtually penniless when their sessions had started but three months into therapy Henry had become a multi-millionaire when the insurance company for the driver who hit Sally settled out of court for her injuries and subsequent death. Sally's family had tried all kinds of maneuvers to attach themselves to some of the money but Dr. Sandler had advised Henry well and Henry's appreciation was reflected in a generous mention of the Sandler Foundation in his will.

David finished putting all the pills back into the proper vials and cleaned off his desk. He grabbed his jacket off the back of his chair and went out of his apartment to the elevator. On the way down he thought about Henry one more time. Henry would never be the same no matter what he did. He had loved Sally with his whole heart and soul. Nothing would ever be good for him again.

Not even having all that money. What was money without love? He was on his way to meet his love, Jenny. He thought that if anything ever happened to her, money wouldn't mean anything either. But now it did. It was the only way he could have her and the kind of life he wanted her to have.

In the underground garage he got into his Trans Am and smiled. He could smell the faint perfume of her from when she had last been in his car. He breathed deeply trying to get his fill before starting the car and driving to Tyson's Corner.

Chapter 54

Tyson's Corner, VA

Jenny was standing in the showroom when she saw David pull his car into a space in front of the showroom. She had some customers in one of the settlement offices so she walked outside to greet him. "Hey, that's a pretty fine automobile you've got there! Any idea where I can get one just like it?" She smiled.

"Yeah, just turn around. There's one behind you."

She turned and looked and sure enough there was a Trans Am on the showroom the same color as his. After all the years of selling cars she had become pretty much inured to the look, feel and smell of new cars. She hardly ever noticed the cars on the floor unless she was showing them to a customer. In fact there had been a few times that she had scoured the lot looking for a particular car only to find it on the showroom floor right outside her office where it had been for days.

David walked up to her and smiled down at her as he put his hand around her waist and led her back inside. "You really didn't know it was there, did you?" he said with a chuckle.

She just shrugged her shoulders and said, "I'm sorry, I just don't see them anymore." She looked down at her bruised shin, "That is until I walk right into them."

David laughed. She was always so much fun to be with, she always made him laugh. Over the last few months he had become less of a customer and more of a boyfriend to her in the eyes of her cohorts so they all nodded or called out "Hi" to him as they passed on their way to her office. It was becoming customary for him to drop by once or twice a week when she was working the late shift.

If she got out at a reasonable time they would go to one of the bars close by. Within two blocks they had a choice between Fridays, Fedora's, American Cafe, Carnegie's and Clyde's. She preferred Friday's because the prices were reasonable. He preferred Clyde's because the prices were outrageous and he could impress her.

He loved to hear about the things that had happened during her day while she was still excited about them. Her face would become animated and she would talk so fast that he just had to laugh sometimes. While her customers where signing papers she told him about one of the new salesmen the dealership had hired a few weeks ago.

His name was Neal Corbette and he was very young, only nineteen. He had come into the dealership and approached one of the sales managers with an enthusiastic grin and a firm handshake and then he had proceeded to boast that he would run rings around their best salesman. He said he needed money for next year's college tuition and he wanted to work for the summer to earn it.

Well, Gary, the sales manager was skeptical to say the least. Here was a brash, young, inexperienced rookie who said he was going to earn in commissions the equivalent of a whole year's income in three months. He started to walk away from him, Neal grabbed his shirt sleeve and said, "If I don't sell five cars by Saturday, you can keep this."

He handed Gary a one hundred dollar bill. Well, this was something you didn't bump into every day, a prospective salesman offering to pay for the chance to sell.

Gary led Neal into his office and after a few more questions and a few phone calls as a background check, Neal was hired. True to his word, he sold five cars by Saturday night. In fact, he sold seven. That had made the rest of the sales force take notice. This was highly unusual. A rookie generally didn't close his first deal for a week or more and then it was more management's doing than his.

Neal needed management's help but not any more than anyone else did. After two weeks, Neal was right up to where Jenny was. It was the 18th of the month and she had fifteen units out. He had fourteen with one set up for delivery in two days. She had nothing working. She was very curious about Neal. She didn't begrudge him his good fortune, but things just didn't add up.

A little nosing around on her part in the deal folders that had been sent upstairs yielded a very interesting thing. All of Neal's deals were short deals. Remarkably short. The cars had been sold for the absolute minimums the house would allow in almost each case. Since Royal was a high volume dealership it wasn't unusual to see deals close to invoice occasionally. But more than ten in a row? Unheard of.

Jenny started to pay more attention to Neal when he was with a customer and though it took awhile she finally figured it out. She was sitting at the up desk one afternoon pretending to look at a new car brochure when Neal had a customer being closed in his office by Gary. The husband and wife who were the customers were seated at Neal's desk. Gary was in Neal's seat behind the desk and Neal was leaning on the wall behind Gary.

Neal's frequent movements caught her eye. He was shaking his head, "no". And then again, "no". Three more times he did this and then he nodded his head, "yes". Gary stood up, reached across the desk and shook the hands of both the husband and the wife before calling out to a passing lot boy, "Get this car ready, will ya Herman? These people would like to take it home tonight." He then tossed Herman the keys to the car Neal had just sold.

Well, well, well. Wasn't that interesting? Jenny thought. Neal was coaching his customers. She snooped a little more and discovered that after Neal helped his customers select the vehicle they wanted he would tell them that he would get them the best deal the house would allow. Then he explained to them that only management could even mention numbers that low. He knew what they were because the stock cards were coded. But he couldn't offer the cars for sale anywhere near that price. But he would let them know when the deal the manager was offering was the deal to take by the nod of his head. And then, he whispered to them, "You have to accept it right away, before he has time to think it over and change his mind."

265

It had worked almost every time. Neal kept using different managers to close his deals, so it didn't seem so odd that all his deals were practically at invoice. Jenny had to hand it to Neal, it was truly ingenious and he had found the only dealership that it would work at and still allow him to make good money. The "per deal" commission was based on a percentage of the profit, with the minimum deal the house would accept paying only $25. All of Neal's deals so far were minimum commission deals. So fourteen deals was only $350.

However, the bonus plan each month was very substantial. First place in units paid $1,500. And, if you sold ten units you got another $500. Fifteen units paid $700 and twenty units paid $1,000 with each additional unit over twenty paying $100 more for each. Should Neal get to twenty-five units, which seemed likely, he would earn $3,000 before the first deal commission of $25 was paid, provided he was still in first place. Not bad for a kid determined to pay his way through college.

Now, what was she going to do with this knowledge? She could alert management but that would be like tattle-tailing and it would look even worse coming from her, the disgruntled star, jealous of the newcomer. She could let Neal know and advise him to give up the gig. Nah, that would only make her look condescending and really, what business was it of hers? Then she hit on an idea.

She went upstairs to Mr. Royal's office. His secretary was out so she knocked on the door and he looked up. He smiled when he saw her and beckoned her to come in. He was eating a peanut butter and jelly sandwich at his desk as he looked over some stock projections. "Jenny, how's it goin' girl?"

She stepped inside and closed the door behind her. "Good. Real good. You got a minute?"

"Sure," he replied, "just let me get this peanut butter off the roof of my mouf." She smiled and sat down at a chair in front of his desk.

266

"I have a favor to ask of you, I want you to do something, but I can't tell you why just yet. This won't make much sense to you now but it will later and you'll be happy you did it."

"Ooookay", he said, "tell me what you want me to do."

"Tonight, when we shut down, have the comptroller go into the computer and change the codes on the stock cards to reflect a $400 over invoice price instead of an invoice price. It will only take a few series of key strokes to change the entire inventory pack so it can be changed back just as quickly when this is over. Make sure you don't tell anyone else what we've done. But just to make certain we don't loose a deal because the price is too high, authorize the managers to accept as much as $300 under invoice if absolutely necessary."

"When do I get to know what all this is about?" he asked.

"When does Janey go back to school this semester?" she countered.

"August 18th. But what does she have to do with this?"

"Nothing, I just wanted to know when Virginia Tech goes back. You'll know way before that, I assure you."

She got up and looked out his window that overlooked the showroom. "I'd better get back down there. I've got some real competition this month." She smiled when she turned and noticed his mouth stuck together again. "No need to reply, I see you're busy." She laughed as she ran down the stairs to the showroom.

Jenny and David were sitting with their heads close so no one else could hear. "That was three days ago and Neal's still going strong. Since he really believes that's the best he can do for his customers, it's easy for him to convince them of that, too. If you believe something's true you can make others believe it, too." David thought it was ironic that she should say that because it applied to his job as well as to hers. "Wait til he sees his commission sheet at the end of the month. A $400 deal pays $125. He just may make enough to pay for room and board too!"

Jenny's customers came out of the settlement office and she showed them all around their new car and continued answering their questions until they pulled out. Then she turned to David, and said, "Let's go to Friday's. I feel like some loaded potato skins and I don't want to use the whole commission on that last car deal to pay for them!" She always offered to pay, but he never let her.

Chapter 55

Tyson's Corner, VA

The crowd at Friday's was loud and it was very hard to carry on a conversation so after they had eaten David drove her back to the dealership so she could get her demo. He was adverse to parting so soon but he knew that she was tired and had to get home to bed. He gave her a few languorous kisses while they were seated in his car but the console in the Trans Am was so wide that it was very hard to hold her and if he didn't hold her she kept trying to move away.

He knew she was adamant about public displays of affection so he reluctantly let her go. He watched her get into her demo and waited until she pulled off the lot before he headed home. This was miserable. He was aching with need for her. This weekend he would be firmer with her. She would agree to marry him and they would set a date, enough was enough!

He shifted in his seat trying to relieve the pressure his manhood was exerting on his zipper. Whoever had coined the expression "blue balls" sure knew what he was talking about. He looked down at the bulge in his lap knowing that if he were able to see his, that they would indeed be blue from all the repeated engorgement with no release in sight. He forced himself to think about something else.

The new patient that he had seen today came to mind. Pete Riddel. Pete was an executive with Virginia Power. His teenage son Robert had died a few months ago from an overdose of an inhalant. He had been at a party and a few of the kids had cajoled him into trying it for the first time. Convinced that his first hit hadn't yielded him anything they encouraged him to try several more times. Within minutes he was vomiting and stumbling around. Then he was out cold. Never to wake up again.

Pete and his wife, MaryAnn, along with their three other children were devastated. Pete had a hard time accepting the fact that his son was gone. When he finally realized it was true that Robert would never come home again, he became obsessed with the safety of his other children.

He carefully monitored their lives, keeping a chart on each of them with their activities and friends listed. He went everywhere he could with them or he sent MaryAnn to accompany them. None of them were allowed to attend any parties or events where there wasn't an adult present at the party, not just somewhere in the house. The nine and eleven year old boys were not as upset by all these changes as the fourteen year old girl was. She complained bitterly to her mother that this wasn't fair. She had only just started dating recently.

Not only did he monitor them as if they were spies from another country, he also did spot checks of their rooms at least three times a week. He would empty out drawers and pull heavy dressers away from the walls, as well as check their videos to make sure that what the label showed was what they were actually watching. He listened to all their CDs before he let them listen to them and he talked to all their teachers every week to see if they had noticed anything unusual in their behavior. In short, he was driving them crazy from the moment they woke up until he personally tucked them into bed each and every night.

MaryAnn was also dealing with her grief in her own way. She was depressed and cried almost all the time she was awake, so she had decided that sleep was her best friend and spent most of the day in bed or on the sofa sleeping or talking on the phone to her many well-wishing friends. She knew Pete was going overboard but she really didn't care. At least someone was keeping track of the kids, she thought.

Finally the complaints from the kids got through to Pete's parents and they talked him into getting some help. MaryAnn had started participating in a group program for mothers who had lost children but Pete was reluctant to meet in a group setting. So his parents set up an appointment for him with a therapist they had heard about. That therapist was Dr. Sandler and he'd met with Pete today.

Chapter 56

Tidal Basin—Washington, D.C.

Betsy's driver pulled up to the curb in front of the monument. Just outside the darkened window of her limousine was a group of tourists posing for a picture and beyond them were several clusters of girl scout troops with their leaders trying to line them up for a head count. She loved coming to Washington on Saturdays. She used to ride in on the Metro line from the University of Maryland when she'd been a student there. Since she'd won the lottery she hadn't had to suffer the rude glances from people because she took up two seats instead of one. She loved the city of Washington. And she especially loved it on Saturdays. There was a different feeling between weekdays and weekends here.

Even the hustle and bustle during the week was distinctly different for each day of the week. Monday's walkers had a just-dragged-in-from-a-long-weekend look and their step was not at all lively. Tuesdays were better and a feeling of resurgent careers seemed to be on everyone's minds as they got serious again about the work of the city. Wednesdays were more productive as work seemed to actually be getting done and faces were a bit more expectant. Thursdays were filled with planning the weekend and the next day's relaxed wardrobe and Friday was the upbeat, havin'-lunch-out-leavin'-work-early frame of mind with everyone smiling brightly anticipating the upcoming weekend.

Saturday was a whole new crowd. Tourists from all over the country and the world clamoring to see the halls of democracy as they lay dormant until Monday morning. People from the Maryland and Virginia suburbs brought their children and relatives into the city for a taste of the culture. And then there were the people like her, there to just experience the influx of all the kinds of people it took to make up the Washington D.C. society she loved.

271

Before extricating herself from the back seat for her weekly people-watching jog around the tidal basin, she swallowed one of her allergy pills that she had shaken out of the prescription vial that she kept in her fanny pack. The Washington parks were some of the most beautiful in the country but to allergy suffers like herself, they paid a big price to admire all the lovely trees.

Her driver helped her step out of her car and she arranged for him to pick her up in two hours. That would be plenty of time for exercise and vicarious voyeuring. The city tended to get very hot very early in the day since it was summertime.

She started out walking at a leisurely pace enjoying the sounds and sights around her. She tried to be oblivious to the obvious stares at her from curious children and rude adults. She knew she looked a sight. Her long dark hair was piled in a large top knot on her head. She did this so it wouldn't get all sweaty and require shampooing again.

Her jogging set was the lightest weight nylon she could find with the unzipped ankle cuffs rolled up to mid calf. Her size 11 Nike running shoes had a wide platform to support her and to spread out the impact of her weight. Her socks had been cut at the top because the elastic was cutting off her circulation and they fell down around the tops of her shoes. Under her unzipped nylon jacket was a T shirt cropped just below the waist to allow for movement of her hips. Adding to the whole mish mash of her attire was her black and white fanny pack snugged up over her nonexistent waist.

She admired the physiques of several young jocks playing a game of touch football in a clearing between some trees. Oh, what she would give to have a body that they would appreciate as much as she appreciated theirs. Her breathing started to get labored but she just chalked it up to her recently incited sexual thoughts. She started to pick up the pace and began a fast walk, arms swinging forward and back with each step.

She was not feeling right, something was off. Suddenly she couldn't catch her breath. When she felt a sharp twinge in her chest she backed off and clutching her hand to her chest she stumbled forward a few more steps until she fell against the side of a large oak tree next to the path. As her fingers gripped the bark on the tree she blinked her eyes trying to shake the dizzying feeling in her head. She was vaguely aware that people had stopped to stare at her as she leaned her head against the tree trunk panting and trying to get her breath.

The next thing she knew she was lying on the sun-warmed grass staring up through the canopy of branches the trees formed over her. People were panicking all around her and she was thinking how beautiful and peaceful the view before her was. The sun was trying to find an opening in the leaves spread out above her and it flickered in and out shadowing her face. A man's face appeared above her and for a moment she thought it was the face of the man on the deck waiting for her at the lake in Vermont. She tried to smile as she lifted her hand to touch his cheek. It fell back to the ground just as her fingers grazed his unshaven chin.

An ambulance came, and from the descriptions of the onlookers, it was assumed that she'd had a heart attack. It had all the classic signs of one. She was seen clutching her chest, having trouble breathing and she certainly did look like a good candidate for one. The paramedics tried to revive her on the ground. When that was unsuccessful they, along with several park policemen, managed to get her into the ambulance.

She was pronounced dead as soon as she arrived at the hospital. Through the prescription bottle in her fanny pack they were able to identify her and determine that she was highly allergic. A cursory autopsy was done several days later and anaphylactic shock was listed as the probable cause of death but the causative agent wasn't pinpointed even though the presence of peanuts was listed as one of several food items found in her stomach.

A detective was assigned to the case and he used the prescription label to track down the doctor who had prescribed her allergy medicine. The doctor confirmed what was in her file.

She was highly allergic to peanuts and knew how dangerous it would be to ingest any.

The detective spoke with the housekeeper who told him what she had fixed for Betsy's breakfast that day and it matched the items listed on the autopsy report. She also told him that she knew about all of Betsy's allergic problems. It was one of the reasons she had been hired. All of Betsy's food had to be prepared from scratch to make sure none of the offending ingredients were used unknowingly. Nuts or any items with any by-products of nuts were not even allowed in the apartment.

Betsy's driver told him that she'd had nothing to eat or drink on the way to the Memorial with the exception of her allergy pill, which she always took right before she left to go walking. The remaining pills had been checked. They were exactly what her doctor had prescribed. The effects of peanuts on her system according to her doctor would have been pretty immediate. Since she had made it all the way to the tidal basin that meant she probably would had to have eaten it sometime after she left the car. There were plenty of vendors in that area and peanuts were usually one of the items sold there. Was it possible this was a suicide? With nowhere else to go with this and no grieving relative pressuring him to find an answer, the detective let the case lay around for a few days and then filed it with all the other unsolved ones this city seemed to generate.

Betsy was buried a few days later. Her housekeeper, her driver and her attorney were the only ones present. There had been no need to post an obituary, none of them knew of anyone else who knew her, but her attorney had done so anyway. It had just seemed like the proper thing to do.

Chapter 57

Fairfax, VA

David was in a vile mood. It was Sunday morning and he couldn't sleep. That was probably because he'd gone to bed at nine o'clock last night, bored out of his mind. He had completely forgotten that this was the week that Jenny, the kids and her parents were going to North Carolina for their vacation. They wouldn't be back until Friday. She had invited him, but she hadn't given him enough notice to keep his schedule clear, so he couldn't accompany them.

He was lonely and he missed them. He was envisioning Jenny in her new two piece bikini, her skin all warm and brown from the sun. He was fantasizing about the things they could do together in the surf late at night when the kids and her parents were asleep.

He was thinking about all the fun he was missing watching Paisley in the pool and playing in the sand when he heard the thump of the Sunday newspaper hit the bottom of the door to his apartment. He got up from the table and went to get it. Well, at least this would occupy his time for awhile.

The Sunday edition of the Washington Post was the equivalent of five weekday papers. There was a little something for everyone in its pages. But, first things first. Since Nancy Meridan's death it had become his habit to check the obituaries daily so he turned to that page first. Not recognizing any of the pictures he was about to turn the page when his eye caught the name Drayton in the lower left hand corner. My God! Betsy! She had actually died! A feeling of sadness enveloped him for a moment but instantly disappeared when he remembered the significance of her death.

He read the small notice. Apparently she had died last Saturday and had already been buried in a Washington area cemetery. There was no mention of how she died, only that it

275

had been sudden. Her obituary was incredibly small compared to all the others and that's when he noticed that the "survived by" names were missing.

He had known that she had no family but it was still hard to realize that there was no one affected by her death. Except him, of course. Now he would just have to see how *affected* he would be. All that money she had from the lottery. He wondered how much she'd left him. He hoped it would be substantial but not so much that anyone would come around asking about it.

His mood was greatly improved with the prospect of some financial relief in the near future and he was kind of thrilled that he had masterminded the perfect murder. He thumbed through the Local section and the Style section to see if by chance there was an article about Betsy anywhere. There wasn't. Her death hadn't been that significant in a city where there were so many every day.

He was curious now. He wanted to know more about how it had happened. He could call her housekeeper after Betsy missed her next appointment but he knew he would arouse suspicion if he called before then. He finally resigned himself to waiting until her missed appointment or until he was notified by her attorney. Then he could find out what had happened without seeming too nosy. It was like being a seven year old waiting for Christmas to come. You knew you were going to get a present but you didn't know what it would be.

Chapter 58

Carolina Beach, NC

Condo Unit Reefs V- 2B

Jenny got up early as she always did when they were at the beach. She quietly dressed in jogging shorts and a favorite tattered old T-shirt, threw on a pair of socks and her Reeboks. Everyone was still asleep so she was especially careful to make no noise as she grabbed a paper cup and filled it with water in the kitchen. She took a few healthy swigs and then grabbed her yellow Sony walkman by the door and left the beach condo they had rented for the week.

This was one of her favorite times of the day. Waking up and getting out just as the sun was coming up and the beach was coming alive with fishermen and joggers and a few romantic couples who, for one reason or another, hadn't made it back to their rooms last night. As she passed the path beside the pool she attached her walkman to her waist, inserted the tiny headphones in her ears and pressed the play button. The sounds of "Hooked on Classics II" made her perk up her steps. She tried to match her pace with the sounds of "Russian and Ludmila", "Czardas" and Beethoven's "Pathetique Sonata", and other than having to dodge the fishing lines from the surf fishers from time to time, she was doing all right trying to keep up.

It was a glorious morning. The sun was promising to be full and hot and was in ready view early in the day. The water was a foamy blue-green, lapping in and out, creating little eddy pools that small children would later play in before the tide went out this afternoon. A few joggers passed her by. She was a walker, not a runner. She could walk for miles and miles but she absolutely detested running.

She had tried running once when a friend of hers had told her about the "runner's high" he got at a certain point in his daily run. He had coached her for three months until she had worked up to six miles a day. Finally after four months she had experienced it. She never ran again. That little rush of headiness wasn't worth the hours of sweat and side aches it had cost her. So she was more than content to wave to the marathon men as they passed, ignoring the double takes a few made as they realized how pretty she was.

As she examined the different tread patterns from the footprints ahead of her, she tried to put some things in perspective about her life. She was reasonably happy. She had two marvelous kids that she simply adored. She had a very successful career and a beautiful home. She had lots of friends and a loving, caring family. Why was there a nagging feeling that she was missing out on something?

She knew it was a stupid question to ask herself. She knew exactly what she was missing. Sex. Love. Adult male companionship. She had heard once that there are only two types of people who walk the beach alone. Those who lament a lost love and those who are looking for a new one. She knew she was in the category of the second. She longed to have the intimacy she saw as she watched the couples walking arm in arm on the beach at sunset. Young and old, they had something she desperately wanted but could not find.

Oh, she may have thought that she was on her way to having it with David, but that was just wishful thinking. She didn't have it and never would with him and she knew it. She felt guilty that he didn't know it, because she'd known it for a long time. No matter how hard she tried to be in love with him, she simply wasn't. He was everything a woman could ask for in a mate and life companion. He was a good provider, he loved her children, he was handsome, tall, gentle and caring. But his kisses turned her off and she couldn't abide the thought of lying in bed beside him doing the things her body was yearning to do, just not with him. But she did miss him. He was a good friend.

As she looked out at the ocean and watched the shrimp boats heading out to sea and then back at the surf foaming a few feet from her, she knew that there would be a man walking out of the water one day onto the beach to claim her heart. She could almost see him smiling at her and reaching his hand out to her. She just had to be patient and look for God's will in her life. If God had wanted David for her, he would have made the chemistry work for them. She resigned herself to that and promised herself that when she got home she and David would talk.

A group of pelicans flew in a line across the first breaking waves about fifty feet offshore. She watched as they soared and then glided and then swooped. God, how she loved it here. She had been coming with her family to this beach since the year Rusty was born. It was a solace unlike any other. Always so peaceful, even when it was crowded. Carolina Beach was a nice family beach and was still years away from the commercialization that was Ocean City or Virginia Beach.

She loved everything they did down here and every year they pretty much did the same things. She even liked going to the grocery store here. The people were so friendly and chatty that she never even minded when she had to stand in line. The cashiers asked her if she needed any help unloading the groceries from her "buggy" onto the conveyor belt and the store manager told her if she ever needed a specialty cut of meat that all she had to do was to "mash" the button at the meat counter. She loved listening to the locals with their southern colloquialisms and twangy accents. It reminded her of the old Shake and Bake commercials where the little girl proudly exclaims, "And I hepped."

Just ahead was the pier and she could see that it was filling up with fishermen setting up their own little areas with their coolers and chairs to spend the day angling for the big one. She knew that by the time she reached the pier the tape would have finished playing "Rhapsody in Blue" by Gershwin, Foster's "Camptown Races", Dvorak's 1st movement "From the New

World" and one of her favorites, Emmett's "I Wish I Was in Dixie's Land." If she was on her usual track it would be time to slap the tall pilings of the pier and turn around just as the "Battle Hymn of the Republic" came to life through the tiny yellow wires running to her ears.

The sun was becoming hot now and sweat was beginning to drip down her neck and between her breasts, but she was exultant. There wasn't anything she'd rather be doing at this precise moment than what she was doing. Strolling, albeit rather rapidly, on a beautiful sunny beach thinking about how God was going to provide her with a perfect love. If she could just hang in there until it was time.

She walked back to their second story condo with the balcony overlooking the pool, and using her key, she entered the unit to find everyone awake. The kids were sitting on the sofa watching cartoons and her mother was fixing breakfast. Her dad had gone to the little shop on the corner to get the morning paper. The kids were already in their swimsuits eager for a morning at the beach and an afternoon at the pool.

Playing with them in the pool and teaching them to swim was one of the best parts of their days at the beach. She also loved the time she spent with her mother in the late afternoon while the kids were napping. They would talk and reminisce while preparing a big delicious dinner. After dinner they would all go back down to the beach to fly a kite or just walk along the water's edge picking up shells. There just wasn't anything she didn't like about being at the beach. One day she thought, I'd like to live here.

Chapter 59

Chantilly High School

Pete Riddel made the loop around the long driveway after dropping his kids off at school. This was a fairly new thing for him because they used to ride the bus. Since Robert died, a lot of things had changed though and as he looked over the intricate grid of his three children's activities attached to a clipboard on his lap he wondered for the thousandth time why he hadn't been doing this all along. Why hadn't he been more aware of his children and their comings and goings before now?

He reflected back to the time when Robert was a staggering two-year old toddler. He had been vigilant then. He had watched him or made sure someone else was watching him the entire time Robbie was awake. He had carefully padded all the sharp-cornered edges of every piece of furniture throughout the house. He had installed child safety latches on every bathroom and kitchen cabinet. He had even tied the Christmas tree to a series of hooks in the corner of the family room to insure that it couldn't be pulled over. When had he let his guard down?

He supposed it had happened gradually as the other children came along and there were more smiling and drooling faces to protect. Then again, Robbie had earned each level of independence, displaying a remarkable maturity for his age as he grew up and helped supervise each younger sibling's tottering stages. When had Robbie become so careless with himself? Pete and his wife MaryAnn hadn't seen it. But then, how hard had they been looking for it?

At the end of the day over dinner they had asked all the appropriate questions, checked out the state of his eyes and speech and smelled his breath whenever they hugged him. But apparently that hadn't been enough. Robbie was lying twenty feet under ground in a double crypt in a cemetery in Falls Church waiting for his family to join him in forty, fifty or sixty years.

At a stop light he made a notation on the chart by Kristin's name. "Help study session in math 3:30-4:30, separate pick up." Fortunately for Pete he was pretty high up in the corporate ladder at Virginia Power and he was able to adjust his schedule to meet the demands of his children. His children didn't think it was their good fortune but they had learned that this was not an issue to get into with their father. They abided by his wishes and obsessive checking up on them hoping that this would pass as he dealt with the loss of his beloved first son.

The concession he made to them was to get some help dealing with the grief. He was on his way to see Dr. Sandler right now for what would be their first attempt at hypnotherapy. He was hoping to have some of the success that MaryAnn was having with her group sessions.

He pulled into the parking garage under Dr. Sandler's office building and after briefly glancing at the kid's schedule for the next event he would be shuttling one of them to, he slipped it under the seat. No one else needed to know where his kids would be later on in the day.

He took the elevator to the sixth floor and entered the door to Dr. Sandler's office. The receptionist told him that the doctor was expecting him and that he could go right in. When he opened the door, David looked up from some papers he was reading on his desk and smiled. "Mr. Riddel, how nice to see you. Please, please come in. Have a seat." He led him over to a long cushiony couch. "How are you managing things this week?"

"Better than I thought I would be actually. I enjoyed our talk about Robbie last week and was actually looking forward to coming to see you. Very few people want to talk about Robbie with me anymore." Pete said shaking his head. "I guess it's just too depressing for us all to remember him right now."

"Well, yes, I'm sure it is. But this is the time you need to talk about him the most. Did you have a chance to do the things I asked you about?" David asked.

"MaryAnn and I went into his room just the other night to try to find the things you asked about. We couldn't find a journal or any letters but we did find a photo album he had started and a yearbook with lots of writing on all the pages. And I took some pictures of his room just like you asked." He reached into his inside suit coat and pulled out a small envelope and handed it to David.

As David walked back to his desk he took the pictures out and fanned through them as he looked at them. One thing stood out to his trained mind instantly. "Your son, he was a pretty big baseball fan?"

"Yes," Pete said, "he was on the school team and whenever we could, he and I went to see the Orioles at Camden Yard or the Prince William Cannons minor league team here in Manassas. He was in the process of teaching his brothers how to play, I think they miss those Saturday afternoons with him at the park more than anything."

"Good with kids, too?" David asked.

"Yes, he was. He wanted to become a teacher. Maybe even a P.E. teacher. God, what a waste!" Pete cried out as tears tumbled out of his eyes and streamed down his cheeks before he caught them with the back of his hand.

"Tell me about the album you found and the yearbook. What did you find out about your son that you hadn't known before?" David said as he sat back in his chair, fingers steepled over his chest.

Pete thought for a few moments and then said, "He was well-liked. Not just by the friends he'd had for years but by everyone, all types of kids. Almost every page had something really nice written about him and signed in the yearbook. And quite a few wished him good luck as a teacher, saying he sure would be better than Mr. So-and-So or Mrs. Dragon-something."

"What about the album? Anything surprising there?" David prompted.

"No, not really. Just a bunch of kids posing together trying to look as ridiculous as possible. Again, I was pleased that he had so many friends."

"Were there a lot of them at his funeral?" David asked.

"I'm not really sure. I was pretty much a zombie the whole time. I think so. It's hard to say," Pete mumbled.

David got up and walked over to the couch. "Here, do something for me. Take off your shoes, and swing your body around this way, putting your head in this well-worn depression." David indicated an end cushion that had over time developed a perfect cradle for a person's neck. Just before Pete laid back to put his head in it, David put a handkerchief over the dent to keep the cushion clean. He walked to the end of the couch and placed a pillow under Pete's stockinged ankles.

"Pete, we're going to try something this morning that may or may not work. But please be open-minded and let's give this a go. If we can relax you and get you focused, I believe we can channel some of your grief away. Are you game?" David asked.

"Sure, Doc. I'm in your hands. Just tell me what you want me to do. I'm anxious to see how this works."

"Close your eyes and think of concentric circles. Visualize them going down, down, down. Spinning into a deep black void. Disappearing but always being replaced by another. Round and round. Down and down." While David was softly crooning these words he placed the tip of his middle finger in the center of Pete's forehead and rubbed it ever so gently in larger circles collapsing into smaller ones. Over and over again until Pete was under.

"You've come to a new place. A place you've never been before. You have a wonderful, light-hearted feeling. Everything is peaceful here. In front of you some big fluffy clouds part and you see a little boy with a bat swinging at a baseball. He misses and hangs his head down. Suddenly from the sidelines comes a young man, a very handsome young man with a brig grin on his face. 'C'mon slugger', he says as he stands behind the boy showing him how to hold the bat without overlapping his hands. 'Now, be sure to keep your elbows out and it'll go a mile!' "

"The young man steps aside and the pitcher sends another ball across the plate. This time the little boy swings out and connects. The ball goes flying way up into the air, disappearing for a few seconds into the baby blue sky before arcing back to clear the fence. The cheers are deafening as the little boy runs the bases, puffing and puffing as he tags third and then slides into home plate. 'Thanks, Coach Robbie. You were right about the elbows!' 'You, my good man, are a slugger of the first caliber,' Coach Robbie says as the little boy beams up at him. As the coach puts his arm around the little boy's shoulder they turn to go back to the dug out. Coming from the middle of their shoulder blades is the faintest shadowing of their gossamer wings deflecting the stadium lights."

David stops speaking and allows the quiet to seep into them. He looks over at Pete who seems to have the most serene expression on his face. He waits a few minutes before walking over to him and removing the pillow from beneath his ankles. He lightly rubs his finger on Pete's forehead in circles going the opposite direction from the ones he had done before. "Now, we are unwinding and the circles are coming back up out of the black void, surfacing and popping like bubbles on the water. One by one they form and rise and pop until there are no more and you are back. Back to this body, back to this couch, back to this office." Pete opens his eyes and stares at the ceiling.

"My boy is exactly where he wants to be isn't he?" he asks.

"Yes, I think he is. Next week do you think you might be up to watching more of the game?" David asks.

"Definitely!" Pete says, "I wouldn't miss it for anything." Pete got up from the couch, shook Dr. Sandler's hand as he said thank you and left to go to work a little less heavy-hearted.

Chapter 60

Fairfax, VA

After Pete Riddel left, David checked with his receptionist about his next appointment. He had half an hour before his next patient. He went down to the little deli on the first floor of his office building and got a cup of coffee and a bagel. On the way back up he thought about Pete Riddel. He was a little surprised that he had taken so well to the hypnosis. At their first meeting he had struck him as a man who wouldn't succumb so easily for some reason. Well, he had, and that pleased David immensely.

After a few more sessions he should be able to do *The Campaign* as he was beginning to refer to it in his head. Once he selected a *death lottery winner*, he then performed *the campaign*. *The Campaign* being the solicitation part of his hypnosis, the *soft touch* for funds so to speak, just as the politicians did it. Hence the idea for *campaign funds*. It was no worse than asking them for a contribution. If people wanted to give, then they would. If they didn't, then they wouldn't. The difficulty here was in accelerating the date for the reading of their will.

Pete would be a good candidate. David smiled at the pun he had made to himself. Candidate, indeed. Pete was a high income earner and because of his obsessiveness over his family it was almost a given that he had a will to provide for them should anything happen to him. And it was highly likely that something could happen to him. What with him being so depressed and all. Suicide seemed like Pete's most direct avenue to Robbie. At least that's how it would seem. No one would doubt that his emotions had gotten in the way of his common sense. Grief could be and often was a double reaper.

David's next patient was Leroy Dressler. Leroy was what most people would call a "neat-freak." Only for him the freak part really applied. He would go berserk if there was any dirt on or around him. He washed his hands constantly, actually wearing out the porcelain inlays in the faucet handles at home long before their time. He was petrified of animals and hardly ever ventured outside his own little realm of sanitized living. He was fortunate that he lived in the city and never had to venture any further into the outside world than parking garages.

His wife had died eight years ago, leaving him quite wealthy. She had been a Washington socialite in her heyday and found Leroy's mannerisms to be cute. Of course then he'd been neat and clean, not fanatically compulsive about it. Her family had owned a chain of Washington area jewelry stores. She'd inherited three of them and Leroy had inherited them in turn. Leroy had found that living in the city afforded him the perfect way to stay clean.

He went from his luxury suite at the Watergate to the parking garage to his immaculately clean Lincoln Continental. From there he would only go to a destination that also had a parking garage. He wore disposable plastic gloves to push elevator buttons and open doors. He only went to locations that he deemed sterile or that he could make that way without compromising the germ barrier he pictured around himself.

He would never go to a movie theater but occasionally he would go to the Kennedy Center just around the corner, if he was able to buy the tickets for the whole box. Then he would give the usher a very large tip to disinfect the area with the supplies he always carried with him in a soft briefcase. He didn't eat out. Ever. He had a cook who'd had to pass some very stringent tests to meet his guidelines to be able to cook for him.

He didn't have to go to work often, since he had some very competent and trusted managers that had been with the company almost from its inception. But he still kept an office in the one jewelry store that was located in the mall of a high rise building on K Street. It was cleaned four times a day. Or that's what he thought. In actuality it was cleaned when the store was closed for the night and then again just before he was expected to arrive.

Of course he knew his behavior wasn't exactly normal, but it had never been a problem to him until recently. In his late sixties, balding and paunchy, Leroy wasn't exactly the romantic type. He wasn't looking for love or companionship when he found it. One night at the Kennedy Center as he was sitting alone in his box waiting for the show to begin, he noticed a very attractive older woman sitting in the front row a few boxes to his right.

She was looking at him and she smiled. He smiled back at her. Throughout the first and second acts of "Sleuth" every time he looked in her direction he found that she was looking at him. He never left his box during intermission but noticed that she was not in hers. A few minutes later an usher appeared with a playbill that had a handwritten message scrawled across the front of it.

He looked at it dumbly for a moment while the usher kept trying to hand it to him. Finally he took a plastic glove out of his jacket pocket, put it on and took the playbill from him. When the usher didn't leave he remembered that the courtesy of a tip would be expected and he laid the playbill down on the seat beside him while he fished in his pocket for some money with his gloved hand.

The message was from a Ms. Margaret Hyde and she said that she had noticed that he was always alone in his box. Would he like some company sometime? Maybe they could talk after the show. When his eyes scanned the seats for her, he was disappointed that he couldn't find her, but after the show had resumed he saw her sitting there, a smile and a shrug indicated that she was waiting for his answer. He just nodded his head and after the show she found her way to his box.

She'd had quite a time adjusting to all his idiosyncrasies at first, but the fact that he was very wealthy gave him a lot of leeway. Fortunately, she was also a very neat and orderly person, just nowhere near the degree that he was. They established a nice platonic relationship but it was obvious that they both wanted more.

Margaret wanted to travel. He said that was out of the question. She insisted on going on a cruise if nothing else and said she'd go with him or without him. He knew that he was in jeopardy of losing her if he didn't accompany her, so he accepted the fact that he had some problems to deal with and agreed to seek treatment.

The sessions were going very well. Leroy was actually walking around without his cleaning kit in his briefcase, but he still hadn't had much to do with places that weren't accessible to the inside directly from his car. He talked about hiring a helicopter to deliver him to the deck of the cruise ship so he could avoid the crowds of strange people.

He had already been assured that their suite of rooms would be cleaned in any manner he chose and that it would be more than all right for his own housekeeper and cook to accompany them to take care of their needs. Leroy could have his meals in their room and then he could accompany Margaret to the dining room while she ate and socialized with the other passengers at their table. He would have been happy to stay in their suite and take his meals there while she dined in the dining room, but he was afraid that Margaret would be approached by many suitors if he wasn't there by her side.

He thought that she was very attractive for her age and he knew he would be jealous if any man so much as approached her. He was really trying to get all he could out of his therapy sessions so they could travel together.

David felt that today would be a good time for *The Campaign*.

Chapter 61

Tyson's Corner, VA

Jenny sat in her office behind her desk massaging her feet, her hot, tired, sore feet. It had been a really rough day. Hot and muggy. Washington's only promise for summer. It had all started with an 8:30 sales meeting to get the sales force all pumped up. "Spot money" had been handed out to everyone with a promise of more to come. The idea behind spot money was to give the salesmen a cash bonus to keep in their pocket with the guarantee that they could keep it if they delivered one unit. At the end of the day if they hadn't sold a car or a truck they had to return it.

Psychologically, this was a very hard thing to do and management knew it. So it usually ensured that the most diligent efforts to deliver a car would be made. If you were lucky enough to sell more than one, you could go back for more "on the spot" money. Jenny had delivered four. The last one was in settlement now and she was trying to rub some feeling back into her toes while they were signing all the papers. The showroom was practically deserted. Most of the sales force had already left to go home.

While she was putting away the car keys to the last six cars she had shown in the key closet, Neal approached her and asked if he could speak to her. She had walked from her office across the length of the showroom to the closet in her stocking feet. Without her four-inch heels, Neal loomed over her and she felt a moment of trepidation as she thought that maybe he had found out what she had done. "Sure," she mumbled, "I'll be right there, just let me put these keys away."

She padded back to her office crossing the now quiet and darkened showroom. Neal was waiting, sitting like a customer in one of the chairs in front of her desk. She took her seat and asked, "What's up?"

Neal reached his hand across the desk as if to shake hers, "Today was my last day, I got my paycheck yesterday and I found that I have more than enough to pay for school. Almost a whole month before I expected to."

Jenny didn't say anything. She just sat there and waited for him to tell her that he knew she had arranged for the cost prices to be adjusted. But he didn't. Instead she was pleasantly surprised when he stood and shook her hand and said, "I just wanted you to know that it's been a pleasure working with you. You're a real class act. Many times you could've made things hard on me but instead you helped me out and showed me the way to be a professional. I have never met anyone as competent as you are at selling cars and to see you do it so well without ever being dishonest to the customer is so refreshing. I will miss watching you and following your example, I just wanted you to know that."

He turned to leave and Jenny called after him, "Neal, it's been great working with you, too. I'm really going to miss the competition you gave me," she said with a chuckle. "By the way, what exactly are you studying in college if you don't mind me asking?"

"Theology," was his one-word answer.

"Theology?" she asked, raising her right eyebrow. "You're studying to be a priest?" she said as if she was stunned by the idea of that.

"No, actually, I'm Jewish. I'm not sure where I'm going to go from here. Next summer I'm going to go work on a kibbutz in Israel and decide if I have it in me to become a Rabbi."

Jenny took a minute to absorb all that and then said, "Well, we're really gonna miss you next summer."

"Yeah, me too. Thanks for the experience," he called as he walked out the front showroom doors.

Jenny sat down hard in her chair. Well! Who would of thunk it? A future Rabbi selling cars. Boy! This business was really opening up.

Just then her customers came down the center hallway and she greeted them with a big smile. "Looks like we're going to be the last ones out of here tonight. C'mon, let's go over your owner's packet while we're waiting for them to finish cleaning your new car."

It was almost 8:30 before she was in her demo headed home. This was her first day back since returning from the beach and it had been brutal. She was hot, sweaty, and she'd never been able to get her shoes back on her feet. She was driving barefoot having removed her pantyhose in the ladies' room before she left the dealership.

She pulled up to her parents' house and got out. She opened the front door with her key and walked down the hallway to the kitchen. Her mother was sitting on the couch crocheting. "Where are the kids?" Jenny asked.

"I just got them down. They were still a little tired from the drive back yesterday and they both were nodding off right after dinner."

This was a little disappointing to Jenny because it meant that they wouldn't be going home with her. Not that she would miss them that much while they were sleeping, but she really did look forward to waking up with them on Sunday mornings when they didn't have any place to be until church at 11:00. She turned back the way she had come and went upstairs to check on them.

Paisley was in her little junior bed surrounded by every kind of stuffed animal conceivable. Jenny moved a little white rabbit aside so she could stroke her cheek. She had been drooling on her pillow and Jenny wiped the corner of her lips where it glistened. She looked down at her beautiful baby girl and smiled. Then she went to check on Rusty.

Rusty was not quite asleep and he opened his eyes when she walked into his room. "Hi, Mommy," he slurred sleepily.

"Hi, Sweetie," Jenny said as she sat on the edge of the bed and brushed a few strands of hair from his forehead.

"I didn't think I'd get to see you tonight," he whispered softly.

"Neither did I," she softly whispered back. "People were lined up everywhere to buy cars today. We actually didn't have enough salesmen for the better part of the afternoon."

"So, you made a lot of money today?" he asked.

"Yesss," she said drawing it out, wondering what his point was.

"Enough to buy me that new Transformer I saw on TV today?"

"Maybe. We'll see. You go to sleep now and we'll talk about it in the morning." But she knew darned well that if she didn't buy it for him, her mother would.

She walked downstairs to where her mother was and leaned down to give her a kiss on the cheek. "Did you eat dinner yet?" She asked. "There's plenty of leftovers in the icebox."

Her mother was the only one she knew who called a refrigerator an icebox. As her mother moved to get up to fix her some dinner Jenny gently pushed her back into her seat at the end of the sofa. "I'm not hungry, Mom. It's too late to eat anyway and besides I had who knows how many pieces of pizza today between deliveries. See you tomorrow. Love ya."

Jenny locked the door behind her and drove to her house just a few miles away. David's car was parked out front but there was no sign of him in it. Great. She really wasn't up to this tonight, but she felt that it would be better to get it over with now than to keep leading David on that there was a future for them other than friendship.

As Jenny pulled into the driveway she noticed that the T-tops were out of David's Trans Am and she remembered when she had sold it to him last year that she had thought he'd probably never take them out. He was always so particular about his appearance that she didn't think he'd like it if his hair got blown around a bit. She wondered where he was. She had never given him a key to her house.

She unlocked the French doors at the top of the driveway and went in through the kid's playroom and then into the family room, turning on lights as she went. She heard a faint tapping on

293

the sliding glass door leading to the deck from the family room so she walked over and pulled the long chain that slid the vertical louvers back. There stood David with a big smile on his face.

She noticed that every hair was in place. She pulled up the safety bar and unlocked the door and stepped out into the beautiful summer night. It was rare to see the stars because there were so many lights in the suburbs, but tonight they were out in all their glory, like little rhinestones on a drop cloth of black velvet.

"Hi! I tried calling you at the dealership but I forgot that the switchboard closes at six on Saturdays," David said as he moved to give her a hug.

"I wouldn't have had time to talk anyway. We were so busy today," she said as she accepted the hug and then moved to the door. "Would you like something to drink? I've had a glass of champagne on my mind for the last couple of hours," she said as she went back inside and headed towards the kitchen.

He followed and replied, "I brought some wine. I'll have some of this," he said as he placed the bottle on the counter and opened a drawer to get the corkscrew.

As soon as he had the cork out, he walked over to where she stood and wrapped his arms around her. He helped her ease the cork out of the bottle of champagne. His breath tickled her ear as he whispered, "I've missed you. It's been a very long week."

He gently turned her around and placing a hand on each side of her head he leaned down to kiss her. His lips gently moved over hers and then when his tongue entered between her lips and sought to seek the sweetness of her mouth the kiss became almost fierce with his desire. As his fingers threaded through the hair at her temples holding her face close to his he kissed first one side of her lips and then the other twisting his face back and forth to match his lips against hers.

It wasn't apparent to him that Jenny was just a sideline spectator in his ravishment of her lips and mouth. When he started to trail little kisses down her throat to her neck, she gently pushed him away saying, "David, I'm all hot and sweaty. I feel

294

so grubby. I really need a nice long hot shower. And this," she said as she turned back to the counter and poured herself a glass of the champagne. She held it up and smiled, "Ah, the elixir of life!" she said taking a nice long sip. "C'mon, let's go back outside. We need to talk." Then she led the way back to the deck.

David didn't like the sound of this. He grabbed his glass of wine with one hand and both bottles by their necks with the other. They sat down at the little round wooden picnic table with the curved wooden benches. Jenny sat facing the backyard and took in the eerie nighttime image of the kids' wooden tree house at the back of the yard up against the tree line that separated her house from the house behind hers.

She smiled briefly, remembering the day she and her parents along with David had assembled it and put it up. David had come over that morning wearing brand new bib overalls with little loops here and there for a hammer and bib pockets for nails and pencils. He always managed to dress for the occasion. He probably had a safari outfit in the back of his closet, just on the off chance that he would be invited to go to the zoo.

But she also remembered how particular he was about making sure the cement was mixed just right and that the holes for the posts were dug the proper depth. When it came to the safety of her children, he was always going overboard. Sometimes when she watched him playing with Paisley, she got the distinct feeling that he thought she belonged to him. It was so touching how he had bonded with her. And now she was probably going to ruin everything.

"David, I did a lot of soul searching while I was away. I thought about my future and what I want out of life for me and the children. And I thought about us." She hesitated and reached for her glass of champagne. After taking a bracing gulp she began again. "I don't love you David. It's not that I don't want to be in love with you. In a lot of ways I do. But the fact is, I don't and you deserve someone who does. You're a terrific guy and I sometimes feel like I'm crazy not to be in love with you. But you can't choose who you fall in love with, can you?"

David just sat there, both hands wrapped around the glass of wine in front of him. As he stared into the pink liquid he was vaguely aware that there was a gnat floating in it on one side. He looked up at her, his eyes unbelievably sad. "If you could choose, would you choose me?" he simply asked.

She thought for a moment. "Yes, yes I would. In fact, I've been trying to talk myself into being in love with you for quite some time. It just hasn't happened."

A sparkle came back into his eyes and he raised one of his eyebrows just slightly, "Really?" he asked. "You have?"

"Yes, yes I have." She took another sip of her champagne.

"Look, I know you're tired. You've had an exhausting day after a very hectic week. Let me help you unwind a little and relax. Come with me to my apartment house. There's a wonderful indoor pool there where you can cool down. The water will do wonders for your spirit, that and a little more of the bubbly," he said with a sideways smile as he reached over and refilled her glass.

The absolute last thing she wanted to do was to get back in a car and drive somewhere. But the look on his face made her feel guilty. He wasn't taking this as badly as she thought he would, so maybe a gradual easing away from him was the way to do this. A nice cool pool did sound nice. "Won't it be too late for your pool to be open by the time we get there?" she asked.

"I have a key. I can go anytime, night or day." He stood up. "C'mon, get your suit and let's go. I'll bring you back home whenever you're ready. This is exactly what we both need. Trust me." He grabbed the bottles and went inside.

David drove through the back streets of Herndon and Fairfax a little faster than Jenny thought he should, but it was obvious that he was enjoying putting the car through its paces so she didn't say anything. The cool night air coming through the T-tops felt invigorating on her face and she didn't even mind that her long blonde tresses were going to be very tangled by the time they reached his place.

She looked over at David several times. It was odd to see his hair going in so many directions and he had an unusual smile on his face. If she didn't know him better she would have thought that he was taking her hostage or something. He turned to her and took her hand from her lap. He raised it to his lips and kissed her knuckles before replacing it. I don't think he understood what I was trying to tell him, she thought.

When they arrived at his apartment building, they took the elevator to his apartment so he could change into his swim suit. While he was doing that, she walked around looking at his apartment. It wasn't the first time she had been there, but she never failed to marvel at his incredible neatness and taste.

The furnishings were impeccable. Jenny just knew that he had hired a top-notch decorating firm and given them carte blanc. The chocolate brown leather sofa in the living room looked as soft as butter and the chrome and glass tables reflected the light given off by the large arc lamp that rose from behind the couch to almost the middle of the room where it hung suspended over the center of the table. There was a large floral arrangement in a cut crystal vase that was one of the most beautiful arrangements she had ever seen. She walked over to see it closer and was surprised to discover the heady fragrance wafting from it. It wasn't silk as she had originally thought. They were fresh flowers. It must cost a fortune to have such an arrangement delivered fresh each week.

David came out of his bedroom wearing a thick terry cloth robe over his swim suit. He hadn't bothered to tie the belt and she had a glimpse of his impressive chest matted with dark hair. He was certainly a handsome, sexy-looking man, that was for sure. He went into the kitchen which was all done in white except for the tiled floor, a checkerboard pattern in black and white.

He opened the refrigerator and took out a bottle of champagne and a bottle of water. He put them in a carry bag along with some plastic champagne glasses. She noticed that the bag was made by Gucci. Where she would have grabbed a used grocery bag, he grabbed a Gucci one. Maybe that was why she wasn't in love with him. They were so different in so many ways.

"Ready?" he asked. She nodded as he held the front door for her. She had put her suit on under her jeans and sweatshirt before they'd left her house.

"Don't you need a towel?" she asked holding up hers.

"They have them down by the pool. You can leave yours here if you'd like." he answered. Not wanting to have another reason to come back up to his apartment before he took her home she hesitated. Then she threw it across the back of a chair by the door. She just knew that he'd have to come back up here to change. There was no way in hell that he'd drive her home without changing his clothes.

When they got to the pool David used his key to let them in and she noticed that he purposefully relocked it behind them. There was no one else around. The echoes of their shoes on the pool apron resounded like they were in a tomb. David led her over to a wrought iron table with matching chairs set off in a corner. He opened the bottle of champagne while she removed her street clothes. He nodded approvingly at her new bikini, remembering all the times this past week that he had dreamed of her in it.

He handed her a full glass and filled another for him with water. "You're not having any?" she asked.

"I still have to drive, remember? Unless of course you'd like to spend the night in which case I'll go get another bottle."

"No," she said. "You'd better drink the water." She took a sip, set down the glass and walked over to the edge of the pool. Ignoring the stenciled sign about no diving, she dove in.

Oh, David had been right. This felt marvelous. She swam several laps and then came back to hug the side of the pool in the deep end where they had put their things. She saw that David had placed her glass beside the pool and she took several deep sips. She looked over to where he was wrestling a silver raft out of a storage closet. He carried it over to the pool and threw it in.

"Here, you can relax on this." He grabbed the bottle of champagne and leaned over to refill her glass. She remembered she hadn't eaten since lunchtime so she reminded herself to slow down and take smaller sips. She tilted her glass on purpose so that some champagne sloshed into the pool and she was reminded of her friend Deanna, in Virginia, who would have called it alcohol abuse. She didn't like wasting it, but she didn't want to hurt David's feelings and she also didn't want to drink too much tonight. David took off his robe and walked over to the edge of the pool where she was still holding onto the side.

Jenny looked up at him and smiled. He sure was tall. And hairy. His well-defined legs were covered with long strands of black hair and the way he was standing she could almost look right up underneath his suit to the dark thatch she knew would be there. Why was she thinking like this? She must just be a bit horny she thought. It had been ages since she'd been with a man. The days of R.J. seemed like another lifetime ago.

David dove into the water, slicing it clean with his muscular body. He swam several laps before swimming over to her. He picked her up with one hand under her knees and one around her back and deposited her on the silver raft. The raft had a built in pillow and was covered with four-inch wells throughout that the pool water was filling because of her added weight. "Lay back and close your eyes. Just relax for awhile. Concentrate on the sounds the water's making overlapping the raft." She did as he suggested. This was nice. Very nice.

David walked her and the raft towards the shallow end so that he could stand beside her. "Do you remember that movie we watched a few weeks ago with Angie Dickinson in it? The one where she falls off the boat in the middle of the night and her husband spends days trying to find her while she's floating around with a life jacket just barely keeping her chin out of the water?" he asks.

"Yeah," she says. "What was the name of that?" she asks.

"I don't remember. Can you remember how she was floating vertically with her body going up and down with the waves, her arms out in front of her?"

"Yeah," Jenny sighs. "Days and Days of just floating in the hot sun during the day and the cold during the nights."

"Try to put yourself in that frame of mind now. Just floating. Feel your body going up, rising slightly up and back down again with each wave." Gently he rocked the raft simulating the movement of the ocean.

He lightly spun her around on the raft pushing her towards the skimmer flapping lightly with the water current. "Hear the sound of the water as it constantly laps over, washing up and receding back, washing up and receding back, over and over and over again." He lightly splashed water over the edges of the raft so she could feel the water licking her body.

"The sun is shining in your face and you have your eyes closed to the sun. But even with your eyes closed you can still see it through your eyelids. It is so bright. It is so quiet all you can hear is the constant lapping of the water over your body. You are miles and miles from anything. The horizon is unmarked for as far as you can see in any direction. All there is, is water and sky. Just a pure blue sky is overhead. Not even a cloud to diffuse the light blue-grey color. The sound of water lapping and floating, floating, floating. That's all there is."

David looked at Jenny's serene face. She's under. He knows she is. But he tests it anyway. He reaches up and moves the straps of her bathing suit off of her shoulders. She doesn't move a muscle. Then he puts his fingers beneath the underwire cups and lifts them up and over the tops of her breasts, shoving them up as far as they will go. He has to stifle a gasp as he looks at her, drinking in her fullness and rosy peaks with his eyes. She is so beautiful and her nipples are so hard and prominent that he shivers uncontrollably as his own body responds to hers.

He knows that he can't touch her. Not yet. There is still work to be done. And he's not sure if he can do what he needs to do with her exposed to his view like this. So he reaches up and pulls her top back down into place.

"Jenny, as you float along in this current, allowing it to take you wherever it pleases, you have plenty of time to think and to realize things about your life that you never knew. It is along about the second day out here in the sun that you come to realize that you love David. You have always loved David."

"You've denied it of course, but it's true. You do. You find him sexy and romantic and you just love being around him. You can't wait to see him and his kisses just thrill you. So, you've decided that next time he asks you to marry him you'll say 'Yes, yes, yes. I adore you.' You will wake up and profess your love to David as soon as you climax."

David looks at Jenny as she lays there, trance-like but very content. He puts his hand on her flat stomach and slowly eases it down until his fingers touch her bikini bottom. He moves his fingers under the elastic band at the waist and spreads his hand wide. His little finger brushes the hairs that begin her woman's mound and he groans.

He removes his hand and placing a hand at each side of her hips, he hooks his thumbs under the waistband and pulls her bikini bottom down past her hips and past her upper thighs. The sight that greets him causes him to become weak at the knees and he has to remind himself that he could blow this if he's not careful.

He manages to get the bikini pants completely off and tosses them to the side of the pool. Panting heavily he takes in the sight before him. She is exquisite. He sees that she's not really as blonde as one would think from the hair on her head. But he is not unhappy about the light auburn curls that cover her woman's flesh so enticingly. He walks around the raft until he is at the end of it.

Her legs are slightly parted so he can just barely see a sliver of the pink gash he longs to be intimate with. He rubs his hands up and down her calves before he exerts the pressure required to open her up fully for his inspection. The sight he sees is almost his undoing. Again, he has to bite his lips to stifle a groan of ecstasy. Never has he been happier or more in love.

Gently he places a hand under each buttock and slides her gently down to the end of the raft where his eager eyes are waiting to examine her even further. With the lightest of caresses he timidly touches her labia and is incredibly pleased when it opens up to him just like a blooming flower.

Beyond lays paradise and he can't wait to experience it. With almost reverent care he leans forward and kisses her there. He feels her tremble through his hands which are now placed on her outer thighs. He can't stop now. If anyone had come in or if there had been a fire in the building he wouldn't have been able to stop.

He kisses her and licks her and suckles on her and as her juices fill his tongue he swallows her. She starts making barely audible moaning sounds and it escalates his fevered lapping. Suddenly she starts to convulse and in his eagerness to please her he finds her engorged clitoris and sucks on it gently. As she spasms out of control she reaches her hand down and runs her fingers through his hair calling out softly, "David, David, David. I love you." The sound of her voice calling out his name as she spends herself so blissfully causes an unexpected reaction in him. With his mouth still between her legs he feels his own explosion as he ejaculates his sperm into the still waters of the pool.

After a few moments when he isn't sure if he is going to fall down into the pool on his knees or climb up onto the raft with Jenny, he removes his mouth from her womanhood. He quickly looks up at her face to see what's going on there. If this didn't work, he was going to have to feign one or both of them being drunk. She just smiled down at him and said, "David, that was wonderful. I am a little embarrassed about where we are though. What if someone saw us?"

"Well, then they won't have to rent a porn movie will they?" he gibed. He took one last look before he closed her legs and then walked around the raft to where her head was laying to one side. He kissed her very deeply on the lips all the while enjoying the musky smell of her on his own lips. When he broke off he asked, "Jenny, will you marry me?"

She looked into his eyes and ran her fingers through his hair. "Yes, yes, yes, I adore you."

Chapter 62

Fairfax, VA

It was early Monday morning and David had arrived at the office extra early so he could prepare Liesel's medication before he met with her. Normally her appointments were on Wednesdays but after the phone call he'd had from her late Friday afternoon upon her return from the Caribbean, he had talked her into coming in today. If what she had told him was true, then today was the last day he could start her on the new medication.

She had explained to him that while she was on vacation with Daniel her Prozac pills had accidentally become wet and had totally dissolved. She was quick to add that she felt just fine and hadn't missed taking them a bit. She actually thought she was happier than she'd ever been in her life. As he quickly counted up the days from the date she said she had last taken one, he explained to her that that was often the case in manic depressants.

They had a false sense of euphoria just before a monumental bout of depression set in. She had to come in as soon as possible. They agreed on Monday morning. She would be his first appointment. David was able to persuade her that going off Prozac cold turkey like that could trigger a massive depression later and that there was a new medicine that he wanted her to take for a week or two to counteract the reaction.

Having prescribed Prozac to his patients for several years he knew that the one drug that should never be taken within ten days of stopping Prozac was Parnate, a monoamine oxidase inhibitor. It would cause the patient to experience headaches, severe muscle contractions, insomnia and an unsteady gait. The other adverse side effect was death.

He would administer today's dose in his office and give her tomorrow's dose to take with her, along with a prescription dated four days from today. She would never have the opportunity to fill it. In the highly unlikely event that it should ever be discovered that it was the Parnate combined with the discontinuance of Prozac that killed her, he would be able to say that according to the dates she had given him she would have been fine to start the new medication the day the prescription was dated for.

The answer to the question of why the Parnate was already in her system would be easy to answer. He had given her a few to take in case she couldn't get the prescription filled promptly, saying he knew that Parnate was not readily available at most pharmacies and would probably need to be ordered. She apparently had taken them days before he had instructed her to. That would be the end of it.

A half hour later he was still waiting for Liesel to show up. It was highly unusual for her to be late. He was starting to get nervous about it when he saw a courier come through the front office door to the reception area. A few minutes later his receptionist walked into his office and handed him a large envelope. Upon opening it he found that it contained a letter from Liesel. It was dated with Sunday's date.

After unfolding it he realized that it was two pages handwritten on both sides and that the stationary was embossed at the top with United Airlines. He settled back into his chair and read it.

Dear Dr. Sandler:

By now I'm sure you've realized that I missed my appointment with you. I am sorry. Things have happened so fast that I hardly know where to start. Daniel made another one of his surprise visits Saturday afternoon. He came to propose, and I accepted. He had decided when we left the islands on separate planes that this wasn't what he wanted for us, so he's going to give marriage another go. He helped me pack my things for shipping and by the time you read this we will be on our way west. You might be interested to know that when Daniel arrived back in Oregon he discovered that Jake had taken his life with a friend's hunting rifle.

The guys at the mill say he seemed to have been losing his mind the last month or so. He was heard mumbling about Anna and how she was haunting him all the time. Daniel says that I got over him a lot better than he got over me. I'm not sure exactly what he means by that other than he's out of our lives for good now. My feelings of guilt died with him since there's nothing I could do now if I wanted to.

I will be seeing a doctor in Seattle as soon as we arrive there to make sure I get whatever it was you said I needed to have by Monday, so please don't worry about me. I'll be just fine. Thank you for all you did for me. I'll never be able express my gratitude. Well, that may not be exactly true. One day your Foundation will still benefit from me. I just hope it's not any time soon!

Very sincerely yours,

Liesel

David just shook his head as he thought, Daniel just saved her again and this time she didn't even know it. He smiled a crooked little smile. He hadn't really wanted Liesel to be one of the "winners" in the "lottery" anyway. He threw the medication and the prescription in the trash can and went down to the lobby for some breakfast.

Later that afternoon when he saw Jessica Tyler he decided that he would have her take Liesel's place, so he prepared her by putting her through the *Campaign.* He had already put everyone else on the list through the *Campaign.* Things were really progressing nicely. There hadn't been any difficulty with any of them completing this phase and his confidence in his abilities to lead them wherever he wanted was bordering on arrogance.

With a cocky tilt of his head he tapped a pencil against his chin. Even Jenny was coming around nicely. She had finally agreed to marry him and although she was not quite ready to announce it yet or to set a date, he knew that his lifetime dreams of having a family would soon be realized.

Chapter 63

Somewhere on Route I-95—South of Richmond, VA

Jenny was enjoying the drive from Tyson's Corner to Newport News. It was giving her a chance to listen to her favorite kinds of music and to be introspective. She was doing a dealer exchange. This was something she did often, but she usually didn't have to drive this far since there were so many Pontiac and GMC dealers around the beltway. It was rare to have to drive over a hundred miles to get a car for a customer. But then again, this was a very rare car she was getting.

It had taken her several days to find it and then quite a bit of negotiating with the other dealer to make the exchange. She was driving down a loaded up Black Trans Am and bringing back a Bright Yellow Fiero GT. Fieros were really hard to come by right now and she'd been very lucky that the other dealer already had a customer for the Trans Am or he wouldn't have made the deal with her.

Right now she was reveling in the power of the big V-8 engine, goosing it every once in a while just to hear the throaty rumble under the hood. She had removed the T-tops before leaving Royal figuring that, as long as she was going to be on the road for five hours, she might as well work on her tan. So here she was cruising down the highway, her long blonde tresses secured in a ponytail listening to Patsy Cline belting out "Crazy", waving her hand through the T-top when a trucker honked his horn at her.

There was something in the back of her mind that had been bothering her and for three days she had been trying to put her finger on it. It just wouldn't come to her. This nagging feeling was pervading through everything she did and it was keeping her from having the bright cheery outlook she normally had.

Now she seemed almost lost in thought all the time, like someone trying to remember what they did the night before when maybe they'd had one too many. Which was precisely when she'd first started having this feeling, when she awoke early Sunday morning alone in her bed wearing a damp bathing suit.

She recalled going with David down to the pool, diving into the pool and floating on the raft. She remembered his proposal and her acceptance and him wrapping her up in his terry cloth bathrobe and driving her home, but she couldn't remember anything in between.

The robe had been thrown across the chair in her room and the pillows she always kept on her bed during the day had been piled neatly on the floor where she usually just tossed them. Apparently David had seen her to her room but had been quite the gentleman and had not undressed her. Boy, she must have been really tired and of course she knew she probably still had too much to drink on an empty stomach, despite continually spilling it into the pool.

She had collected the kids from her parents' house after showering and dressing and taken them to church. Then she had treated them to lunch at Fuddrucker's and went home to work on her laundry. When David came by later that afternoon they talked about their engagement, which was one thing Jenny did remember agreeing to Saturday night.

She didn't feel as happy about it as she thought she should. A woman accepting a proposal should be walking on air and thinking about her betrothed almost constantly. She wasn't doing either. She felt like she loved him, but not quite the way she knew she was capable of. The uncertainty of her decision was chasing her thoughts like a bad headache throughout the day.

She asked David to give her some time to get adjusted to the idea of getting married again, hoping these feelings would even out soon. She asked that they not announce their engagement or set a date yet and even though he wasn't happy about it, he agreed. They postponed shopping for a ring until she was ready to wear one, but he insisted it be soon.

They took the kids to the park and Jenny fixed a big Sunday dinner. Then they all settled on the couch to watch "The Little Mermaid" on video. After getting the kids bathed and settled into bed Jenny told David that she was still tired from staying up late last night and was going to go to bed early. David walked to the door with his arm slung over her shoulder and at the door he gently lifted her onto the first step of the stairway going up to the second floor.

This made them almost the same height. David put his arms around her waist and pulled her against him as he gently kissed her on the lips, letting his lips slide over hers as he tenderly contoured them to fit against his. It was a nice kiss and she wondered at the time just why she was anxious for it to be over. He lovingly fingered her hair as it cascaded down her back and looked deeply into her beautiful green eyes. He smiled and kissed her on the cheek close to her ear. "Sweet Dreams, my beautiful bride," he said before turning to go out the door.

Jenny locked the door and went upstairs to check on the kids. Then she settled into bed with her pillows propped up behind her to read for awhile. Ten minutes later she was sound asleep. The book she had been reading having fallen from her hands to the floor.

Now it was Wednesday and she was pulling into the dealership at Newport News. The yellow Fiero GT was already out front ready for her inspection. She went inside to meet the sales manager she had arranged the dealer exchange with. As usual he was surprised at how young and pretty she was. They always were.

The stereotyping for car salesmen was bad enough, but the stereotyping for women car salesmen was even worse. She guessed that people assumed that they were the dregs who couldn't make it anywhere else. I mean what kind of a woman would want to be around a bunch of smoking, cursing, lying, cheating, womanizing men all day and night anyway? Geez, talk about stereotyping!

Even people in the profession didn't have the elevated sense of self worth that they should have. Why should anybody else think highly of them? This was the attitude that Jenny fought so hard to change by being the most professional and knowledgeable person she could be. By the look in the sales manager's eyes she knew the image he'd had of her was not the one he had now. When he offered to take her out to lunch she politely declined saying that she had to get back to deliver the Fiero early this evening.

She put her dealer tag on the back of the Fiero while the rest of the sales force watched through the large plate glass window. She'd learned how to stoop down and put tags on without revealing anything, but it was still a provocative position and guys still hoped for an intimate flash. She tried not to accommodate them. Then she opened the door and very carefully eased in being especially mindful of keeping her skirt from hiking up too far.

She stopped at the first gas station she saw to fill up and then drove through a McDonald's drive through window to get some lunch. She sat in the Fiero eating her lunch thinking about her newly fiancéd status. Damn! What in the world was bothering her about this? She popped open the sunroof, put a Patsy Cline tape in the tape player and pulled back onto 95. She belted out the songs with Patsy, feeling the music get into her soul.

Chapter 64

Washington, D.C.

Shawn let himself into his apartment near Dupont Circle. He had just come from his weekly session with Dr. Sandler and he was very pleased that he and the doctor had become so close these last few weeks. Hell, he was actually getting better and enjoying everything about the process thanks to Dr. Sandler's trust in him. As he flung his shoulder bag onto the kitchen counter he called out to Jeremy. "Hey, Jere! Where are ya?"

"Back 'ere," was the reply he got from his young Brit.

Shawn walked down the dim lit hallway to the back bedroom where there was a light flickering from the television screen. Jeremy loved American soap operas. He watched them all. Those he couldn't watch because he was already watching one, he taped to watch later in the evening when Shawn really would've preferred to watch some sitcoms. But that was Jeremy. You had to take the good with the bad. And he was about as bad as they came when it came to sex. Just thinking about the rough play acting they did together sent shivers down Shawn's spine.

When he reached the doorway he saw Jeremy propped up in bed. A grimy tan elastic tourniquet was still wrapped around his upper arm where he had just injected himself. "Christ! Jere! I thought you said you were going to do this program with me! You promised!"

"Yeah, yeah," Jeremy muttered, his eyes beginning to glass over. "Next week, okay? I got this really good stuff, I just could na pass it up."

Shawn looked around the room. "And what did you hock this time to pay for it?" Shawn asked through barely clenched teeth.

Jeremy pointed with a wave of his limp wrist to the open closet on the wall in front of him. Shawn walked over and looked inside. Scanning the contents it only took a few seconds for him to notice that his favorite snake-skin cowboy boots were not there. When he spun around to confront Jeremy the blaze burning in his eyes caused Jeremy to cower. As he drew his knees up to his chest he rolled himself over onto his side into a ball and started weeping, saying over and over and over, "I'm sorry. I'm sorry. I'm sorry."

Shawn knew it would do no good to try to talk to him for quite a few hours. He'd just shot up. He'd be in his own little world, shutting Shawn out as he did every night with the soaps. Shawn kicked the bed post as he walked through the room to the hallway, causing it to jostle its lone occupant almost over the side of the bed.

His father had given him those boots many years ago when he felt that his son's feet had stopped growing. Forty-two hundred dollars was a lot to spend on a pair of boots if they weren't going to fit in a year. That was when things were good between them, before his father found out that he was gay. It sickened him to know that Jeremy had probably gotten less than a hundred dollars for them and now that was probably gone too.

Shawn went back to the kitchen and fixed himself a Healthy Choice TV dinner and sat in front of the television in the living room while he alternately folded laundry and made a shopping list. After awhile he went in to check on Jeremy. He was still lying on his side all curled up but he was staring at the blinds covering the window like they were the most engrossing thing he'd ever seen.

Shawn covered him lightly with a sheet and went back to the living room. It was time for his treatment so he took the bag from the kitchen counter and went into the bathroom. He emptied all the syringes into an old shoe box he kept under the sink leaving one on the counter. After administering the injection he went to lay down on the bed next to Jeremy.

When Jeremy woke in the middle of the night he was his old aggressive self. And he was horny. This didn't bother Shawn at all. This was the Jeremy that he loved. The rough, masterful male animal, sure of his domain and his possessions. At times like these Shawn felt as he believed a treasured wife would feel, adored and irresistible. Jeremy's frantic clutching and clawing only served to reinforce Shawn's idea of his own desirability to his mate. And mate they did. Repeatedly.

Jeremy's insatiability was due largely to the drugs in his body and their enhancement made him crave more and more of the same. Sadly it was like a dog chasing after its tail. The level of enjoyment would never be as good as the first time, each successive culmination bringing less feeling and intensity ultimately causing Jeremy to discard Shawn from him with a violent shrug.

Shawn was exhausted but totally unfulfilled himself. Jeremy was truly a brutal husband. He cared only about his own gratification and Shawn was miserable in his love for him. He realized with some shame that he was a lot like the housewives you heard about all the time, taken advantage of by their brutal husbands.

Ten days later when Shawn came home from his new job as a clerk in a video movie rental store, he found Jeremy lying across the bed, dead from an overdose of whatever it was he had taken. Shawn was shaking as he called 911 as much from fear as from grief. A month earlier and that could've been him lying cold and wide-eyed on their rumpled sheets.

Waves of pain washed over him as he sat on the bed next to Jeremy's body stroking his hair away from his forehead. His beloved Jeremy. They had talked of so many things for their future, even the possibility of traveling to Canada for their wedding. Now he felt as if his core had been ripped out. Jeremy had been his reason for getting straight. Jeremy who needed someone to take care of him and protect him.

Feelings of inadequacy and guilt began to overcome him as he cried and sobbed, rocking back and forth on the bed with Jeremy's body between his outstretched legs. It never occurred to Shawn that there wasn't a syringe anywhere in the bedroom. He'd seen the tourniquet still wrapped around his arm and knew that heroin was Jeremy's drug of choice whenever he had the money for it.

When the ambulance and the police arrived, Jeremy was taken from him and after a cursory examination of his eyes and his pulse he was lifted to a gurney and covered with a sheet. Shawn had been spared the additional agony of watching all of this as two police officers had taken him aside for questioning as soon as they had arrived.

When one of the officers found a trash can full of used disposable syringes Shawn had to shake himself out of his grief to explain that they were Methadone treatments he was taking. When they asked where he had gotten them he told them he had bought them off of a junkie who had stolen them from a clinic. They took him in for questioning along with the four remaining unused syringes as well as the trash can containing the used syringes.

After six hours of questioning and detainment they let Shawn go. Shawn had adamantly told the same lie over and over again about the junkie. He was not going to get Dr. Sandler in trouble for this. The officers figured that they weren't going to gain any brownie points by charging the son of a famous actor with possession of Methadone to cure his well-known drug addiction. Besides the law was very vague on the possession of Methadone. No one knew how much it took to constitute illegal possession since it was not generally available on the street.

Shawn was very relieved to get out of jail without having to call his father for help. He was now focused on trying to get the money he would need to get Jeremy out of the county morgue and to bury him decently. It was several days later that the police department received the results of the lab tests.

Jeremy had died from a lethal dose of morphine, not heroin as everyone had suspected. In the trash can there had been one syringe containing traces of morphine, all the others had been Methadone. There were no wrappers and the police detectives assumed that since the wastebasket had been right next to the toilet that the wrappers had been flushed along with the normal course of events for the two roommates.

It stood to reason that if what Shawn Vanscoy said was true, that he bought the Methadone syringes from a junkie who'd stolen them from a clinic, that it was quite possible that in the junkie's haste to grab and get out when he'd somehow found the opportunity, that he'd grabbed a morphine syringe along with the Methadone syringes and neither Shawn nor Jeremy had noticed the difference. How the morphine dosage had become a lethal one, they hadn't a clue.

Shawn had told them that Jeremy hadn't started the treatments yet, but that he kept promising to. Well, as far as they could figure, Jeremy picked one hell of a time to start. When they went looking for Shawn to report what they had come across, they found that he had moved out of his apartment and taken Jeremy to his hometown in England to bury him.

Figuring that it probably didn't matter to Shawn to know whether his "boyfriend" Jeremy died from heroin or morphine they let it go. He had enough problems to deal with now that the media was right in his face with a camera everywhere he went asking how he was handling the death of his gay lover.

Chapter 65

Herndon, VA

David and Jenny were standing in line at the Giant Food store in the Elden Street Marketplace waiting for their turn to be rung up when David spotted the headlines on a tabloid. "Shawn Vanscoy's gay lover dies in love nest from drug overdose." There was an accompanying picture of Shawn and a young blonde man exiting a movie theater taken sometime in the winter. As the realization hit him about what he was reading he smacked his fist down hard on the conveyer belt causing it to momentarily skip a beat in its continuous cycle of dumping groceries by the scanner window.

"Damn!" was all he said in the way of explanation to Jenny who had never seen any violence or temper erupting from David.

When he repeated the one-word expletive again, she turned to stare at him. "David, what's wrong?" she asked with concern.

Well he sure as hell couldn't tell her that his plans to murder one of his patients had somehow gone awry now, could he? He leaned down to whisper in her ear as he nodded his head in the direction of the newspaper.

"Shawn Vanscoy is one of my patients and this is really going to set him back." When her eyes widened with surprise and curiosity over David's revelation of his patient's celebrity he quickly leaned back down and said, "Shh. I wasn't supposed to tell you that."

Jenny turned back to the cashier as her order was being rung up and it gave David a few minutes to get himself under control. Without being too obvious he tried to scan the substance of the article to try to see if he could glean any more information. The gist was that Shawn had come home to his Washington, D.C. apartment and found his lover, Jeremy, dead from an overdose of what was believed to have been heroin. Because of Shawn's notoriety and recent drug problems his apartment had been searched. Some drugs were confiscated along with drug paraphernalia for testing. Shit! They found the Methadone. He just knew it.

He helped Jenny load the groceries in her car as he tried to go over the repercussions in his mind. He should have known that Shawn wouldn't keep the drugs he had given him a secret. Now somehow his boyfriend had chanced across the lethal injection meant for Shawn. If Shawn told them where he had gotten the methadone, he would be sunk.

It wouldn't take much to connect the murder to him once they discovered it was morphine that had killed him instead of heroin. Unless of course, he had really died from heroin. In which case he'd better make sure Shawn didn't take anymore Methadone treatments. Two overdoses would surely be looked upon as queer. Oh that was funny, he thought.

As soon as they got to Jenny's house and David had helped unload all the groceries onto the kitchen counter, he made his excuses, saying he needed to get in touch with Shawn to see if there was anything he could do for him. Jenny thought it was sweet of him to be so concerned and accepted his apology for changing their afternoon plans.

The kids were at a birthday party for one of their cousins with their grandparents. They were going to go pick them up in a few minutes and take them to the park. Just before he went out the front door, he turned and called back to her. "Jenny, please make sure you don't mention this to anyone. The fact that Shawn was seeing me is very privileged information."

She smiled back at him and said, "Don't worry, I won't."

David drove to his office and reached for his rolodex. None of the numbers he had for Shawn worked. The apartment number just rang and rang with no machine to pick up and the cell number had a recording that the number was no longer a working number. He knew that Shawn had just started a job a few weeks ago at a movie rental place, but he had no clue which one.

He grabbed the phone book and started to call the ones closest to where he lived before he realized that Shawn would never have used his real name. He had no way to find him unless he tracked him through his father. Seeing no other way, he dialed the number he had been given months ago when he had been first contacted about Shawn's care.

The woman who answered the phone knew all the right questions to ask. The media must have been driving them crazy. After ascertaining that he was really who he said he was and not just an inventive reporter, he was connected to Shawn's father. He was informed that Shawn was in England seeing to Jeremy's funeral. They had spoken several times over the last few days, mostly about him attending the funeral.

Shawn was very disappointed that his father wouldn't come but he understood the reason given, even if it wasn't the true reason. The last thing Jeremy's family needed now was a media circus. After thanking David for the progress his son was making he gave David a number that Shawn could be reached at.

Again he had to go through a verbal gauntlet before Shawn was put on the phone. "Dr. Sandler!" Shawn exclaimed happily. "It's so nice to hear from you. This has really been a rough few days for me, I'm so glad you called."

They talked for a few minutes about his lack of sleep, how awful it was to have found Jeremy like that and how wonderful everybody was treating him, except for the press of course. Before David could ask him Shawn volunteered the information he was looking for. "The police found the treatments, but don't worry I told them I got them from a junkie on the street who stole them from a clinic and they believed me. I think there were only four left anyway. I think I'm okay now. I'm not fighting any cravings, even with everything I've been through I haven't wanted anything stronger than a cigarette. I think I'm cured, Doc. Seeing Jeremy like that made me realize how easily it could've been me."

David's reply was a simple, "Yes. It could have been." Silently he was screaming in his head that it should have been.

Shawn told him to hold his appointment for next week, that he'd be back to continue their sessions. And then hung up.

As David replaced the phone in the handset he realized that he had been gripping it tightly, so tense from anger. $350,000 just waiting for him to pick it up and he'd blown it! This should've been one of the easier *lottery winners* to take the ticket from. His day ruined, he drove home to his empty apartment and did something he hardly ever did. He took a nap in the middle of the day, trying to dispel the anger that was festering in him.

Chapter 66

Fairfax, VA

Two days later David was cheered by two things. He'd received a letter from Betsy Drayton's attorney announcing her bequest to him in the amount of $100,000. The check would be in the mail to him by next week. He had been hoping for more but the way things had been going he was happy with that. And, he'd managed to switch the pills he had prepared for Pete Riddel with the real ones he had found in Pete's briefcase when he was under hypnosis.

The prescription David had written for Pete several weeks ago was for Sinequan. It was an antidepressant that was indicated for psychotic depressive disorders and anxiety. The pills Pete had been taking were in 50 mg capsules and his instructions were to take two of them twice daily, once in the late morning and once again just before bedtime.

David had carefully separated the light and dark pink capsules that he had at home and refilled each one with the contents of two of the bright blue Sinequan capsules he also had at home. They were 150 mg each. So instead of Pete getting a combined dose of 100 mg each time he took two pills he was going to be getting 600 mg each time he took two pills.

Anything over 600 mg a day was dangerously overdosing. 1200 mg would definitely look like someone committing suicide. He had made sure that Pete was at the end of his prescription so that there wouldn't be any pills left to examine. If anyone were to count how many pills there had been and the days since the prescription had been filled and realized that there wouldn't have been enough left to overdose on, it could be explained very easily.

Manic depressives often saved up doses to take at one time if not carefully monitored. He would state that he didn't believe Pete had been in a manic depressive state and assumed that he was taking his medication properly. It would only be a matter of time now before he'd have more money flowing in. And he needed the money now more than ever.

He'd finally convinced Jenny to announce their engagement and to pick a date. Now he wanted to build a new house for them to live in, a big house in Great Falls with lots of land for the horses he planned on buying Paisley. Everything was finally starting to work out for him. All his planning and preparing was paying off. Only one thing was a little disappointing. It had never occurred to him that once he and Jenny became engaged that she'd still refuse to have sex with him.

She said she'd never had intercourse without the benefit of marriage and she wasn't planning on doing it now. She was okay for a little light petting on the sofa, but she was adamant that they were going to wait until their wedding night to couple. He remembered the long-drawn out groan he had given her when she'd said that and then he'd used her argument right back against her as a way to get her to commit to a real engagement and to set a date.

They finally agreed to surprise her family with the announcement at Thanksgiving dinner. Although he doubted that anyone would really be surprised. They had been seeing each other for quite awhile now, and anyone who saw him and Paisley together just knew that they should be father and daughter. No one thought it odd that he and Rusty were not as close. It was a common thought that boys bonded to their mothers and girls to their fathers.

Jenny wanted to be married in June, David didn't want to wait that long so they compromised and settled on April 1st. April Fool's Day. That would be an easy anniversary to remember David thought. Not that he'd have any trouble remembering the day when Jenny would become his wife and Paisley would start calling him *Daddy*.

He was startled out of his reverie by the arrival of his next patient, Leroy Dressler. Leroy was starting to have headaches brought on by the stress of planning and executing the cruise he was going on next week. David had already planned out his medicine for the trip also.

Chapter 67

Tyson's Corner, VA

It was 7:30 on a rainy Thursday evening and the showroom was deserted. Jenny sat in front of a computer at the up desk checking the stock that had come in earlier that day. She was expecting a factory order for a customer who really wanted to have it by the weekend. She looked up and saw one of the salesmen walking towards her saying, "D'you do the puzzle today?" Tom Kickingbird had almost the same obsession with the Post's crossword puzzle as she did. She cut it out of the paper every morning and carried it around with her all day until she finished it. Today's had been fairly easy and she had it finished a few minutes after she'd started on it.

"Yeah," she said. "It's over on my desk. Help yourself. It's another one with names of Czechoslovakian rivers in it."

A few minutes later another salesman came up to ask her if she wanted anything from Taco Bell. The days that had a lot of down time seemed to be filled with eating. But actually a few soft tacos sounded good to her so she got up, went to her purse and gave him some money.

When Freddie got back 20 minutes later she joined all the hungry participants back in the lunch room. When it was slow like this you just knew something unusual was going to happen. All these creative thinkers having to keep their energy at idle didn't last long. Among the banter and hilarity going on somebody generally became the brunt of a practical joke.

Jenny typically was a spectator in these things. Only rarely did she stick her neck out to chance management's wrath. And she never was involved with anything crude or hurtful to anyone. Tonight something tripped inside her and she felt just a tiny bit devilish. Tom Kickingbird was covering the showroom while everyone else was in the lunch room chowing down. When someone mentioned that he didn't like hot stuff, which was why he hadn't ordered anything, she smiled. Tom never turned down free food and she knew he loved tomato soup. He was always asking her to get some for him whenever she went to Spring Road Deli.

She took a Styrofoam coffee cup and dumped all the unused salsa into it and then opened all the hot taco sauce seasoning packets and squeezed the contents out into the cup. Carefully she stirred it up while everyone was guffawing and snickering. "Now, don't say anything or look at me. You'll make me laugh and I won't be able to carry this off," she instructed before she stood up and carried it out to the showroom.

Tom was sitting at her desk working on his puzzle, using hers as a guide. She sat the cup down beside the blotter on her desk as if she was going to sit down and eat it when he got up. She sat on the corner of her desk as he asked, "What's that?"

"Just some tomato soup I had left over from lunch. I just heated it up. But I'm a little full now from eating those tacos. You want it?"

"Sure!" he said greedily and snatched the cup up.

He took the cup, put it to his lips and tilted it almost upside down as he attempted to down it in one big swallow. As soon as the cup left his lips his entire face and neck went red and his eyes bulged. He stood up so fast that the chair fell over in his mad dash to get to some water.

Everyone who had been watching from the corner, hidden from view, started laughing uproarishly. After a few minutes Tom came back around the corner with a sheepish expression on his face. Jenny smiled at him and said, "Well I did tell you I had just heated it up!"

He smiled and patted her on the back and said, "I owe you one."

Now it was Jenny's turn to smile sheepishly and say, "I was afraid of that."

He would make her wait for weeks suspecting every noise and movement until he took his revenge. Idle minds, she thought shaking her head. The car business. Never a dull moment if we can help it.

While everyone was gathered around her office she proceeded to tell them about the most hilarious joke that had backfired on one of the finance managers years ago. His name was Mike and he was a card. He was always keeping everyone in stitches. He reminded her of Michael J. Fox. He was an impeccable dresser, short and athletic and had one-liners for everything going on.

One night he was getting ready to do a settlement in a back office when he had a brainstorm. He pulled the tanish-gray glue strip off of the top of a note pad and rolled it up into a ball and placed it under his nose on his mustache. It looked just like a big bugger hanging there. The salesman came in with the deal folder. His name was Larry and he was the funniest hell raiser. Always up for a good time. Well when Larry saw Mike he started laughing and couldn't stop. But then he thought, hey, let's let the customers come in and sit down and see if they get up the nerve to say anything.

Mike agreed and Larry went to get the customers, trying to keep a straight face as he walked them back to the finance office. Meanwhile Mike is imagining what the customer's reaction will be and in his fit of laughter he manages to snort the glue ball up into his nostril. When Larry rounded the corner and ushered his customers into the office they all saw Mike banging his head on the desk and trying to blow the glue ball out of his nose while holding the other nostril closed making all kinds of snorting and wheezing sounds.

That didn't seem to be working so in his panic he jumped up, opened the center drawer of his desk, grabbed a sharp pencil and shoved it up his nose. That only managed to push it up higher and he fell onto the carpet in a kneeling position with his head down between his knees snorting and hitting his hand on the floor while he tried to blow the thing out. Finally he got it out.

Then he stood up, straightened his clothing and put his hand out to the couple saying, "Hi, I'm Mike, I'll be doing the settlement on your new car." And then he indicated the chairs in front of his desk and said, "Won't you please have a seat, this shouldn't take long at all." As if nothing had ever happened.

Everyone laughed until one of the mangers walked out in the showroom and said, "What's everybody doing? If there's no customers let's go home!" Everyone scurried to get their stuff together and get out. Jenny grabbed her purse and walked to the showroom doors.

Tom Kickingbird called out after her, "Don't forget! 'Cause I won't!"

Jenny turned in time to see his smile. "Oh, I won't," she answered. "Just make sure it's a good one," she taunted. "Something they'll talk about for years to come."

Chapter 68

Fairfax, VA

Pete Riddel died in his sleep two days later. David found out about it when two Fairfax County Police Officers came to question him at his office. He was informed by them that the coroner suspected suicide by an overdose of the pills the doctor had prescribed for him. David shook his head feigning sadness and disbelief. The officers seemed very matter-of-fact about their investigation and only seemed to be verifying information they already knew.

When they asked him about the medication he prescribed for Pete, David stood and took a folder out of the mahogany file cabinet behind his desk. Even though he knew everything in it by heart he pretended to scan the page for his notes and then he read them the medication he had prescribed and the dosage directions.

He was asked about Pete's condition and his treatment. David told them that his patients were entitled to confidentiality even after death unless the court ordered the records opened. But he didn't want to ruffle any feathers and send anyone off on a campaign so he added, "I can tell you that he was very depressed over the death of his son a few months ago and that I thought he was making progress. I am shocked that he considered suicide an option. I thought he was managing his grief fairly well the last few times we talked. But the death of a child triggers very intense emotions and often they are not fully expressed even after years of therapy."

The officers seemed satisfied with the doctor's answers and said they would be in touch if they had any more questions. When David finished ushering them out through the front office door, he let out a deep drawn out sigh. Only he knew that he had been nervous and perspiring heavily under his shirt. Now that they were gone he allowed himself a few minutes to calm down and get the inner shaking under control. He waited until late in the afternoon to call and talk to Pete's wife.

The shock and surprise of all this was still in her voice as she said over and over again, "I just can't believe he would have done this to us! We have three other kids he's left behind! And he was terrified of what would happen to them if he didn't watch over them. It's just so hard to believe that he would have taken his own life like this!" She didn't sound exactly angry, just helpless and unsure of the future.

"MaryAnn," he said, "I am so sorry that I didn't see this coming. He seemed to be managing everything so well the last time I saw him. I guess he just couldn't take the pain anymore. Either that or he saw this as a way to be with Robbie."

MaryAnn was sobbing uncontrollably and after a few seconds another voice came on the phone.

"Dr. Sandler, I'm MaryAnn's sister, Ruth. She can't talk anymore. This is just tearing her apart having to bury her husband so soon after her son. But we appreciate you calling."

"Ruth?" He asked just as she was removing the phone from her ear.

"Yes?" She asked.

"Have the funeral arrangements been made yet? I would like to attend if you think that would be all right."

"Pete's family is coming down from New Jersey to take him back there to bury him but we're having a memorial service tomorrow afternoon at St. Andrew's Catholic Church. If you can come, I'm sure MaryAnn will appreciate it."

He really didn't want to go, but he thought that he should. People would probably be looking at him as if he'd handed Pete a loaded gun, but it would seem very calloused if he didn't even show up. He didn't want to go alone and he didn't want to ask Jenny. The less she knew about his patients dying the better. So he asked his receptionist to accompany him, on the clock of course, and she said she would.

The next afternoon, as he sat in one of the rear pews with Glenda by his side, he observed the stunned family as they proceeded to the front of the church. The men were stoically supporting the women with their arms under their shoulders and the children were walking behind them like zombies, unsure of the protocol expected of them.

MaryAnn was brought forward last between two hulking men, one he supposed was her father by his age and the other probably a brother. They half carried half dragged her to her seat as her knees buckled every time she looked ahead and saw the coffin. Throughout the service she sobbed and wailed, unmindful of the decorum she was supposed to be exhibiting for her children. And the more she cried, the more they cried.

As David listened to first one relative and then another eulogize Pete's life he actually felt pangs of remorse that he had been the instrument of destruction causing all this sadness and grief. The looks of misery on the children's faces caused him to get a little teary-eyed himself.

They left the church as soon as the service was over and went back to the office. He tried to get out of the funk he was in by recognizing that he couldn't undo anything so he might as well make the best of it. He began mentally envisioning the house he was preparing to build for him and his family with some of Pete's legacy.

Chapter 69

Great Falls, VA

Over the next several weeks David used all of Jenny's free time dragging her all over the countryside of Great Falls and McLean looking at houses and lots. They spent hours touring model homes and looking at floor plans. David and Jenny didn't generally argue very much about things but they certainly didn't see eye to eye on what they wanted in a house.

David wanted a big, looming mansion on a hill with land all around and stables. Jenny wanted a nice little cozy cottage with a very small yard. She was not fond of yard work at all. And she wasn't crazy about having horses around. She'd only been riding once in her life and had been petrified the whole time.

The only thing they seemed to agree on was the kitchen. Jenny loved to cook and needed lots of storage space for all her kitchen equipment. David also wanted a large kitchen, suitable to handle all the entertaining they would be doing. Especially as Paisley grew older and needed to have more of a social life.

The more homes they went in and out of the more they disagreed. Every home seemed to be bigger and more expensive than the last. When they saw one that had a beautifully paneled billiard room with a long bar at the end Jenny knew from the look in David's eyes that he wanted it. She felt that they were way out of their league.

"David, this house is too big! We don't need all this space and I don't want to clean a house this big. That's all I'd ever be doing!"

He took her hands in his and smiled down at her, "Jenny, you won't have to clean anything. We'll have a maid. And a gardener. And probably one or two part-time stable hands to help out with the horses."

Jenny just gaped up at him, her mouth slack with surprise. "David, we can't afford all that! This is just way too much!"

"Jenny," he said in soothing tones, "we can afford all this. I'm a very good doctor. I make lots of money. Believe me, by the time the house is ready, we'll be able to pay cash for almost all of it."

Jenny looked down at the brochure she had in her hand. "David, this house is $450,000!" she bellowed.

He gathered her in his arms and put her chin on his shoulder as he looked around the room. "I know. Don't worry about a thing. I'll take care of it."

That afternoon David signed a contract with the builder, leaving him a check for $100,000 to secure the land and to start building. Jenny was mesmerized as she walked through the model home again. She couldn't believe that she was actually going to be living in a house like this.

She had originally wanted to stay and live with David and the kids in her home in Herndon after they were married but David wouldn't hear of it. Now as she walked around the rooms daydreaming, she was getting caught up in the excitement of building a new house. She had never dreamed that she would ever live in a house as magnificent as this.

On the drive back home it was decided that they wouldn't sell Jenny's house. They would rent it out and use the money to pay the mortgage and to put a little aside for the children's college fund. By the time they were ready for college the mortgage would be paid off and they could sell it and have enough to put them through any school they chose.

The money side of David was one Jenny hadn't seen before and she was relieved to know that he would be taking over all the financial and investment decisions for her. Money had a way of just slipping through her fingers. Here was a man who knew how to save. He actually had $100,000 in his checking account! She was starting to look forward to the idea of being able to lean on David for the security he could provide for her and the children. Maybe some day she wouldn't have to sell cars and she could be a stay-at-home mom, taking care of her family.

Chapter 70

Chantilly, VA

MaryAnn was sitting at her kitchen table talking with her best friend, Cindy Policki. The last few weeks had been extremely hard for MaryAnn. Managing the kids on her own, handling all the financial details of life that she hadn't paid a bit of attention to before and lying down to bed at night alone knowing it was going to be like this forever. Pete would never be coming back and she missed him.

They had been high school sweethearts and had married during Pete's last year in college when they had discovered she was pregnant with Robbie. Although the passion hadn't been there in the last few years as it had been in the first few, they had a companionship that was envied by a lot of couples. They were united when it came to decisions regarding their kids and they were devoted to each other in ways that no one else could ever see.

They recorded each other's favorite programs without being asked to. They each got up early once a week to fix a special breakfast for the other. This was something they had started when the kids were babies and had discovered that the only meal they could eat together in peace was at 5:00 a.m.

They took such joy in doing the most menial things together. Switching summer and winter clothes from the basement cedar closet to the master bedroom closet became a game as they passed each other on the upstairs staircase placing passionate kisses on a newly revealed naked stretch of flesh. These biannual traipses often left them gasping for air on the landing, having spent their passion among winter wool suits and flowery spring dresses. Their second child was believed to have been conceived during one exceptional bout of spring cleaning.

MaryAnn was suffering from not only losing her husband and helpmate but from the greatest loss of all. She was suffering because her companion hadn't told her that he was choosing to leave.

Cindy had been MaryAnn's childhood friend. There hadn't been a week in her life that they hadn't seen each other, not even when they were on their honeymoon. Cindy and her husband Frank had married the same week as MaryAnn and Pete and they all stayed at the same hotel in Cozumel. Cindy had since divorced Frank and had gone from one bad relationship to another in the last six years. She was now in a lull and they were both bemoaning their lives without men.

"I don't see why a man has to keep lookin' when he already has what he wants. How can they say they 'love you' and then go around smilin' and flirtin' with every little thing in skirts?" Cindy was saying between bites of coffeecake.

MaryAnn just shrugged as she poured them more coffee.

Cindy looked up at her and said, "Well, of course you never had that problem. Pete was as loyal as the day is long. I don't think I ever saw him look at another woman, ever."

"Nope, I don't think he ever did." MaryAnn said.

MaryAnn sat back down and looked at her. Cindy had stopped by on her way to work as she often did. She was in the blue and gray uniform of the Fairfax County Police Department. A little gold plate above her pocket identified her as C.Policki. She was not an unattractive woman, but somehow she wasn't attractive either. A lot of it had to do with the chip she had on her shoulder and some of it was just her size.

She was bigger than most guys liked their women to be. At six foot she was an imposing presence. She didn't strike you as a woman who needed coddling. But MaryAnn knew differently. Cindy was like a little kitten running around waiting for someone to tenderly stroke it.

"Cindy, I found something yesterday that's been bothering the hell out of me," MaryAnn said.

"Yeah, what's that?" Cindy asked, swallowing a big gulp of tan-colored coffee.

MaryAnn reached around her to the counter behind her and grabbed a clipboard. "I found this under Pete's side of the bed."

Cindy reached for it and looked at it. Not recognizing what it was she shrugged. "What is it?"

"It's Pete's schedules for the kids. Every night he'd plug in all their activities for the next day so he'd know exactly where everyone was and when to pick them up," Mary Ann replied.

"So?" Cindy asked.

"So look at this. The night he took all those pills he'd carefully filled in all the times and places he'd have to be the next day. Why would a man who was going to kill himself go to all the trouble to make a chart he'd never use?" Mary Ann asked.

"Gee, that's a pretty good question, Mere," Cindy said, looking thoughtfully at the clipboard and all the papers it contained.

"I don't think Pete killed himself," MaryAnn said. "I never thought that he'd killed himself and this only makes me believe that more."

"So what do you think happened?" Cindy asked her.

"I don't know," Mary Ann replied. "I just don't think he killed himself."

"Have you spoken to anyone else about this?" Cindy asked.

"No, I just found this yesterday and who would I talk to anyway? Everybody thinks I'm crazy," Mary Ann sighed.

Cindy thought for a moment and then said, "I know this guy. He just retired from the force. He's been written up a few times in the paper and stuff because he's some kind of super detective, leaves no stone unturned so to speak. He's solved a few cases for the department that they had filed away as hopeless. He's turned private now. Maybe you should talk to him."

"Yeah, maybe I should. This is bothering me so much I can't think of anything else. And besides, if there's any chance at all that I can get rid of the stigma of this suicide hanging over us, I should try it. Especially for the sake of the kids. What's his name?"

Cindy popped the last piece of coffee cake into her mouth as she stood up. "C. G. Scott" she mumbled as she chewed. "Colin Gregory Scott. I'll get his number for you today." Out the door she went, tucking her cinnamon colored hair under her hat.

Chapter 71

Fairfax, VA

It was Leroy's last appointment before he left for his cruise tomorrow. David had asked him all about his plans so he would know where he'd be on which days. And he knew that early tomorrow he and his companion Margaret, along with his housekeeper and cook, would be driven to La Guardia Airport in New York where a helicopter would be waiting to take them to their cruise ship docked in the harbor.

From there they would travel to the Virgin Islands. The cruise line had hired a private tour specialist to accompany Margaret anytime she chose to leave the ship. Leroy had insisted that the agent be female and close to Margaret's age so that she would have someone to talk to.

There were no special facilities for the cook to use in the large crowded galley but he was invited to supervise the preparations of their food for each meal. Leroy would try to eat in the main dining room but they all knew that it would be more likely that they would eat in their stateroom, except the nights Margaret was invited to dine at the Captain's table.

This would be David's only opportunity to switch the pills he had prepared for Leroy with the ones Leroy already had in his sports coat pocket. Instead of an overdose or a dangerous combination of drugs, David had decided that for Leroy the best plan was to deprive him of a drug he desperately needed. Without him knowing, of course.

David knew that Leroy had Congestive Heart Failure and that he was being treated with Lanoxin, a digitalis glycoside. Without this medicine his heart muscle would not be able to pump properly or control its beating rhythm. A normal dosage for a man his age would be around 0.125 mg daily.

The notes in his chart along with a careful examination of Leroy's prescription bottle on his initial visit to him had indicated that Leroy was taking a slightly higher dosage, 0.25 mg daily, 0.125 mg twice a day. That meant that he really depended on the drug to keep his heart pumping and also that he couldn't handle the full dose at one time because of his susceptibility to adverse effects being as old as he was.

It had been really tricky trying to figure out which pills had been prescribed since they were available in so many dosages, until he had remembered that the pills he had seen were white. The only white Lanoxin found in his Physician's Desk Reference were 0.25 mg. That meant that they had to be cut in half. Just guessing, knowing Leroy as he did, that Leroy would have cut them all up at one time if the pharmacist hadn't already done that, he searched through his book for a pill that looked like the Lanoxin when it was halved.

Capsules sure were easier to plan around, he mused as he thumbed through the book trying to find a pill that would look like Lanoxin and would be safe for him to take. Ha! That was a laugh! Safe in this case meant not leaving behind any unusual telltale traces. Finally he found one. Tavist. At least during his final days he would have a clear head and no chance of hives. He wrote out a prescription for Michael Smith, the name he always used, and took it to a pharmacy he had never been to before.

It would probably take at least two maybe three days of missed digitalis before his heart would begin to fail and by that time they should be well out to sea. The ship's doctor wouldn't suspect the wrong medication even if he looked closely. They were remarkably similar and the code numbers would not be able to be read once they were cut in half and abraded a bit in the vial.

By the time they realized that they couldn't help him it would be too late to get him anywhere where they could. And by the time an autopsy was performed, if it was required, the toxology levels wouldn't be accurate anyway, the digitalis tended to be removed mostly by the kidneys instead of the liver. This was going to go so well. He just knew it.

When Leroy got there, David took his jacket from him and went to the closet to hang it up as he did every time Leroy came.

While David was hanging it up for him and while Leroy was washing his hands in David's private bathroom, David switched the pills he had prepared, for the pills Leroy already had.

After the session David gathered the pills that were loose in his jacket pocket and flushed them in his toilet. Then he threw away the prescription bottle with the name Michael Smith on it.

Chapter 72

Chantilly, VA

Colin bent his six-foot-two-inch frame in thirds trying to get behind the wheel of his new Mustang convertible. He cursed his stupidity for having bought such an impractical car for himself. Not only did he not fit in it unless the top was down but also his golf clubs didn't fit in the trunk unless he took the clubs out of his bag.

When his wife of seventeen years separated from him four months ago, he did what every newly unattached male in his early forties does. He traded the family mini van in on a sports car that much more suited the image he was now trying to live up to. Single, carefree, happy-go-lucky, when it was actually anything but.

As soon as he was able to get his right thigh under the steering wheel and his leg positioned over the proper pedal, he started the car. If it wasn't so damned hot, he'd put the top down. He also hadn't known when he'd bought this car that he probably wouldn't see much top down action until October. It was just too damned hot around Washington until after September.

Driving down Route 50 to his new apartment he thought back to the events of the last few months that had changed him from being a married man driving a mini van home to his suburban house complete with dog and kid to a bachelor driving an over-priced sports car to his sparsely furnished apartment with no one there to greet him when he got there. Not even so much as a house plant was breathing out oxygen for him.

The years of police duty had struck down another marriage. Twenty some years ago when he'd been just a cadet at the Academy, he and his classmates had been instructed not to take the job home whenever they managed to get back there. Being the dutiful officer that he was he'd done just that. He'd never shared the stresses of the job with Lynn.

She never knew about the times that he was scared at night pulling cars over or the times that he had to check out completely blackened buildings because an alarm was going off. Or the frustration he felt when he made a good case that couldn't be prosecuted because of a technicality or favors the prosecuting attorney owed.

She never knew about the auto theft ring he'd uncovered after eight months of mind-numbing boredom during late night stakes outs or the drug dealers that had almost killed him. She never knew how hard he worked at his job to put the bad guys in jail even though the Commonwealth of Virginia didn't seem to want to keep them there for very long. She never knew because he'd been told not to tell her.

The less the wives knew, the less they'd worry, and they were women after all. They didn't need to hear about all the gruesome things that went on. It was the man's job to shield them from the harshness of the world, even if it was a part of their day to day life. So, through the years the officers leaned on each other for support and established a bond between them that would never be broken. Through tragic deaths and jubilant honors they shared their emotions with their police family, giving the best of themselves and the worst of themselves to the men and women in their unit instead of to their spouses.

Over the years Colin couldn't even begin to count the number of marriages that fell by the wayside because two people stopped communicating about the things that really mattered the most to them. He didn't know when he and Lynn had started to drift apart. He only knew the day the marriage crashed, there in the parking lot with people stopping to gawk as a part of him died.

It wasn't until many weeks later that he realized that the part of him that had died was his pride. He should have been able to see it coming. She was having an affair for Chrissake! He was a detective! He was known for his keen sense of observation. How had he missed all the signs?

It was of little comfort to know that the Academy now advocated an open relationship between officers and their spouses, sharing the emotional ups and downs of their lives as if they were in this together. What a novel idea, he thought bitterly.

The day Colin had chanced to see Lynn coming out of a restaurant arm in arm with her boss he had practically wrecked his cruiser turning around to get to her. The confrontation in the parking lot had been pretty ugly and as he had escorted Lynn to the patrol car he had vaguely realized the anger he was feeling was not so much with her, as it was with himself.

That night they talked like they hadn't talked in years. They talked about everything they'd been avoiding and where they should go from here. Even though it pained him to say it, he was willing to forgive her affair. He was jealous and angry but he still loved her. When she told him that she loved him, but that she was no longer in love with him, he was crushed. She was in love with someone else now and wanted to be with him. He suggested counseling and a hundred other things. She said no to them all. As far as she was concerned it was over and had been for a long time. He was the only one who hadn't known it.

She asked him to move out so she could get the house ready for sale and the next day they sat down with their son Adam who had just recently turned fifteen. Adam had always been more Lynn's responsibility than Colin's because for the first seven years of Adam's life, Colin had worked the graveyard shift, working at night and sleeping during the day.

The times that he had any real interaction with Adam had been mostly holidays and vacations and one or two summers when he'd coached Adam's baseball team. Colin liked to spend his days off playing golf with his buddies and then falling asleep on the sofa in the afternoon watching golf and drinking beer. Adam had his own friends now and the news that his mother and father were divorcing was accepted without a lot anguish.

When the dog got hit by a car a few months later, Lynn hadn't even bothered to tell Colin. Colin found out about it from his mother who'd been told by Adam. They really didn't need him anymore and it hurt him to realize that they hadn't for quite some time.

Since then he'd tried to keep busy. He went to the officer's gym every other day and worked out, although he didn't need to for bulk, he already was very muscular. Still it was good therapy to sweat out his anger and to deal with his heartache as he passed some time away. He was on his way home from just such a session. The tank top he was wearing showed off his very broad chest and strong tanned arms, both covered with thick brown hair just beginning to become interspersed with silver-grey threads in places.

Years of exercise and strenuous police training had kept him firm and toned. He had a golfer's tan on his face, neck, arms and legs. He was always nicely tanned because he went golfing whenever he could all year long. He was very athletic and loved to be involved in team sports. He was on the Police Department's softball team, which was usually good for keeping him occupied two or three nights a week during the summer.

He had just retired a few weeks ago after 25 years on the force at the age of 43. He planned on doing some private detecting work for a few banks and insurance companies while he worked on perfecting his golf game. He was hoping to become good enough to qualify for the Senior's tour by the time he was fifty. There were also several southeastern tours in the Carolinas he could qualify for when he turned forty five. Since everything else in his life was changing he felt this might be a good time to make a career change too.

He pulled into a parking space in front of his apartment building. As he was walking up the outside steps to his second floor apartment he saw two young women in bathing suits walking towards the pool. Maybe there were some benefits to this apartment-living lifestyle after all. He let himself into his apartment and quickly put on his bathing suit.

He assessed himself in the bathroom mirror. He curled his arms together down to his waist with his hands fisted. He flexed his muscles causing the muscles on his chest to pump up also. Even he, with his self-esteem as low as it was right now, had to admit that he had an impressive physique. He put his teeth together and smiled, baring his lips to the gum line to check his teeth. The image that was reflected back was of a very handsome man with a mixture of thick silvered blonde hair and bright steel-blue eyes under expressively arched brows.

His chiseled features gave him a rugged quality while his mustache lent a rakishness to his smile. His full sensuous lips were framing perfectly white teeth as he relaxed his lips back to normal and smiled back at himself. His smile was a devastating one to the females and he knew it. Next to his 9mm Glock it was his most powerful weapon. "Time to go check out the pool," he said to his mirror image as he grabbed a towel and headed for the door.

Chapter 73

Fort Lincoln Cemetery

Washington, D.C.

Henry Blocker knelt in front of the small brass plaque that identified Sally's place of eternal rest from the hundred or so in front of him. This particular section of the cemetery, The Garden of the Apostles, was always so quiet and peaceful. He looked forward to coming here for his daily talk with Sally. His head was beginning to get a bit stuffy again so he took the nasal spray Dr. Sandler had given him out of his pocket and took two quick squirts in each nostril.

When Henry had been in his office last week complaining of his congested sinuses Dr. Sandler had offered him some of his own personal medicine from his desk drawer. He said he used it all the time during the late summer and fall to keep his head clear and offered Henry one he hadn't even opened yet to try. He was such a nice man. He was also practically the only friend he had other than his co-workers at Burger King.

Even though Henry was pretty well set for life since the insurance settlement, he still chose to work. Without his job he just didn't know how he'd ever get through the days. The nights were bad enough as it was with the night terrors and insomnia keeping him surfing the TV at all hours, although the medicine he'd been taking was helping a lot.

Shortly after Henry's wife had died, Dr. David, as Henry called him, had called Henry's physician, Dr. Wilson. He suggested that Dr. Wilson prescribe a mild antidepressant like Sinequan for Henry's sleep disorders and eating problems, saying he'd prefer his regular doctor prescribe all his medicines for him since he was more familiar with all the other medicines Henry was taking for his mental problems. The other doctor understood and appreciated the professional courtesy and immediately issued a prescription for the Sinequan. This was one of the things that had so endeared Dr. David to Henry. He went out of his way to take the best care of him and at the time he wasn't even getting paid.

He told Sally about his day at work and then he told her about the Fidelity Magellan account Dr. David had helped him establish. He loved watching the points go higher every morning when he used one of the courtesy papers at the restaurant to track its progress. A few times it went lower but Dr. David said not to worry it would always go back up and it always did. He also told her about the scholarship fund he had established in her name at the community college where they had met. That had been Dr. David's idea too. He said Henry should give some of his money away now so that there would be less for Sally's family to argue over later.

He bent down to the ground to kiss the "Mrs." in front of Sally Blocker's name on the brass plate. He'd had to insist on adding that. Not only did Sally's mother not want that, she also didn't want Sally's married name. She wanted her marker to have her maiden name. Henry wished he'd known then how much money he was going to have now.

He would have liked to have seen Sally have one of those large marble monuments with a beautiful angel carved into it. And a seat for him to sit on. But they didn't allow those in this garden. His knees were starting to bother him from all the kneeling. Or was it all the weight he was gaining from the fast food he was now eating for breakfast, lunch and dinner. When Sally had been alive she had insisted that he could only have one meal at the restaurant. The others she would fix for him. He missed that.

Henry walked to the top of the hill and to the bus stop at the entrance to the cemetery. At least Sally would be pleased with the exercise he was getting. Fort Lincoln was sprawled over many acres of immaculately kept lawns. The Garden of the Apostles was a little over a mile from the gates. He took a bus to the metro which took him to Vienna, Virginia and then another to Fairfax to Dr. David's office. He walked the last few blocks taking in all the sights and ignoring the stares of the passersby as he took out his new inhaler and deeply inhaled the vapors.

David was ready for Henry when he got there. He'd taken the pills he'd already prepared and put them in his sport coat pocket. They were in an open little plastic baggie. Pink and fuschia capsules filled with Sinequan and Nardil. Sinequan was a tricyclic antidepressant that should never be combined with a monoamine oxidase inhibitor, which was exactly what Nardil was.

The combination would cause a high fever, convulsions and death. The phenylproprandamine in the over-the-counter nasal decongestant, along with the ingredients in the Dexatrim diet pills he had encouraged Henry to start buying and taking, would add to the fatal combination of drugs in his body and would ultimately turn out to be the culprits blamed for his drug reaction. There would be so much of the others that they wouldn't even look for the Nardil.

Unfortunately Henry's death would not be quick. He would suffer headaches, fever, double vision and other visual abnormalities before the eventual muscle contractions and convulsions shut down his system. The ingredients in the nasal spray and the Dexatrim combined with the other drugs, would trigger a hypertensive crisis and his blood pressure would soar until the marked elevation killed him. Then he would be with Sally and David's foundation would inherit the funds from the Fidelity Magellan Money Market account as the beneficiary.

When David ushered Henry through the door he said to him, "Did you see that Fidelity was way up again?"

"Yeah!" Henry said with his eyes glowing, "up 16 points from yesterday. We're gonna be rich!"

David just patted him on the back and walked with him over to the sofa. He didn't even know that he already was rich. "Henry, I was thinking about calling your doctor. Dr. Wilson is it? To tell him that I think you're about ready to come off the

Sinequan. What do you think about that? How many do you have left anyway?"

"Whatever you say, Doc," Henry said as he fished around in his front pants pocket for his pills. Since he never knew what shift he'd be working at the restaurant he always carried them with him. "You're the boss. But I do like not having those night-time terror things. They won't come back will they?"

"Well then let's not take you off of them just yet. How many do you have there?" He asked as he reached out and took the bottle from Henry.

He walked over to his desk and dumped them onto his blotter making sure several fell onto the floor. "Oh, I'm sorry Henry," he said, bending down to pick them up. "Just make sure you wash each one before you take it."

With his other hand he reached into his pocket and pulled out the baggie and dumped its contents onto the floor with the other pills, replacing the empty baggie back in his pocket. When Henry came around to the other side of the desk to help him he saw Dr. David putting the pills back into the bottle one by one, counting them as he went.

"Twenty-six. At three pills a day that's a little over a week. I think that's good. Let's plan on stopping then unless you have any more problems, okay?"

"Okay," Henry said as Dr. David handed him back his pills.

"Sit down and tell me about your day, Henry. I always love to hear what's going on at the restaurant."

Chapter 74

Chantilly, VA

Colin sat at the little dinette table in MaryAnn Riddel's kitchen. It would have been comical if the situation hadn't been so serious. He looked like a man sitting at a little girl's tea party. His long legs were sprawled out in front of him as he slumped in the seat, the dainty round seat of the chair unable to hold all of him.

Colin was looking at the clipboard MaryAnn had placed in front of him. "Tell me again, exactly what this represents," he said softly.

Wiping her red nose and eyes with a tissue and tucking a lock of stray mousy brown hair behind her ear she looked back down at the chart. "Every night Pete would plan out the next day. We have three kids now since Robbie died and Pete wanted to make sure that he knew where each one was every minute of the day."

She flipped through the pages to the last one where there was a laminated sheet showing three columns. "Each column is a separate class schedule for each kid. From homeroom to last bell at 3:00." She let the pages fall forward again to the top sheet.

"If there was to be any deviation from the normal schedule, like a field trip or an extra band practice the kids were to tell him the night before and he would put it on their chart."

"What is this notation here for?" he asked, referring to a penciled in symbol of something that looked like a peace sign, a plus sign and the number four.

"That," she said pointing to the peace sign, "is a steering wheel. It means car pool. The driver plus four kids. He would have been picking up our kids plus Andrea, a girl who lives six houses down. She had to stay for basketball practice," her finger followed the grid to where there was a picture of a basket ball at 3:30 below Kristin's name, "with Kristin, our daughter." Her finger traveled to the right and landed on a small horn also sketched in pencil, "Josh had band practice," her finger went to the next column, "and Keith had detention." Her finger landed on a capital D with three exclamation marks after it.

"Pretty good system, huh?" Colin asked, impressed with the detail.

MaryAnn shrugged, wiping her red-rimmed eyes again as she replied, "It worked for him. He never missed a pick-up or left anybody behind. But most importantly he always knew where each child was, every minute of the day. That's why I have such a hard time believing he would have gone to all the trouble of filling this in the night before if he was just going to swallow a bunch of pills to end his life and never need to use it!"

There was no doubt she was bitter. And he didn't blame her. This was not the way you cared for a loving family. You didn't desert them. His own guilt crept up on him a bit when he realized that he had no earthly idea where his son was right at this moment. But he hadn't deserted his family. They had deserted him.

"How long did it take to make this every night?" Colin asked as he gestured toward the clipboard.

MaryAnn thought for a moment and then said, "About half an hour or so. First he'd have to track down each kid to see what they would be doing the next day and then he'd sit in front of the TV and pencil in the after school events and the times for everybody to be picked up."

"And he did all the driving?" Colin asked incredulously.

"Usually. He didn't let the kids ride home with their friends unless a parent was driving and he didn't trust most of the parents to be on time, so he usually did it himself," Mary Ann said.

"Didn't this conflict with his work? All this running around in the afternoon?" Colin asked.

"No, his office is right up Route 50, just a few blocks from the school. He didn't take a lunch hour and they understood that this was something he had to do. Any important meetings were

350

scheduled in the morning or right after lunch. It was never been a problem as far as I know."

Colin tapped his pen against his lips. He had to agree with her. It did seem like Pete had gone to a lot of trouble just minutes before taking his medication and going to bed if he knew no one would ever see it. Could it have been an accidental overdose? "Where did Pete keep his medication?" He asked.

"He carried a briefcase with him wherever he went. It had his cell phone in it and papers he needed to read for work whenever he had time to kill. He kept his pills there."

"Did he always take them on time?" Colin asked.

"Yes," MaryAnn remembered, "as far as I know, he was pretty punctual about everything he did."

"Had he been taking them for long?" Colin asked

"About two months, I think."

"Did he talk about the future with you during the last two weeks or so?" Colin asked as he studied her.

She looked exhausted and just about ready to crack at any time. "No. Nothing more than commenting on the school basketball playoffs he was looking forward to going to."

"Any references to where things were, like bills he paid, life insurance policies, or retirement accounts?"

MaryAnn sighed and grimaced. "No, he didn't. As a matter of fact I have had a hell of a time finding everything. He kept some stuff at work, some in his night stand drawer and just yesterday I found a safety deposit box at our bank that had all our legal stuff in it."

"Anything surprising?" Colin asked.

"No, all the bills had been paid up to date, the mortgage and car payments are paid automatically and all the others were paid at the same time a week before."

"Did he say anything fatalistic that might have indicated he was tired of living?"

"No," MaryAnn said emphatically.

"Did he give anything away to anyone, hand something down to one of the kids as a memento or anything?"

"No," MaryAnn said. "I've gone over everything he said and did. There was nothing out of the ordinary, absolutely nothing."

"And there was no note, right?" Colin asked beginning to feel sorry for all the questions he was asking.

"No. No note," MaryAnn responded, her voice flat.

There was silence for a few minutes while they just stared unseeing at each other. Finally Colin broke the silence. "Okay, if Pete didn't purposely overdose, what happened? Who would have wanted him killed and why? What would a motive be?" MaryAnn just shook her head.

"Was there anyone he wasn't getting along with, maybe at the office?"

"No, everybody loved Pete. He was gentle and kind to everyone. I've never heard anyone ever say anything bad about him in all the years I've known him."

Colin stood up and paced around the kitchen. "MaryAnn, I have to ask some questions, and I don't want you to get mad. But they have to be asked. I didn't know Pete, so you have to tell me everything you know, no matter how insignificant you think something might be. Okay?"

"Of course, Colin. I want to get to the truth of what happened to Pete much more than you do."

Colin turned to face her. "Okay, good. How was your sex life? How often were you and Pete intimate?" Colin stepped back expecting some sort of tirade. Instead he just got a glare.

"Our sex life was just fine! He wasn't seeing somebody else if that's what your asking! Talk to Cindy. She'll tell you. Pete never even looked at other women, or men, if that's where you're going with this!"

Colin put his hands up in mock surrender. "Okay, okay. I had to ask." He took a deep breath, jutted out his lower chin and blew out his lips causing his mustache to twitch. "People kill other people because they're jealous or they want something that they have. Seems like you're sure there's no scorned woman anywhere around. So what did Pete have? Any secret formulas, inventions, dirt on somebody?"

"No, his job wasn't like that. He worked with Consumer Affairs and Customer Assistance Departments and he handled all the training programs. If he knew something he shouldn't, he'd keep it to himself. He'd never betray a confidence," MaryAnn said.

"Well then," Colin said, clearly frustrated, "how much money did he have? Anything substantial?"

MaryAnn laughed. "That's a joke! We're not broke, but we're just making ends meet." She slumped down into one of the chairs. "Pete made good money and I do all right, but we spent almost every dime we had every month. Our mortgage is close to $2,000, we have two car payments on new cars, we have three kids who like to wear designer clothes and one whose funeral we'll be paying for until next year. Our savings has less than $1,000 in it and our retirement accounts can't be touched for twenty-three years. Other than that we have what you see."

She turned and spread her arms out indicating all that was beyond. Colin looked where she was indicating and saw a comfortable family room with a large screen TV and a large sectional sofa in off-white leather with big Navaho style pillows on it. They lived nicely, but not excessively.

"What about life insurance? Anybody take out a policy that you know of?" Colin asked.

"That's all getting worked out right now. He had a policy at work and we had a policy that we started when Robbie was born. That's going to be the only thing keeping us in this house. I could never afford it on my own. We didn't have mortgage insurance."

"Do you know how much the policies are worth and who the beneficiaries are?" Colin asked.

"Yeah, the one at work is for $75,000 and the one we got is for $150,000. The kids and I are the beneficiaries."

"Did Pete have a will?" Colin asked.

"Yes, he did. It's at the lawyer's office. He's on vacation for a few weeks so we're waiting for him to get back to handle everything," MaryAnn stated.

Colin could tell that she was getting tired of all the questions so he closed his notebook and stood up. "Do you mind if I talk to the kids for a few minutes? I'll be careful to be discreet and it'll only take a few minutes."

"No. Do you want me to call them downstairs or do you want to go up and see them in their rooms?" she asked.

"I'd rather go up if it's all right. It'll be easier to talk to them in their own environment. And I'd like to see Pete's briefcase, the bathroom he used and the bedroom, is that all right?"

She nodded. "Does this mean you're taking the case?" MaryAnn asked hopefully, leading him to the stairway.

"There's not much to go on, but I'll see what I can do. Let me know if there's anything else you can think of that might help, or anything that you forgot to tell me that bothers you, okay?"

"Okay," she smiled, "and thanks."

The kids were polite and he enjoyed talking to them but they really couldn't help him very much. The night before Pete died had been just like any other. No one thought anything was strange. Pete hadn't had any private conversations with any of them that had involved personal reflections, plans for their future or advice that he was passing along. None of them had received any kind of token or present from him in the last few weeks. It was almost as if he hadn't known he was going to die.

The case was beginning to intrigue him. After talking to the kids he called down the stairs asking if it was okay to check out the things in their master bedroom. MaryAnn hollered back up from the kitchen, "Sure, go ahead. I'll be up in a few minutes."

Colin walked down the hallway to the master bedroom. Everything was neat and clean, as it had been throughout the house. He found Pete's briefcase on the floor of the walk-in closet. He thumbed through the papers and agreed with MaryAnn. There certainly wasn't anything there anyone would covet.

The pill bottle wasn't there and he knew from reading the police report that the officers had taken it with them that morning to the coroner's office. It had been empty. The only other items in the briefcase were pens and pencils, index cards and paper clips. The cell phone was on the dresser.

He opened it and pressed the redial button. The number that came to the screen was the number MaryAnn had given him for Pete's office. He pressed the speed dial numbers. Again it flashed the work number. The second speed dial number was the home number. He closed the phone and placed it back on the dresser.

He went to the master bath and poked around opening drawers and cabinets. MaryAnn came up behind him and stood in the doorway. "Pretty standard stuff, huh?"

"Yeah," was Colin's only reply. He removed the back of the toilet tank, a favorite hiding place for all kinds of things and found nothing.

"MaryAnn, where were you that last night when he took his pills?"

"Downstairs making sandwiches for the kids and Pete." Apparently she'd already been asked this question.

"The bottle was empty after he took his pills, where did you or the police officers find it?" Colin asked.

"It was in the trash can," she said pointing to the matching mauve colored wastebasket beside the sink.

"So, if we assume he had been taking the proper dosages, he was out of pills and would have needed some for the next day."

MaryAnn walked over to her nightstand and produced a prescription slip. She showed it to Colin. "I was supposed to pick it up for him the day before but I forgot. He hadn't even asked me yet where I'd put them."

Colin studied the form. The handwriting was scribbled as expected but he could read the word Sinequan and under that 50mg. Sixty was the number of pills prescribed and it looked like the instructions were for two, twice daily. He could almost read the signature but the imprinted letterhead at the top of the form said: David L. Sandler, MD ABPN.

"Who's this?" Colin asked.

MaryAnn looked where he was pointing and answered, "His psychiatrist. After Robbie died we both needed help. Dr. Sandler was helping Pete deal with his grief. I thought he was doing a wonderful job with Pete."

"And the medicine? How was that working?"

"Okay, I guess. He didn't seem as depressed or agitated. It kind of mellowed out the hard edges of the things he was dealing with."

"Mind if I keep this for awhile?" Colin asked.

"No, help yourself. I certainly don't need it anymore."

"Do you have the phone bills for the home phone and the cell phone for Pete's last few weeks up until the day he died?"

"I think so. I'll go see." MaryAnn turned and went downstairs.

Colin went through the nightstand drawers and then through the dresser drawers that MaryAnn had said were Pete's. In the night stand drawer, under a Bible he found a small paper drugstore bag. Inside was an anniversary card from a husband to a wife, it hadn't been signed or put into the envelope yet. He took it down the stairs with him.

He took the phone bills out of her hand and handed the bag to MaryAnn and watched as she took the card out of the bag and read it. Before she had turned the front flap tears were streaming down her face. "When was he supposed to give you that?" Colin asked softly.

MaryAnn sniffed and wiped her eyes with the back of her hand. "The day I found him dead in our bed was our 17th anniversary. We had a babysitter all arranged and reservations for dinner at L'Auberge Chez Francois."

Colin recognized the name of the trendy restaurant in Great Falls that required a month's notice to get a reservation. "I am so sorry, MaryAnn. I will do my damnedest to find out what happened."

He reached out and squeezed her shoulders and then let himself out the back door so he could stop in the garage to check out Pete's car. The only thing he found there was a stale pack of

356

crackers in the glove box and an old baseball mitt. The name "Robbie" was written on the front in black permanent marker. He hadn't known Pete but he felt like he knew enough about him now to know that he didn't seem like the kind of guy who would give up on living with this kind of life to come home to.

Chapter 75

The Atlantic Ocean

"What a glorious day!" Margaret exclaimed as she entered the stateroom she shared with Leroy.

He was sitting on the sofa in front of their big picture window staring out at the ocean and the people milling around on the deck below.

"Yes, the skies are an unbroken blue as far as you can see. And boy, you sure can see far. I can see how the old mariners came to believe that the earth was flat. It does look exactly like you could drop right off the edge of the water. So you had a good time at the pool?" Leroy asked.

"Yes, it was very nice. The people on this ship seem to be tripping all over themselves to make me happy. I'm afraid I may have accepted one or more *Yellow Birds* than I should have." She was referring to the popular tropical drink served at all the shipboard bars. The sweetness of the fruit juice masked the strength of the rum.

The reason it was so popular was that some people actually thought they were drinking a healthy drink because of all the fruit juice and fresh fruit skewered on top. Others thought it was a good value since you got to keep the souvenir glass it came in. Margaret liked it because it was her favorite color and she liked the song "Yellow Bird" that the Caribbean bands on board were playing all the time.

Leroy liked them because they relaxed Margaret. And when Margaret was relaxed she let him do anything he wanted, and he wanted her now. He followed her into her bedroom and watched her in the mirror as she removed her jewelry. Her eyes caught his in the mirror, "You should have seen the dancing competition they had by the pool. These people can really tango and samba and do the limbo. It was great fun. I wish you'd come down and join me sometime."

He came up behind her and kissed the back of her neck, "I'd like to *join* you now." His hands undid the sarong tied around her waist and let it fall to the floor. Then he moved the strap of her bathing suit off of her shoulder pulling it down to her waist until he had bared one large pendulous breast. One hand reached around to cup it while the other hand bared the other breast.

As his eyes met hers in the mirror he murmured against her ear, "You are very lovely Margaret. Let my eyes feast on you while my mouth devours you!"

He gently spun her around to kiss her on the mouth as he gingerly removed the rest of her bathing suit. Margaret gave a long sigh as she fell into his arms in submission, a part of her groggy euphoria recalling the hero in her pool side paperback gothic romance novel. "Yes, yes, I'll be yours to do as you want with me. Just please, please, don't hurt me."

Hours later Leroy was still having trouble getting his heart beat back to normal. He took his medicine two hours earlier than usual trying to get things right. His pulse was so fast that he could feel himself shaking internally. Just as if he'd had too much caffeine. Way too much caffeine.

When the Captain arrived to escort Margaret to dinner Leroy came out of his bedroom to greet him. But as soon as the door was closed behind them, he fell into the chair beside the sofa. Staring out at the darkened ocean with only the deck lights reflecting off of it, he wondered about this feeling he was having.

Something wasn't quite right. His breathing was becoming labored and there was a pressure in his chest that was coming and going. When his cook arrived with his dinner, he just picked at the exquisitely garnished plate and then had him take it away, complaining of heartburn. He left a note for Margaret saying he was tired and wouldn't be up when she got back, hoping after a good night's sleep that he would be himself again in the morning.

Margaret and Leroy had breakfast together in front of the bay window the next morning and Margaret commented on the paleness of Leroy's complexion. She was embarrassed to mention the sheen of perspiration that seemed to coat his facial features but she did say she thought they should call the ship's doctor.

Leroy quashed the idea saying that ship doctors were incapable of diagnosing anything other than seasickness and sunburn. They were many miles south of Bermuda and due to be in St. John early that afternoon. Leroy promised that if he didn't feel any better when they docked he would allow the ship's doctor to have a look at him.

They docked at St. John around two in the afternoon. The tour guide provided for Margaret, a matronly lady named Constance Walker, came around asking if Margaret would like to disembark to see a few sights. Leroy saw the glimmer of excitement in Margaret's face and sent her off to enjoy herself, assuring her that he would call the ship's doctor if he didn't feel better by dinner time.

After Margaret left, Leroy opened a bottle of wine that he found in the mini-bar. He poured himself a tumbler and sat in front of the window. He had a melancholy feeling and the wine was mellowing him even more. He finished the bottle and tried to take a nap. Sleep just would not come. He was so jittery he just couldn't settle down.

He was so tired by dinner time that he didn't have the strength to call the doctor. When his cook arrived with his meal and found Leroy disoriented and experiencing shortness of breath he called the ship's doctor. Two hours later the ship's doctor arrived, woke Leroy up and did a cursory examination and proclaimed Leroy drunk.

He asked Leroy when the first symptoms had begun and Leroy told him that he hadn't been able to regulate his heart beat since he'd had sex with Margaret. The doctor snickered and called Leroy's cook back into the room. The doctor, along with the cook, managed to get Leroy into his bed and then left him on top of the covers, snoring.

Constance Walker had been a tour guide on St. John twenty out of her thirty years in the business so she knew all the places to take Margaret where they would be assured to have a good time. It was 2:30 in the morning before they got back to the ship and when Margaret looked in on Leroy she was so inebriated that she didn't even notice the pallor of his skin and that his lips had started to turn blue.

The next morning when she finally did awaken it was almost eleven in the morning. The cursory check of Leroy before she headed for the shower caused her great alarm. He was blue and breathing as shallowly as humanly possible. A frantic call to the ship's doctor brought an intern who in turn ran to get the doctor. The doctor found his medication and forced two pills down his throat.

In the middle of the panic Margaret passed the picture window and noticed that they were moving. They had left St. John at 10:00 am heading for St. Maarten. They were not due to arrive for another hour. Even she knew that Leroy needed a hospital right away. An hour would be too late. And it was. After interviewing everyone involved it was determined that Leroy died of heart failure brought on by excessive sex and excessive alcohol.

Because of Leroy's age and known heart condition, and since a doctor had been in attendance at his death, the government of the Virgin Islands did not insist on an autopsy. But they did require that his body be embalmed before allowing it out of the Virgin Islands.

Constance helped Margaret arrange for Leroy's body to be shipped back to Washington, D.C. where his children would have him picked up. Margaret saw no reason to accompany his body as she figured she'd arrive back in Washington at about the same time as Leroy's body if she just continued on with the cruise. So she invited Constance to share her stateroom and the two of them mourned Leroy's passing sitting at the pool with *Yellow Birds*.

Chapter 76

Fairfax, VA

The Washington Post reported the death of Leroy Dressler on the front page of the Style section. Since he had been such a prominent part of the Washington social society in his heyday it was newsworthy to note his passing.

David came to attention from the slouched position he was in when he recognized Leroy's picture. As his eyes scanned the article he slowly exhaled his breath. From all he could glean from the article everything had gone as planned. He was elated with the success of his plan and almost regretted not being able to tell anyone about it. He was beginning to feel powerful and so very, very clever. They had no clue. No one was on to him. How heady this feeling was. He wanted to celebrate. He wanted to be with *his girls*. He picked up the phone and dialed Jenny's number.

Jenny was always at work these days. She had so many clients demanding her time that he was often shut out of her schedule for days. It was the fall, model change-over time. People were coming in to get the latest cars and trucks off of the assembly lines and others were looking for the best deals on last year's leftovers. It would be this way for her until the beginning of November. They paged her several times for him and finally he left a message.

When she returned his call an hour later she explained that she had been on several test drives with customers. He started asking her about her customers. Lately he wanted to know who she was with, all alone in a car.

They'd had several discussions about her going on test drives alone with men. Jenny felt that she could not do her job and properly demonstrate her product without the all-important test drive. Usually the deal was closed by the time they pulled back onto the lot or at least she knew what it would take to close it.

David felt that Washington being Washington, it was unsafe for her to go on rides with absolute strangers.

She assured him that she always took a photocopy of their driver's license and left it on her desk for the manager to see just in case she didn't return within the normal time frame. She had never told him that she had been abducted almost seventeen years ago. The first year she had started selling cars.

She had been so eager that first year. She really wanted to do a good job. So she'd gone on a test drive at around 8:00 in the evening in a brand new Ford LTD with an older man who smelled a little of whiskey. She was explaining all the options and telling him all about the new features, remembering to explain the benefits to the customer not just the features, when she noticed that they had traveled a little farther than her normal test drive route.

"I think we should turn around now," she said timidly. Adding, "The dealership will be closing soon, we really should be getting back," when he didn't seem to hear her.

"Not takin' you back," was his simple reply.

"I beg your pardon?" she asked, beginning to tremble inside.

"You heard me. I ain't takin' you back. I like the car. I like the woman. You're stayin' with me." Jenny looked out the window and realized they were going way too fast on Route 1 in Alexandria for her to roll out of the car without getting hurt.

"You know, they're going to come looking for me, probably already have since it's closing time."

"So? The hell with 'em! I want to have some fun! Where ya wanna go? We could drive all the way to Las Vegas if you want."

Something inside Jenny made her realize that the only chance she had to get out of that car safely was to play along with him, so as loathsome as it seemed she raised the arm rest separating them and scooted over on the 60/40 split bench seat.

363

"You know, you're right. I've been working too hard lately. A little vacation would be nice. I've never been to Las Vegas. How far is it?"

He turned his head and smiled at her. His yellowed tobacco-stained teeth looked eerie as they reflected in the lights of the neon signs up and down Route 1.

"Couple days maybe, if we don't stop."

"Well, where's the fun in that?" She asked. "I don't want a grueling road trip," she reached her hand down and stroked his inner thigh with her finger tips. "In fact, I'd like a drink. Let's stop and get a few drinks at one of these bars," she indicated the pull-ins to several local taverns, "to sort of celebrate the start of our trip."

She could not believe it when he actually pulled into one and stopped the car. She was out of the car so fast that he hadn't even had time to come around to her side to see her out. He'd only made it as far as the trunk before she was running into the bar. As soon as she was inside she made her way across the smoke-filled lounge to the bar and screamed for the bartender to call the police.

Things had been sorted out pretty quickly that night at the police station and Jenny drove the LTD back to the dealership where the manager was waiting for her. These were the days before she worked for Royal Pontiac. She was working for a Ford dealership owned by a group of men who had no use for women in their dealership.

Had the manager known the day he had hired her how much grief he was going to take on her behalf he would have slammed his office door in her face before she crossed the threshold with her application in hand. She shrugged off his efforts to hold and console her as she hastily gathered her things together.

"You know, I could make this job a lot more profitable for you if you'd just be a little friendlier to me," he said as he followed her through the darkened hallways.

She shivered visibly with her revulsion. She grabbed her purse and briefcase and stormed by him. "Don't you think I've been through enough tonight? Can't you leave off with the constant harping, I'm not interested in doing anything with you and if you don't get the message soon, I'm going to give it to your wife!"

Normally she was pretty docile and put up with the constant flirting she got around here but she'd had enough for tonight. She went through the glass showroom doors to the parking lot and to her demo. She put the key in the ignition and when it roared to life she sped off the lot pealing rubber like a banshee.

The next day she was called into one of the owner's offices on the second floor. It belonged to a Mr. Thompson that she'd only met one time before, shorty after she had been hired, when everyone had been in such an uproar over her. There was a woman sitting in a chair in front of his desk. She looked old-fashioned in a dowdy kind of way. Her hair style looked like one from the forties, large curls the size of sausages pulled away from her face with combs. Her long dark brown dress was gathered at the waist with a matching belt although you could tell it hadn't been washed as many times as the dress had.

On her feet she had the type of shoes that had been worn during World War II, if you could believe the old movies. They were dark brown with polish over the scuff marks and had uneven heels from many years of use. She was introduced as Mrs. Walker. At first she thought she had been called up to take care of a house deal, a deal that is generated by upper management and given to a salesman for him to do all the leg work on in exchange for the board count and commission.

"Mrs. Walker is married to Tom Walker, the man who you took for a test drive last night."

Jenny did not like the way that was phrased. It made her sound like she was the one who had dragged him off the street and kidnapped him.

"She wants to talk to you."

Jenny turned to face her, her eyes incredulous. The woman had a tired face that looked like it had once been pretty, now it was pale with washed out brown eyes looking up at her. The lips outlined with red lipstick applied by a shaky hand gave a tentative smile.

"I came to apologize for my husband's actions last evening. I knew when he left the house that he'd had too much to drink, but I wasn't able to stop him. Please believe me when I say that he has never done this type of thing before. He is really quite a nice man when he isn't drinking."

When she turned her head slightly, Jenny saw a yellowish bruise on the side of her neck that had almost faded away. "I've come here to plead with you not to press charges against my Tom. We have three children who live in this area and it would be really hard on them if their Daddy had to spend any time in jail, or if this became public in any way."

Just then Mr. Thompson came around the front of his desk and looked hard at Jenny. "Mr. and Mrs. Walker have decided to buy the car he test drove last night." he smirked. "At full list price of course," he added satisfactorily, glancing at Mrs. Walker who nodded her head.

"A nice big commission for you and a great deal for the house." Jenny could tell that she wasn't being given an option.

"Why don't you go get it ready for her while I start the paperwork?"

She was being bribed to forget all about this, to drop the charges and let everything go. She would never have done it if it hadn't been for the sad, haunted look in Mrs. Walker's eyes. She could stand up to her greedy owner but she couldn't refuse the pleading look those tired eyes were giving her.

She knew she would regret this and to this day she did. She always wondered if she had caused someone else to suffer the same way she had or possibly even worse, much worse. She prayed that Mr. Walker had gotten the help he needed and that the police officers who had come to her aid had forgiven her for not standing up and doing the right thing as they had expected her to. Two months later she received a phone call asking her to come sell cars for a brand new Pontiac dealership opening up at

Tyson's Corner. She leapt at the chance to get away from the depravity that was at some dealerships in those early days.

Coming back to the present, she assured David again that she took precautions and that she didn't go on test drives with just anyone who asked her to, mentioning that most of her customers these days were repeats or referrals. And she reminded him that she always had her pepper mace attached to her demo keys. Still, she could see that this was an argument he was never going to let up on.

"Other than giving me such a hard time about my job, what did you call me for?" she asked sarcastically.

"Oh, I just wanted to see if you wanted to grab a bite and maybe a drink after work," David said.

"No, I can't tonight. I'm swamped. It'll probably be after ten before I get out of here tonight," Jenny replied.

David gave a long sigh of disappointment. "You are working way too much these days. You are averaging over sixty hours a week!" David sputtered.

Jenny was a little surprised that he kept track of her hours. "David, you've always known that this is how the car business is. You can't make any money working 9 to 5. Most of the customers come in on the weekends and evenings!"

"Well, you're going to have to make some adjustments! This is not good for the kids. They hardly ever get to see you and when they do, you're exhausted. I make plenty of money. When we get married you're cutting back on your hours!"

Jenny had never heard him talk like that before. It set her ire up another notch. "Oh, yeah, we'll just see about that!" And she hung up on him.

When she walked out of the dealership at quarter til eleven David was waiting by her demo. It was a warm night so he was just leaning against her car, his navy blue blazer flapping in the gentle breeze. As she walked toward him she assessed him as a woman who had never seen him before would. He was impeccably dressed. His bright white shirt was open at the throat revealing a deep vee of curly chest hairs descending downward to his khaki trousers with a razor sharp crease and stylish front pleats. He wore navy and tan argyle socks, which she knew to be cashmere costing more than most of her dresses, finished by shiny cordovan loafers from Johnston and Murphy. David was definitely classy.

At six foot he was almost a head taller than she was. He didn't exercise a lot but he really didn't need to. He had no paunch or any extra weight and at the same time he wasn't spare anywhere either. If a woman was going to pick a groom to walk down the aisle beside she really couldn't do much better in the looks department.

"Hi!" She called out. When she got closer she said under her breath, "I'm sorry about hanging up on you. It was very rude of me." In answer he just opened his arms to her. She set her briefcase down by the car and walked into his embrace. They stood there for a few minutes just holding each other.

"Let's go get something to eat," David suggested.

But Jenny was too tired and had to be back to work at eight the next morning for a sales meeting. "No, I'm not really hungry and I've got a hectic day again tomorrow."

"We will have to make some adjustments after we're married," he said softly, "I can't have my bride and the mother of my children being one step from exhaustion all the time."

Jenny just nodded as she leaned over to pick up her briefcase. He opened the car door for her and waited til she was settled into the bucket seat of the Grand Prix she was driving this month.

He leaned into the car and kissed her thoroughly on the lips while his left hand massaged the side of her neck. "I love you Jenny," he whispered as his lips slid towards her ear. "I can't wait til we're married and I can be at home when you get there, ready to take you to bed with me."

He gave her another lingering kiss on the lips and then closed the door for her. He waited until she started the car and drove off the lot before he got into his car for the lonely drive home.

Jenny drove down the toll road fighting to keep her eyes open and trying to shake the feeling that she had every time she thought about her impending marriage. David was such a great guy and a remarkably "good catch" as the girls at work would say. What was the problem here? She asked herself.

Chapter 77

Chantilly, VA

Colin drove to the Fair Oaks police station to track down the two officers that had responded to MaryAnn's frantic call the morning that she had found Pete dead in their bed. They were also the same two officers sent to talk to his doctor, Dr. David Sandler. He had run out of ideas so he was beating the bushes trying to find a lead to follow.

Because of his association with several of the local banks, he handled fraud cases and insurance investigations whenever they needed him, he was able to use the computers in the Fraud department to check on Pete and MaryAnn's bank accounts. He found nothing out of the ordinary there. They were the standard upper middle class family trying to show the world they were a little more prestigious then they really were. It appeared that they paid their bills on time and true to what MaryAnn had said, by the end of any given month they were scraping the barrel to buy bread. The microfilm of the checks written for the last year showed him nothing he could question.

He'd visited Pete's place of employment, Virginia Power, and talked to many of his associates. It seemed that Pete was well-liked and greatly missed. Almost everyone expressed the idea in one way or another that they thought Pete could have committed suicide right after Robbie's death, but that they had a hard time believing he was capable of it now, months later. He was always talking about his kids and the things they were up to. He was very proud of them and he acted like he was their personal champion to steer them away from the temptations that had taken Robbie from him.

In Colin's mind, suicide just wasn't adding up. When he arrived at the substation he walked around saying "hi" to everyone while he waited for Kenny and Dan to show up for their shifts. He saw Cindy Policki standing at the end of the hallway talking to an officer and waved to her. It was because of Cindy that he had taken this case.

He and Cindy had been partners for about two weeks while he taught her the ropes about auto theft. A smile came to his face when he remembered the first time he told her to lay on the ground and get under a car to verify a serial number.

He remembered distinctly what she had said, "The only way I'm gonna lay on this dirty ground is if you're gonna lay on top of me."

He'd laughed and then given her a look that said he wouldn't stand for a refusal. "Equal pay, equal duty. It's your turn to get grease in your eye."

Since then they'd been pretty good friends. When she was on the co-ed police softball team he'd captained last year he'd counted on her several times to bring the runners home. She was an unusually strong power hitter. For a woman.

Cindy walked away from the man she'd been talking to. "Hey, Colin! Did ya come by to roll in the dirt with me?" She joked.

"No," he said, "but down and dirty with you does sound nice. I came to see Kenny and Dan about Pete Riddel. They were the officiating officers for the death report. How are ya?" he asked.

"Okay, I guess," she answered glumly. "Got dumped again last week. What's it take to find somebody faithful around here these days anyway?"

"Yeah, I hear ya." he said.

Cindy grimaced, "Sorry, Colin. I forgot about your old lady. So how'd it go with MaryAnn?"

"Oh, she seems to know her man all right. Everything I find verifies what's she's been tellin' me. What do you think about all this? Could he have had a little honey on the side do you think?" Colin asked as he waved to Kenny and Dan who'd just come in.

"No way! He was the last faithful man made in America. MaryAnn never had a thing to worry about with him. He didn't even look at trouble. He was the most devoted husband you can imagine. You're gonna have to look someplace else, 'cause that's not where it's at. Hey, I gotta go. My partner's waiting. Give me a call sometime. Maybe we can have a drink, drown our sorrows and talk about who's gonna be on the bottom in the dirt, okay?" she said wistfully, because she knew he'd never call her. Men that good looking never had a problem finding women that were that good looking too.

"Sure. And thanks for recommending me for the case," Colin called as he turned away from her and faced the two officers standing in front of him.

He put out his hand and shook each one's hand in turn as he greeted them. "Kenny, Danny, good to see you. Can you spare a few minutes to help me on a case?"

"Not a problem," Kenny said and they lead him across the aisle to an empty interrogation room. "What's the case?"

"A Mr. Pete Riddel. His wife found him taking a permanent sleep. You responded and filed a report."

"Yeah, I remember," Dan said. "The wife couldn't even talk to us; we had to go back to interview her that afternoon."

"Just a few questions if you can think back that far. Do you remember where you found the prescription bottle?"

"It was in the trash can, next to the sink."

"Anything else in there?" Colin asked.

"An empty can of shaving cream and some used tissues is all I can remember," offered Kenny.

"Was there anything that you thought was odd, or anything that would make you think the guy intended to be awake in the morning?"

"His cell phone was being recharged on the dresser," piped up Kenny.

"That's probably more habit than anything," Colin said as he discounted that. "How about clothes laid out or anything like that?"

"Nope. Just the man in his pajamas lookin' for all the world like he was just asleep," said Dan.

"When you went to see the psychiatrist, what happened there?" Colin asked.

"Just routine. He seemed pretty straight up," Kenny said.

"Was he surprised?"

"He wasn't surprised and he wasn't not surprised. He was pretty matter-of-fact. Said this happened all the time with these kinds of cases."

"What kind of cases?" Colin queried.

"Don't know, he wouldn't say. Started talking about confidentiality between him and his patient."

"Anything about him strike you as odd?"

"No, just your regular ol' well-to-do shrink, takin' it all in stride. I don't think he'll miss the patient or the money," Kenny mused.

"Did the department send anyone to photograph the funeral?" Colin asked.

"Not that I know of. Once we filed the report I don't think anybody paid any attention to it. It seemed pretty routine. Isn't it?" Dan asked.

"Don't know yet. That's what I'm tryin' to figure out. His wife doesn't believe he offed himself. She hired me to check everything out. I gotta get out of your hair so you can get back on the street. Call me if you think of anything, and thanks." He shook their hands again and walked out of the station house.

Chapter 78

Fairfax, VA

Colin was bench pressing 220 pounds in the gym at the Police in Fairfax when his pager went off. He placed the bar on the rack and reached for the vibrating black box clipped to his waistband. It took him a few moments to recognize the number flashing at him. It was MaryAnn Riddel's home phone number. Damn! He was going to have to give up his position in front of the glass doors to go phone her.

This was the coveted position that afforded the viewer an unobstructed view of the women's Jazzercize class. Just as well, the women parading in front of him now weren't doing a thing for his libido. The painted and coiffed hair and the carefully matched exercise outfits all designed to attract the bees to the pollen were far from the type of woman that appealed to him. But it was still fun to watch the blatantly sexual gyrations they came up with to amuse the officers as they worked out.

Colin grabbed his towel from the bench and wiped the sweat from his face as he walked down the hallway towards the pay phone. Unclipping the pager from his workout pants he punched in the numbers displayed on the screen. MaryAnn answered on the first ring.

Instead of saying hello, he heard her anxious voice say, "Colin?"

"Yes," he replied, his voice soft and concerned.

"I've been cleaning out Pete's side of the closet and I found something I thought you'd like to know about," she said.

"Yeah?" he asked, interested in anything that would move this case forward again.

"In the middle of his suits I found a sports coat still hanging in the dry cleaning bag." The significance of this escaped him until she continued, "The receipt stapled to the bag is dated the day before he died. He must have brought it home and put it in the closet while I was cooking dinner in the kitchen."

It didn't need to be said. They both knew that a man saving pills to commit suicide would never take the time to stop by the dry cleaners to pick up a jacket he never planned on wearing again.

"I'll stop by in a few minutes if it's all right. We've got to figure some things out about those pills."

After being assured that was fine with her, Colin went to the locker room to shower. On his way he passed the Jazzercize class as they were snaking their way around the hallway, jogging to the beat of some seventy's tune. They all gave him a wide encouraging smile as he walked past them. The last one in their conga line ran her dragon lady acrylic fingernails down his arm. She blew him an exaggerated kiss and winked at him. He shivered with revulsion. My God, the woman must have been seventy!

On his drive over to MaryAnn's he pondered the things about this case that really bothered him. There sure were a lot of them. Starting with the carefully filled out schedule, the special anniversary dinner and now this seemingly normal dry cleaning ticket. Then there was something else, something he hadn't even bothered to mention to MaryAnn; men generally did not commit suicide with pills. It was emasculating. A coward's way out. A man like Pete, if he had really contemplated suicide would probably have used a gun or hung himself. Not overdosed.

He pulled into MaryAnn's driveway and looked up at the large colonial styled house. Pete would have had to have been a fool to have tried to get away from all the love he could feel emanating from this house. He was painfully reminded of his own family and the love that had once been, but was no more, when his wedding band smacked against the car door frame as he slammed the door shut.

MaryAnn was waiting at the door for him when he came up the steps. She looked like she was trying to put herself back together. It certainly was an improvement from the last time he had seen her. When she smiled at him he noticed that she had pink lipstick on her front teeth. Well at least she was wearing makeup and it looked like she had styled her hair into some sort of a flip, reminiscent of a sixty's style.

"Hi!" she called cheerfully as she opened the door for him.

"Hey there," he said as he stepped through the doorway and into the foyer.

He waited for her to close the door and then followed her down the hallway back to the kitchen area. Hanging from the top of an open pantry door was the dry cleaning garment, the plastic reaching almost to the floor. He inspected the tag then lifted the plastic to check all the pockets.

Finding nothing, he turned back to MaryAnn and said, "Did he wear this coat often? Was it a favorite of his by any chance?"

"No, I don't think so. He liked to wear it when he knew he was going to watch one of the boy's home games. He wore it with khaki slacks so he would be wearing the school's team colors, navy and gold."

"So it wasn't anything he would have wanted to be buried in?" he asked.

"Oh, no!" she replied. "He always said he wanted to be buried in old jeans and a T-shirt and that's what we did."

"So, it's safe for us to figure that he planned on wearing this jacket to another home game some day?" Colin asked.

"I would think so. Wouldn't you?" she asked.

"Yes, I would," he said with a deep sigh as he took a seat at the little dinette table. He remembered that she had told him that the playoffs for his son's team were due to start two weeks after Pete had died. Pete had probably planned to wear the blazer to every game.

"Okay, let's figure out who had access to those pills." He took out a little note pad and pen from his coat pocket. "Starting from the pharmacist. Pete kept them in his briefcase right? Which he took where?"

MaryAnn shrugged. "I guess he took it everywhere he went. His briefcase also had his cell phone and some work papers he read whenever he had to sit and wait for the kids. So it was either in his car or at work or here."

"Then I guess that means I need to know about all the people in his office and all the people who've been in his car and all the people who've been in this house since he had the prescription filled. What day was that?" he questioned as he flipped back in the book trying to find that date.

"What good would that do? Shouldn't you be looking at some other way that he could've died? Maybe they missed something in the autopsy, an aneurysm or something?" MaryAnn seemed confused. Colin hesitated before bracing himself to tell her flat out what she needed to know if she was going to be any good to him.

"MaryAnn, he died from the pills. That's a fact. If he didn't take too many on purpose or by accident, which doesn't seem likely, then somebody had to make him take too many without him knowing it."

"What! How could that be? And why would anybody want to do that?" she almost screeched.

"That's what we need to try to figure out. Now, tell me about all the people you had in the house the whole week before he died." Colin sat with pen poised waiting for her to search her memory. An hour later they had a list that comprised almost a hundred people.

"We definitely are going to need to narrow this down some," Colin said with a wry grin, "this list would take a whole task force to investigate. Can you think of anyone who could have had the motivation to see Pete out of the picture? Who was in line for his job?"

"Phil Bertonski. But I heard that he didn't even accept it when it was offered to him after Pete died. It was a thankless job that everyone knew wasn't easy. Pete was perfect for it. He didn't even mind all the after hours reading it required. He had to read every training manual that they handed out, for every single department. I don't think job envy is the motive you're looking for," MaryAnn mused.

"Okay. Let's check out the most predominate motives for murder, namely greed for something, usually money. Then love and or fear. Who stood to gain anything by Pete's death?" Colin asked.

"Me. Everything becomes mine. I'm the only one he's left anything to. I go see the attorney tomorrow, but I can assure you, it's not enough for anyone to contemplate murder over."

"You and Cindy have assured me that Pete couldn't have been involved with another woman. Could there have been someone who would have been angered if he had rejected them? Someone whose advances had been spurned once too often?"

"Colin, I honestly don't know. He never mentioned anyone coming on to him and I never saw anyone hanging on his every word or movement. Pete just wasn't that type of guy. He was all right looking, but not someone you'd set your sights on unless you were into meek, mild, slightly overweight, balding older men. Pete was Pete. He thought about sex once or twice a month when I thought to remind him about it. I don't think that's your motive either."

"Was he possibly a threat to someone? This incident with Robbie awhile back. Did he ever threaten legal action against someone? Did anyone get charged with anything? The other kids involved, did they have any reason to be mad at him?" Colin's brow was deeply furrowed. He knew he was grabbing at straws. He couldn't figure out why he couldn't get anything to connect.

"Pete wouldn't harm anyone. Ever. And everybody knew it. Pinning blame or making a profit out of Robbie's death wouldn't have helped anyone and Pete knew it. He did make sure all the kids at that party had drug intervention sessions with the counselors from the school but nobody, including the parents, had objected to that. I think that's what everybody wanted also. Are you absolutely, positively sure that it was the pills that he died from? It couldn't have been anything else? A broken heart, maybe? He still missed Robbie tremendously."

"Well, he could have died from a broken heart, but it was helped along by a large overdose of Sinequan," he said stubbornly. "It was in his body. The question is, how did it get there?" Colin gritted the question through his clenched teeth.

Frustration was beginning to set in and he was tired of sitting around running into dead ends. He grabbed his note pad and stood up suddenly. "I'm going to start from the beginning. I'll go see the pharmacist who filled the prescription. Maybe something he says will click."

MaryAnn got up also. "Colin, don't let this beat you to death. We may never have the answers. Just the questions."

"That would be sad, because I'm as convinced as you are that Pete didn't do this. Someone's getting off scot-free." He went out the door and down the driveway to his car. Checking his notes again he found the page that had the drug store address he was looking for. It was just down the road in the Greenbrier Shopping Center.

As luck would have it, the pharmacist who filled Pete's prescription was in. His name was Robert Jones and he reminded Colin of Dennis the Menace's father, tall and wiry with dark hair and dark heavy spectacles. When Colin introduced himself and gave his reason for being there he came out from around the counter and shook Colin's hand.

"I read about Mr. Riddel's death in the newspaper and I always wondered why no one had come out to talk to me. Not that I know anything mind you, just curious."

"Well, I guess you weren't a suspect then, and you aren't now," Colin hastily added. "I'm just at a stalled point in this investigation and I thought maybe you could help me out. Do you have a few minutes you could talk to me?" he asked.

"Sure, don't know that I can help you out any, but I'll try," Mr. Jones replied. And then added, "It wasn't suicide as they said it was, was it?"

"I don't know. I don't think so. But I can't get anything to point in any other direction, either," Colin stated.

"I waited on Mr. Riddel many, many times over the last few years, and he just didn't seem the sort of man to do that," Mr. Jones said as he shook his head slightly. "Almost always had his kids in here with him. Bought 'em just about anything they asked for. Last time he was here gettin' that prescription refilled he bought them each a new toothbrush and whatever kind of tooth paste they wanted. He told me that one brand wasn't any better than another if they didn't use it. So he let them pick out the ones they wanted. He spent ten bucks just on toothpaste!" Colin smiled at the thought and then frowned as he realized that he had no idea what kind of toothpaste his son used, or his wife either for that matter.

"That refill was for sixty Sinequan pills, right?" Colin asked.

"Yeah. Sixty. 50 milligrams each. But they weren't pills," he said matter-of-factly. "They were capsules."

"Meaning?" Colin paused to look over at Mr. Jones' dark studious eyes.

Mr. Jones motioned with his hand for Colin to follow him and he led Colin around the edge of the counter to a long elevated work surface under shelves and shelves of bottles and small boxes. Mr. Jones reached up and pulled down two bottles. Opening them he dumped a few pills from each onto the counter.

"This," he said picking up a light and dark pink pill, "is a capsule. It comes apart." He demonstrated by pulling the two halves away from each other and pouring the white powder onto a small piece of paper on the table. "This is Sinequan, 50 milligrams."

Then he reached for a capsule from the other pile. "This is also Sinequan." He held up a bright blue capsule for Colin's inspection, "150 milligrams." Again, he took the capsule apart.

He placed the two halves in front of the powder from the pink capsule and took the two pink halves and placed them in front of the powder that had come from the blue halves. There was a difference, but you could see that it would fit quite easily. In fact, the powder from two of the blue ones would fit in the space a pink capsule allowed. Colin felt that this was what Mr. Jones was trying to tell him without using any words.

Colin stared at the drugs on the counter for a moment, trying to remember something he had written in his note pad a few days ago. "Why sixty? A month's worth?" He went back to their previous conversation.

"No," Mr. Jones said. "Sixty for fifteen days. Two pills at a time, twice a day. 100 milligrams each time."

"Mr. Jones, from what I've been able to find out, the normal dosage of Sinequan for an adult would be less than 100 milligrams a day. Is that not true?"

"Yes and no," Mr. Jones answered thoughtfully. "Sinequan, also known as Doxepin, is effective in different dosages. It's up to the prescribing doctor to determine the proper dosage for each patient. Generally a senior adult can be maintained on 50-75 milligrams a day. But it's not unusual for the amounts to range from 75 up to 200 milligrams a day for a younger adult."

"Why sixty instead of enough for a whole month?" Colin queried.

"Antidepressants are administered to people who are having a lot of trouble in their lives. It wouldn't be prudent to give them too much of a temptation for a way out."

"Which is exactly what I'm trying to prove did not happen," Colin mused. Stepping back to the piles of powders and pills he did some mental math. If there was the equivalent of two blue capsules in each pink one, Pete would have been getting 300 milligrams with each pill, 600 with each dose, 1200 for each day.

"Are these capsules easy to reassemble?" Colin timidly asked, almost daring not to be heard.

Mr. Jones picked up the small piece of notepaper under the powder, gathered the powder in the center and rolled the paper into a skinny tube. He then coaxed the powder into the darker half of a pink capsule by thumping it with his thumb. When all the powder was in that half he took the light pink side and inserted it into the edge of the darker pink one. Placing his thumb on the bottom and his index finger on the top of the capsule he held it up for Colin to see. It looked exactly as it had before. Only Colin and Mr. Jones knew that the capsule now contained six times as much medicine as it should.

Colin shook Mr. Jones' hand and thanked him for his time. Mr. Jones smiled up at him and grasping his hand with both of his said, "Good luck to you. My curiosity sure could stand some appeasing in this matter." Colin walked out the front door of the store into the hot muggy oppressiveness of late summer. Folding himself back into his car he felt a sense of some accomplishment. He still had no clue who could've killed Pete, but at least now he had an inkling of how it might have been done.

The list could now be narrowed to people who had some access to the drug Sinequan and as far as he could remember, there wasn't anyone on the list who did. Their suspect list had dwindled from 96 to none in less than an hour.

The next afternoon when MaryAnn called to tell him that Pete's will had been changed almost two months before he had died and that Dr. Sandler was now one of the beneficiaries of Pete's life insurance policy, Colin realized that *his* name hadn't even been on the list. His next thought was that Dr. Sandler had access. From his little prescription pad he had access to any drug available in the world.

Chapter 79

Fairfax, VA

The letter from Nancy Meridan's attorney arrived at Dr. Sandler's office in the middle of the week and just as he'd expected, it was a letter telling him he was a beneficiary in her contested will. Although his part of the settlement was not being contested, until everything was determined in court, the proceeds from her estate would be held in testate. Nothing he hadn't known, but it sure didn't make it any easier to deal with. He did wonder how much she had left him, but it was really moot right now if he wouldn't be getting it anytime soon.

There was good news today, though. Good for him anyway. Henry Blocker had been found dead in his apartment after missing work for two days. The apartment was over a garage in the city and had been closed off with no air conditioning in the sweltering summer heat, so his body had already started decomposing pretty badly. David was grateful for anything that would camouflage his misdeed.

He had learned of Henry's plight from the Channel 5 news on TV as he dressed early that morning. They were always looking for a story relating to the severe weather and so far the death was believed to have been caused by the extreme heat. They also believed he was indigent. He had scornfully knocked the media as he sat on the edge of his bed putting his shoes and socks on. In their haste to get a story on the air they weren't being very thorough. Nothing new about that though. His elation was tempered by a genuine sadness. He really had liked Henry. Maybe it was just a case of always cheering for the underdog.

If it weren't for Sally's family, he feared it could be a long time before Henry's money would be discovered and distributed. But those greedy parasites were probably already knocking on his attorney's door claiming the money was theirs. Boy, they would be in for a rude surprise. Ol' Henry in his slow, dimwitted way had out smarted them and he was sorry Henry wouldn't be around to see their faces when they found out they were disinherited.

All he was waiting for now was to hear from Pete and Leroy's attorneys to learn how much they had left him. Even though the weather was not conducive to an outside lunch he decided to call Jenny to see if she could meet him at their new homesite to check on its progress and have a picnic lunch in one of the framed in rooms.

It had been his habit to drive by every afternoon after work to see what had been done from day to day. He had been very pleased last night to see that the roof trusses had been delivered. Tomorrow he and Jenny were supposed to go pick out the brick.

Jenny was in a meeting but the switchboard operator promised to give her the message as soon as she came out. Twenty minutes later she returned his call. There was a tinge of excitement in her voice and she eagerly accepted his suggestion to meet at the new house. She said she had something she wanted to talk over with him.

David went down to the Deli and picked out a few sandwiches from the display case along with some Dr. Brown's cream soda and some chips. He already had a blanket in the back of the Trans Am, so he got behind the wheel and drove from Fairfax to Great Falls. Since it was lunch time and there was a fair amount of traffic, it took him almost an hour. Jenny was already there walking around the perimeter of the house and looking into the big hole in the ground that would soon be a swimming pool.

"Hi!" he called as he stepped out of the car. Jenny turned to look at him and marveled at the handsome sight he made. His starched white dress shirt was rolled up from the cuffs and the first few buttons had been undone but other than that he looked very GQ with his dark blue dress pants, cordovan belt with a stylish gold buckle and designer socks slipped into matching cordovan loafers. He was very overdressed for a picnic, but then he was always very overdressed.

Jenny waved to him as she looked down at her very simple straight skirt and sleeveless shell sweater. On her feet she had the spare set of shoes she always kept in her desk drawer, a cream colored pair of Minnetonka moccasins. Her black patent leather high heels would have never seen her up this steep incline.

He walked up the dirt hill and leaned over to give her a kiss on the cheek. Most of the workmen had left for lunch but there were still a few here and there so he deferred to her sense of modesty and public decorum. What he really wanted to do was to throw her down on the blanket he carried and make her moan and scream his name so loud that she frightened away all the birds that were singing in the tree branches just over head.

"You looked like you were ready to take a dip in the pool," he said softly into her ear.

She laughed at him and said, "Oh, if it were ready for me to take a dip, I'd jump in right now, clothes and all. It is so hot, I'm sweating inside my ears!"

David laughed at her as he swatted her on her bottom, "C'mon, let's go see if we can find the dining room, I want this to be a formal lunch!"

The firmness of her derriere sent a pulsing leap of electricity from his palm to his groin. If there weren't so many workmen hanging around he might have seriously considered trying to take her here in their new house on the sub flooring.

While they were placing the blanket in front of the fireplace in the dining room, Jenny looked over at David and said, "David, there's something I need to talk to you about. It's about this morning's meeting. I met with Ron Royal for over an hour this morning. They want me to become the new General Sales Manager."

David stopped emptying the bag containing their lunch and turned to look at her. "Geez, Jenny, aren't you already working hard enough?"

"Well, yeah, I guess I am. But being a sales manager doesn't necessarily mean I'd have to work harder. I'd just have to work more for the common good instead of just for myself," Jenny replied.

"But you'd have to work more hours, right?" he asked pointedly.

"No, not really. A manager works more hours than a salesperson, but right now I work more hours than most managers."

"So you're saying this position will require less work and less time?"

"No, not exactly, probably about the same. The difference will probably be in the money. A top salesman makes more than a top manager. Generally."

"So, you're considering a job that will require you to work for other people, just as hard and as long as you're working now, for less money?" he asked.

"Well, when you put it that way, it sounds pretty stupid." She took a few minutes to try to figure out what she was trying to say. "Ron needs me. There are some problems that need addressing. We need a good closer and a good trainer and I know that I'm good. Maybe it's the challenge of the job that is attracting me. To take a sales force that's not at all cohesive and make them work as a very productive team. There's so much I think I can do for the dealership and for the sales force. I think I can make us one of the best Pontiac franchises on the East Coast. And of course I'm quite flattered that Mr. Royal thinks I can do it, too. It's not always about the money, you know."

"Sounds like you've already made up your mind. Are you sure you want all this added responsibility at a time when everything else is changing for you?" he asked with concern.

"I've been offered management positions before with Royal, but a sales manager is very different from a general sales manager. I'll have control of all the front end departments. That's huge! If I want to give away a car at cost to pick up the finance money, I'll be able to. If I want to put more money on a trade-in being booked into the used car department to make someone's deal, it'll be within my power to do so. All the deals I see go out the door for one reason or another might be able to be put together if someone who can see the whole picture gets in there and manages it right. I think I can do the job. I think I'm the right man for the job!" she stated emphatically.

He stood up and came over to her and wrapped his arms around her shoulders. "Well I can certainly see that you believe this job is for you, but I have to disagree about you being the right *man* for it."

She turned a puzzled face up to his as he added, "You are all woman. *My* woman."

With that he wrapped his hand around the back of her neck and brought his lips down to hers. His passion was fierce as he moved his lips over hers, beckoning hers to open for his entry. Then he lifted her up into his arms and gently laid her down on the blanket. The sound of more workers returning from their lunch break necessitated him pulling away from her, that and the heat. It was scorching hot in more ways than one. He was on fire and he needed to put it out. Soon.

They gathered up the untouched lunch and blanket and headed for the cool comfort of his air conditioned car. They ate in companionable silence as they watched the workers hook up a crane to a truss and slowly maneuver it over to the top of the house. It was very exciting watching their house being built. Jenny was contemplating all the exciting things going on in her life these days and David was contemplating his exciting Jenny.

Chapter 80

Chantilly, VA

Colin left his apartment and drove to his old office at the Criminal Investigations Building in the heart of Fairfax City. He went to talk to some of his old cohorts about the loan of some surveillance equipment. When he got there he was greeted warmly by his previous police family.

"Hey, C.G. Scott!" a woman officer called from her desk. This woman officer had been his partner on many a fugitive assignment.

"Judy!" he called as he came over to her, lifted her out of her chair and gave her a great big bear hug. It had only been a few months since his retirement party, but these were people he'd seen every day for over ten years.

"Ya wanna go down to Bob Evans for some breakfast?" she asked.

"Na, I already ate two of those bear claws you got me addicted to a few years ago. Couldn't resist when I drove by the ol' bakery down the street."

Judy had as healthy an appetite as he'd ever seen on a woman, she generally could out eat him. But that was okay, she was a good partner, strong and athletic. Just the type of partner you'd want fighting beside you in a brawl. She could eat all the carbs she wanted, as long as she could still pick a 180 pound man up with one hand and throw him down on the ground.

"What brings you our way?" drawled Steve Brisbane as he sauntered over with a cup of steaming hot coffee in his hand. "I didn't think I'd ever see you within these four walls again." He snickered.

Steve was one of the reasons Colin had decided to leave the force. Too many detectives not pulling their weight around here. And he was definitely one of them. Colin had never seen a man as lazy as Steve who, at the same time, whined for not getting enough money or slaps on the back.

Colin gave him the kind of put down he'd never been able to give him before when he was still on the force. "I just came over to see if they ever found a case you managed to finish by yourself."

Steve's eyes went wide with shock in his pudgy face. His bottom lip came up to cover his top one and he turned on his heel and stomped away. Judy laughed hysterically.

"Really," she asked, "what did you come by for?"

"I came by to see Rudy. I need some help with a recording device for a case I'm working on. Have you seen him this morning?"

"Yeah, he's down in his work shop working on some new spy stuff."

"Well, I'd better go talk to him before ol' pinched-face finds the boss and tattles on me," Colin smirked. "See ya later, okay?"

"Yeah. Colin? You know you can still hook up with us at Lucia's every Friday night like old times. You don't have to disappear completely for months at a time."

He gave her a quick smile as he said, "I know." And walked off down the hallway to find Rudy.

Judy'd always had a bit of a thing for him and he knew it. She didn't want a relationship though, just an experience. He wasn't really drawn to her at all but he would have liked to have seen her topless just like all the guys on the squad. She was vavoom in the chest area.

He walked into Rudy's workshop and watched for a minute as his dear old friend sat tinkering with what appeared to be a mantle clock of some kind.

"Hi ya Rudy!" he called after a few moments. "How's life treatin' ya?"

Rudy looked up from his project and displayed a huge grin. "Colin." He stood up to wipe his hands on his pants and put his hand out for Colin to shake. "How the heck are ya!" He pumped his hand up and down several times like he was reluctant to let it go.

"I'm great. This retired life is wonderful. I get to sleep in and play golf whenever I want and not have to worry if the Captain's gonna find my cruiser in the country club parking lot!" He laughed. "And you, what's new with you? How's the family?"

"Oh, we're good. Amanda took the kids to visit her mom this week so I'm kinda batchin' it. And work is work. There's always plenty of it."

Rudy was in charge of a department whose total focus was on watching and listening to people without them knowing it. And he was very good at his job. He alone had designed several miniature cameras that had been instrumental in breaking quite a few important cases, some of them Colin's.

"Whatcha workin' on now?" Colin asked as he pointed with his chin at the clock.

"Oh, this is going to be really neat," he said with boyish enthusiasm. "It's an Anniversary clock," he showed him the four balls as he rotated them around with his finger. "Each one of these balls has a miniature camera in it, and they're timed in sequence so that we can view a whole room at one time as they spin around and around. If it's placed on a mantle it's at just the right height to get everybody's faces. Should be great for surveillance."

Rudy was, in Colin's mind anyway, a virtual genius. He could be making three times the money in the private sector if he hadn't been so dedicated to fighting the cause of good over evil. Colin admired him a lot and for some reason, Rudy felt the same way about Colin.

"Surveillance is exactly why I'm here my good man," Colin mimicked an English accent, trying to emulate *007* conferring with *Q*. "I have need of a miniature tape recorder that can record for at least an hour without making a sound in a very quiet room. Got anything along that order?" he asked.

Rudy walked over to another worktable and took a box off the shelf above it. "Here ya go. This should do the trick. 75

minutes, no tape sounds, picks up everything, even breathing noises. But it does have a slight click when the tape runs out, so ya gotta watch out for that."

"Perfect. Can I sign it out? Or would that get you into trouble?" Colin asked.

"Fightin' bad guys?" Rudy asked.

"Yup," Colin replied.

"Then it's no trouble. Just bring it back when you're done with it."

"Thanks Rudy. You're the best." Colin picked up the box with one hand and shook Rudy's with the other. "I'll get it back as soon as I can." He turned to leave.

"Oh, Colin?" Rudy called after him. "Need any of these?" In his hand he held a few mini tapes.

Colin gave him a sheepish look, "Yeah, I guess that would help, wouldn't it?"

Rudy also gave him a handful of small batteries and Colin took his new toy home to experiment with it before putting it to work in the field.

MaryAnn really wasn't able to tell Colin much about Pete's sessions with Dr. Sandler, only that Pete had seemed much better with each succeeding visit. Since Colin now had someone with a motive and a method he was reluctant to tip his hand.

If this Dr. Sandler had indeed doctored up the pills he had prescribed for Pete then he didn't want him to have any inkling that he was being suspected of anything by anyone. So he had opted to go undercover as he had done so very many times over the years. He started setting the stage to become one of Dr. Sandler's patients.

He started by first trying to secure an appointment. MaryAnn had tipped him off that Dr. Sandler had had a waiting list when Pete first inquired and it had taken him almost a month to get his first appointment. Colin was able to get an appointment two weeks away for Mason Williams, the name he usually used when he went undercover.

Then he set out to learn as much as he could about Dr. Sandler. Cindy and Judy helped him with the police computer work since his password no longer worked. He found out where he lived, that he drove a late model Pontiac Firebird, all about his clean driving record and even some fairly current credit information. He went to the library to check out the information in Who's Who in the medical profession which led him to check out the Washington society books on prominent citizens. He also went to GW University and checked out all the information he could find there. He spent the day scanning old yearbooks and transcript files. He was very grateful that he was able to flash his old badge and shield without any one looking to see that the date had expired.

From the credit file he had uncovered an inquiry from Custom Home Builders in Great Falls. That led him to the builder's trailer where he found a sign saying he was working on site and could be paged. The door was open so he went in and looked around. On the wall behind a desk was a big map of the planned community the builder was developing.

On several sold lots there were little yellow flags with names on them. He quickly found the one that said "Sandler" and wrote down the lot number. He followed the roads with his finger and memorized the street names. Then he got back in his car and drove to the site. Colin didn't want anyone to know why he was really there so he thought he'd investigate on his own. Sometimes construction workers were more observant and more willing to talk without explanations than most people would be.

When he pulled up in front of a house that was probably only one third built he was duly impressed with its size. He got out of his car and walked around, trying to pretend that he belonged there. After a few minutes one of the men carrying some wood called out to him. "Can we help you with anything?"

Colin waved to him and sauntered over. "Yeah, I spoke with the builder awhile back and he said I could look around at some of the houses under construction. My wife and I are looking at a lot just up the street."

"Oh. Well help yourself. If you have any questions, Brad over there is the foreman. I'm sure he can answer them for you." He indicated a shirtless man hammering something on a saw horse.

"Well, the only question I really have is what kind of neighbors I might be settling down with. That's very important to me. I've really got some lousy neighbors where I live now. Know anything about the people buyin' this house?"

"Not much," he answered. "They were just here this afternoon looking around and being all lovey dovey. Tried to have a picnic lunch there in the dining room, but either the heat of the day or the heat of their bodies made 'em call it off. I think he's some kind of doctor or somethin', and she's a looker, umm umm, if you know what I mean. I wouldn't mind her for a neighbor." Colin laughed along with the man.

The man wiped the sweat from his brow. "Hey, I gotta get back to work but if you want to meet this guy he usually comes by everyday in the late afternoon, some time around 4:30."

"Thanks," Colin said and he continued to look around for a few minutes pretending to look at the quality of the construction before he got back in his car and drove off.

So, Dr. Sandler had a girlfriend. Figured. According to the court records he'd combed through he'd been divorced well over a year ago. Statistically most divorced men remarry within two years of their divorce, usually to the woman who had caused it. His smile quirked a little. When his divorce became final who would he marry? His future held no such promise for him and it saddened him to think about it.

He drove home to thoughts of Lynn and Adam planning their new future with her new paramour. It seemed like everybody had somebody and it really grated him that somebody had just walked into his life and taken his wife and child away from him without so much as a "how do you do." How long had he been asleep at the switch? He wondered. He should have seen it coming in time to stop it.

When Colin got back to his apartment he unloaded the books he had checked out from the library. Everything he could find on hypnotherapy and some on psychiatry in general. He was going to have to come up with a condition, something that could be treated with pills. He went to the kitchen and fixed himself a drink, a big vodka tonic with a lime slice in it. His drink of choice was actually Canadian Club and ginger ale, but the only problem with that was that he knew he would just keep drinking it until he passed out, judging from the mood he was in right now. Tonight he had work to do and drinking alone was really starting to depress him.

Chapter 81

Tyson's Corner, VA

Over the next several weeks Jenny found herself immersed in her work. She had accepted the General Sales Manager position and all the work it entailed. She was busy defining new policies and procedures and setting up new follow-up systems. She wanted this new sales floor to be the most professional one anywhere. Smoking was banned throughout the building, not just in the showroom but in all offices throughout the dealership.

Profanity was outlawed. No longer would a customer have to chance onto a conversation filled with lewd remarks as they turned a corner in the building. There were training meetings twice a day, one for each shift, and sales meetings twice a week at 8:30 in the morning, a half hour before the showroom opened. Jenny was determined that none of the stereotypes for new or used car salesmen would apply at Royal.

She was redoubling her efforts to close deals, trying everything she could to appease the customers and bring them back in the door to buy again if they weren't closed the first time. She backtracked each deal to make sure everything was done right before it went into settlement all the while still trying to make sure her own customers were being treated properly and personally. Jenny didn't want them to feel like they were being handed off as house deals, even though that's exactly what was happening.

As a manager she couldn't collect a deal commission any more but she insisted that each retail deal have the benefit of a salesman and the salesman the benefit of the commission. That way the customer would always have someone to come to if there was ever a problem and the salesman would have the impetus to help them out.

The stresses of her new job, along with the extra hours she was devoting to make sure things were running smoothly in the transition period, were beginning to show. She was always tired and seldom up for any of the things David suggested they do, preferring to have dinner with her parents, tuck the kids into bed and fall exhausted into hers. Her days were filled with waking the kids, getting them dressed and fed, taking them over to her parents, going to work, coming home, getting the kids, putting them to bed and starting all over the next day with the same thing. The cycle never seemed to end until Sunday when she didn't have to go to work.

David kept reminding her to take her vitamins and often brought a "pill-pak" of vitamins from the 7-11 convenience store to her with some carry out food. David was keeping busy following the progress on their new home. He spent hours at the site every afternoon making sure things were done to his specifications and making modifications daily, driving the builder a little crazy.

Money was coming in now, almost with weekly regularity. Leroy Dressler's estate had netted him $80,000 and Henry Blocker's a whopping $300,000. The day he received the check from Pete Riddel's attorney, he was so incensed that he had almost torn it up. A measly $15,000! That wouldn't even be enough to buy the billiard table for the new house! He had been livid. His receptionist wondered about all the ruckus as he slammed drawers and hit his fists against the desk. He had taken the greatest risk with Pete and look where it had gotten him! He should never have considered anyone who had the future of young children to think about. He resolved then and there that he would only focus on the truly wealthy patients who had no children as potential heirs. Going back to his list of candidates he crossed Donna Bristol off his list and circled Jessica Tyler's name. He had enough for the house, but now he wanted to furnish it and buy a few horses for Paisley.

Chapter 82

Chantilly, VA

Colin had instructed MaryAnn not to object in any way to the settlement of the $15,000 to Dr. Sandler, to go ahead and encourage the attorney to send it out as soon as possible. He didn't want any waves to be made over it. MaryAnn agreed for the sake of Colin's investigation but she was sorely angry at Pete for stipulating it. $15,000 was a lot of money to them, especially right now.

After reading for practically two days Colin felt he knew a little bit about hypnosis now, certainly a whole lot more than he'd ever known before. And his original plan had to be thrown out the window. He heard that a lot of people went to hypnotists to be cured of smoking. Apparently that was just hearsay and not at all true. Hypnosis won't really help you get rid of a habit that you don't really want to give up and most smokers really don't want to quit or they would have found a way to. The success rate is so low that most hypnotists don't even like to try it. Well, in a way he was kind of glad that wasn't going to be his problem. The thought of making himself reek with putrid tobacco had been unpleasant, he was glad he wouldn't have to do that. He'd been a non-smoker since 1978 and he intended to stay that way.

His other thoughts had been something along the lines of pain management or anxiety attacks but the more he read the more he realized that he would not be the one in control in that doctor's office, Dr. Sandler would be. To have the best chance at being believable he'd better pick something a little closer to home, also a little closer to Pete's problem. When he seriously sat back and analyzed his feelings, he realized he actually was somewhat depressed and suffering some pain from his soon-to-be divorce. Also self-esteem and inadequacy doubts were always nagging at him now. Might as well get some useful advice as well as bring some real problems to the couch.

He had no idea what would go on in these sessions but it was a cinch he'd be put under at least once or twice, in fact he was counting on it. He wondered what it was like, and if he'd really be able to be put under. He kind of doubted it, but who knows? Better stick to as much truth as possible, just in case.

So he was going to see a psychiatrist about his marital problems, specifically his grief over losing his wife to another man. When he thought about it he knew that he could come up with some genuine emotion for Dr. Sandler to see but he really didn't think that he had it as bad as you would need to, to seek outside help. Given a few more months he was sure he'd work things out for himself. But it was either that or anxiety attacks and he wasn't sure he could pull that one off.

He'd read that the more fully you imagine something the more real it seems to the brain and the greater amount of information sent to the nervous system. Kind of like a wet dream he thought. The better you could visualize those breasts the sooner you could get off. What in the world could he be anxious enough about to need help? He doubted that Dr. Sandler would be interested in treating his sexual frustration problem or if he did his solution would be a referral to a massage therapist down on K. Street.

Hypnosis was also used for pain therapy. He'd read that it was used for women in labor and in dental offices for all kinds of procedures and even by some surgeons who had actually done complete operations with patients anesthetized by hypnosis alone. It was a way of filtering out information that you really didn't want to have. You have to pay attention to something for it to hurt you, so you can lessen or remove the pain entirely by turning down the attention to it. What pain was it he could come up with that would be convincing? He couldn't think of any. I guess grief by way of marital separation was the only avenue he could take, he thought, ending the debate with himself.

He drove to the section of town where Dr. Sandler's office was located. He drove around the block several times noting all the banks that were close by. Then Colin went to the fraud office at First Virginia Bank, one of the banks that retained him. Using the computer and an attractive computer technician he had flattered into submission, he checked the accounts for anything in the name of David Sandler personally and professionally.

He found nothing. Going to the list of banks he had written down he saw that there were two other possibilities. He had a friend at one of them, maybe he'd get lucky. He went into the nice cool lobby and looked around for the pimple-faced girl he'd known since high school. She didn't have the scourge of acne any more, in fact she was quite lovely and very happily married to one of his best friends. He spotted her in one of the glass encased offices. The nameplate on the open wooden door announced that this office was hers. Debbie Scarpagio, wife to Frankie, once bitter nemesis, now best fishing and golfing buddy. "Hey Deb," he called as he poked his head into her office.

She looked up and smiled at him. "Hey, yourself you big galoot. Where you been? We haven't seen you in ages."

"Oh, I've been around. Just busy I guess. You got a minute?"

"No, but for you, I'll make one. Have a seat." She gestured toward the chairs in front of her desk.

"I guess you heard about me and Lynn, huh?" He asked.

"Yeah, I was real sorry to hear it too. How are you doing with it?"

"Okay, I guess. Coulda been worse, she could have taken my Harley instead of my kid," he joked.

Debbie laughed, it was just like Colin to make a joke about something so serious. "What can I do for you, I know you didn't come here to spill your guts to me."

"I got a case I need some help on." He didn't bother informing her that he was no longer with the department, just in case she didn't know. As an officer if he needed information he could get it with a search warrant and she knew it, so this was just a more direct approach saving them both time and paperwork.

"I just need to know if the account is here and if so, if a lot of money has been going into it lately."

She turned to her computer and typed something in. "Okay, what's the name?"

"David Sandler, or Dr. David Sandler or any kind of professional organization or association with that name," he replied.

"Dr. Sandler!" She whispered in a long drawn out hiss. "I know Dr. Sandler, he comes in here all the time. What's he being checked out for?"

Colin gave a deep sigh and shook his head. It figured that she'd know him, now what? He didn't want her to know what was going on, it would be so easy for her to change her attitude towards Dr. Sandler and he would be sure to detect something amiss next time he came in.

He lied. "I'm not checking him out. I'm checking out his secretary, he suspects her of embezzling some of his funds." He whispered back to her. God, he hoped she didn't know who his secretary was, whoever she was. "And you can't say a thing to anybody, not him, not her, not anybody. Understand?"

"Yeah, Colin. I understand. I wouldn't ." She turned back to the computer eyes all alight over being instrumental in a police investigation.

"Here it is. Actually there are three accounts. One personal, one business and a new one just opened recently under the name of The David L. Sandler Foundation. It's got a lot of money in it, too." She turned the screen around so he could see the account. The balance was just shy of $400,000. He scanned the credits column. The last deposits, all in this month were for $300,000; $80,000 and just yesterday one for $15,000. Bingo! Pete's money. He'd bet anything on it.

On the other side of the screen were the debits. There was only one withdrawal recently. $100,000 had been taken out almost two months ago and transferred into his personal account.

Debbie got called away by a teller so he took the opportunity to copy everything he saw on the screen. When she returned to her office she sat back down and with a puzzled expression on her face she asked, "I don't understand, if there's so much money in the account how can his secretary be embezzling? Is he supposed to have more than that in there?"

"Well," he hedged, "I think maybe he's confused and she just put it in the wrong account, maybe it all should have been deposited in the operating account." He wanted to see Dr. Sandler's personal account but Debbie was starting to ask too many questions. "I've never seen her, what's her name?" Debbie asked.

Man this was getting deeper and deeper. He surreptiously pressed the button on his pager and it instantly started its high pitched beeping. "Oh, I gotta go, that's my partner letting me know we got a call out. Thanks for all your help, you're a peach." He quickly jumped up and as he was turning to leave she called out to him, "Come over to the house sometime, I'm sure Frankie would love to see you!"

"Sure, I will," he called back.

Adrenaline was pumping through his veins, he charged out through the glass double doors and ran to his car. He was on the verge of cracking a murder case! He slid behind the wheel and turned into traffic before he remembered that there were other deposits recently, substantial deposits. Much larger than the deposit from Pete. Where had they come from? They couldn't also have come from death benefits, could they? Wouldn't it be a little unusual for that many psychiatric patients to die at one time? Lord! The thought blazed across his mind like lightning in the sky. Had he stumbled onto a serial killer? His hands shook on the steering wheel and he had to grip it tightly to keep in his lane.

He tried to calm down. Think rationally! He admonished himself. There must be a reasonable explanation for such large amounts of money. Maybe the Foundation had owned some property that it sold. Maybe it wasn't as he was thinking. $300,000... $80,000... that's some pretty hefty change. Then another thought came to him, maybe Dr. Sandler was blackmailing his patients.

This was getting scary. Maybe he should get some help with this. He drove to the Association Hall to work out. He needed some time to think, some time to sort things out. And he needed to get rid of all this charged energy pumping through him. He felt like a horse at the starting gate, pulling on the reins, raring to go.

After a grueling workout where he was besieged with hundreds of unanswered questions, he decided that he really didn't have enough to go on, no evidence whatsoever. He could just be imagining all these scenarios. So the guy had money, big whoop. Lots of foundations had money, that's what they were all about. Collecting money and using it for their purposes.

The next step was to find out about the money the foundation had collected, namely those deposits. They were most likely checks since the amounts were so large and if he could find out who issued them then he could find out why. What the money was being used for was something he needed to find out also. One step at a time he told himself.

This was more than he could saddle Debbie with, he'd have to go to the main office to see copies of the checks, this he already knew from previous experience. Maybe he could use his credentials from the fraud department at First Virginia Bank to get someone at First Union Bank to show him those checks. It was worth a try anyway. He had to get more substantial proof of his suspicions before he involved anyone else. He didn't want to cry wolf when there wasn't one. He'd had a pretty spotless career up to this point, it would be just like him to retire and then make a fool out of himself on his first private case. But somehow he didn't feel like that would be the way it would turn out. His instincts told him that this might be his most challenging case ever. Something deep in his gut told him to go slow and methodical.

Chapter 83

Tyson's Corner, VA

Jenny plopped down into the chair in front of Tammy's desk. Aside from David and her sister, Tammy was Jenny's best friend. From the very first day that Tammy had come to work at Royal a few years ago they had clicked immediately. They were work mates and soul mates. They didn't see each other often outside of the dealership but they confided everything to each other all day long, every day, while they were working. Tammy was Royal's finance manager.

It had been the first promotion Jenny made when she had accepted her new position. Up until then Tammy had been a settlement clerk but Jenny had seen much more potential in Tammy than anyone else and every day Tammy was proving Jenny right. Jenny looked over at Tammy's face and gave her a smile that zig zagged as she said to her, "The most embarrassing thing in my whole life just happened a few seconds ago."

Tammy looked over at her and said, "Now Jenny, how can you possibly say that? You still have lots of life ahead of you, you're only in your thirties!"

"Wait til you hear what happened and then tell me that!" Jenny wailed.

"Okay, what happened?" Tammy prodded. It was a busy Saturday afternoon but they were between deals right now and she had a few minutes.

"I had a lull between closing a few deals and I thought I should take the opportunity to change my tampon before it became a problem. You know how heavy I bleed the first few days." They really did know practically everything about each other. "And you know how I stick a tampon up my sleeve to carry it to the bathroom since it's rather obvious to the guys if I drag my purse out ten times a day to go to the ladies' room?"

"Yeah," Tammy nodded. She knew Jenny didn't like the guys making fun of her cycle and telling her she was PMSing every time she went on a rampage about something. "Go on," Tammy said with an outward roll of her opened palm, wanting her to get on with the story.

"Well, just as I passed Chuck Binder's office he called out to me, 'Miss Miller, I'd like you to meet Mr. and Mrs. So-and-so, they just drove one of our Bonnevilles and were very impressed. I told them you like to say hi to everybody before they leave.' So I walk into his office, I stand beside him behind his desk and as I reach my hand out to shake theirs to greet them, the tampon falls out onto the desk. Right there it lays on the desk in front of us. No one says a thing. I very calmly pick it up and put it into my pants pocket which has a slit in it where it attaches to the waistband with a button. Well, wouldn't you know, it goes through the slit, falls all the way down my leg and onto the floor. This of course is missed by no one, you could hear it drop for Pete's sake! So I pick it up again and excuse myself. And here I am mortified beyond belief and I know the worst is yet to come when Chuck tells everyone what happened!"

Tammy stared at her wide-eyed for a few moments and then started laughing so hard she was crying by the time Jenny jumped up and stalked away in a huff.

Several hours later when she and Tammy were locking up, Tammy came over and gave her a hug. "I gotta hand it to you, I never thought you'd top the one when the customer you were drooling over caught you on your hands and knees in a short skirt with your high heels up in the air, trying to open the safe."

"Well I was trying not to scratch my shoes on the cement and I was not drooling! He was very good looking. But I was not drooling!"

Tammy was referring to the time during the recent remodeling of the finance office in the back hallway when part of the carpet had been pulled up and the safe had been right in front of the doorway. She had fancied this particular customer until she'd found out that he was married. But the look he'd given her at that moment when he chanced upon her in such a compromising position had pretty much indicated that, married or not, he would have joined her right there on the floor if they'd been the only ones around at the time.

Jenny pulled back from Tammy's embrace and looked at her sweet face with the sparkling blues eyes misted with tears. Then they both started laughing and it was several minutes before they wiped their eyes and turned off the lights.

As Jenny was driving home she thought about Tammy. Next to her sister she was really her closest friend. She knew more about her than anybody. She had held her hand through many trials at work and she'd been there to advise her about every man she'd dated or thought about since R.J. Tammy had worked with R.J. once at a Chevy dealership and there certainly was no love lost there. So she was able to commiserate with Jenny over her failed marriage with genuine sympathy.

Tammy was single and without any prospects at the time. Jenny longed for Tammy to get involved with men so that she could turn the tables and get to hold her hand for awhile. She wanted to listen to her gushing with excitement over a man and hear her stories of disaster dates for a change.

But Tammy was incredibly shy and over the years she built a wall around her heart to protect it from the pain it had experienced when she was in her early twenties and happened to discover her live-in lover being unfaithful. The wall took the form of extra weight and it was an extremely effective barrier against unwanted male advances.

Try as she might Jenny could not get Tammy to eat right, exercise or wear any makeup. It just wasn't important to her, not that she needed a lot of help. She had natural beauty with her beautiful, fluffy natural blonde hair and her sparkling blue eyes. She had all the necessary beginnings, a lot more than most women were born with, she just needed a little attention to detail. Jenny never gave up haranguing her about her avoidable shortcomings but she also never stopped appreciating her for her sunny disposition and quick mind. Smart as a whip, she was like

Jenny's right hand and sometimes when they were very busy, her left one, too. Royal never had as loyal and as dedicated an employee as Tammy and Jenny wanted the very best for her. She was always hoping some very intuitive guy would appear one day and see all the goodness in her and whisk her away to his castle. Jenny always had hope even though Tammy didn't.

When Jenny arrived home she was surprised to see David waiting for her. She had finally given him a key and he was already inside waiting for her, as evidenced by his unoccupied car parked in the driveway. The kids were sleeping at her mom's house since she had left work so late in the evening.

As she let herself in through the French doors at the top of the driveway she called out teasingly, "Hi, honey! I'm home. What's for dinner?"

David got up off the sofa in the family room where he had been watching television and came to meet her. His big smile and open arms met her as she entered the family room. "Hi! I'm glad you're home. And you're what's for dinner. I'm going to eat you all up!" With that he grabbed her and started making growling noises against her neck. His lips, moving over her throat as he pretended to eat her, were wet and sticky against her skin.

"Well, that's not going to do me any good, what's for me to eat?" she asked playfully. He lowered her down his body and as her thigh grazed his she gasped at his hardness pressing into her. "I see you found your dinner," he said smiling down at her.

His forwardness scared her. She wasn't ready for this, not tonight. "Really," she said, "I'm starved, don't we have something more substantial." She purposefully accentuated the last word and turned away from him going towards the kitchen.

He raised his left eyebrow at her mockery and followed behind her, "Oh, yeah, don't think I'm substantial enough for you do you?" He whispered against the back of her neck. "Let me show you that there's more than enough of me to accommodate you." He breathed against her ear.

"Can't," she said simply. "I'm having my period."

His reaction actually surprised her. He quickly spun her around and she could see the rage in his face. "I think you're lying to me, I think you're stalling me and I don't like it! It's not like you're some kind of virgin or something, you know! Show me! Show me you're having your period, I don't believe you," he hissed. He felt around her waistband trying to find a zipper. When he found a button instead on the seam side of her trousers he unbuttoned it. He pushed her pants over her hips until they fell in a pile at her feet. All the while Jenny stood there stunned at his outburst and frozen in disbelief. When he put his hand in her pantyhose to pull them down, she jerked awake and grabbed his hand to stay it. "I knew I was right," he growled as he jerked her hand away from his and pulled her hose and panties down at the same time past the top of her thighs. While she stood there in the middle of the kitchen, he quickly knelt in front of her and put his hand between her parted thighs. When he saw the string hanging there he pulled on it and it came out of her body. His only words were, "Jesus, Jenny I'm sorry." As he stared at the bloody tampon swinging on the string held between his thumb and finger tip.

If Jenny thought she was mortified today, that was nothing compared to this. She started to tremble and didn't know what to say as she feebly reached down and pulled her panties up and then her pantyhose. She stooped down to the floor and grabbed the waistband of her pants and as she gingerly pulled them back up she said through clenched teeth, "I think you should leave now."

"Jenny, I'm sorry. I'm so sorry, I shouldn't have done what I did and I shouldn't have doubted you. He wrapped the tampon in a paper towel and opened the compactor with his foot. He dropped the little package into it and closed the door, glad to be done with the offending thing. "I don't know what got into me, I guess you're driving me a little crazy, I want you so badly and I'm tired of waiting. Jenny, I ache for you continually. Please forgive me."

"What you just did to me was despicable, I don't care what your reasons were," she said sounding hurt. As she watched him go over to the sink and squeeze a generous amount of dish soap into his hands before he turned on the hot water and soaped them up, she felt an inner shiver as if he was somehow conveying to her that she was dirty and he needed to rid himself of her germs. "I don't want to see you for a few days. And I don't ever want an inspection like that again! We had an agreement! The wedding night? Remember!" She screamed at him.

"Okay, I understand," he said as he dried his hands on a dish towel. "I'll go. I'll call you tomorrow." He walked over to give her a kiss and she turned her cheek away from him, side stepping any contact with him. He let himself out and after she heard the door close she walked over and locked the top lock behind him. Then she sat down on a chair at the kitchen table, put her face in her hands and cried.

Chapter 84

Fairfax, VA

Colin sat on a silk covered armchair in Dr. Sandler's waiting room filling out a customer profile sheet. As instructed he had come in fifteen minutes before his appointment to fill out the necessary paperwork. For most doctors that would include insurance forms but in Dr. Sandler's case those patients needing insurance reimbursements had to apply for them themselves. If you couldn't afford to front the money, you couldn't afford him.

Carefully scanning the forms he filled out the required lines with information he had previously prepared. Trying to profile himself somewhat after Pete, he knew he had to be well-to-do and willing to take drugs. Under the occupation line he neatly printed, Bank V.P. and under the name of the company he printed Bank of America. There were so many branches, he'd never be able to check them all.

Where it asked about marital status he checked the divorced block and gave a date one week from today's. The line that asked about current medications and specific dosages he filled out using information he had copied from a friend's prescription bottles. Listing high blood pressure as the cause, he noted three medicines in the blank spaces: Cardizem CD 300mg once a day, Prinzide 20/25 once a day and Prinivil 10mg, once a day. That ought to show him he'd be willing to take almost anything Dr. Sandler wanted to prescribe, he thought.

He used his pager number as his phone number noting that he was never at home at the Regency Park address he had listed with a PH notation behind it. It was Colin's perception that Dr. Sandler would probably understand that to mean the penthouse suite exactly as he wanted him to.

After completing the form he handed it to Dr. Sandler's receptionist, Glenda Jameson, as her nameplate indicated. He went back to his seat to review in his mind the information he had made up and to keep reminding himself to answer to Mason or Mr. Williams when addressed that way. He fingered the mini recorder in his pocket and was ready to flick the on button as soon as he was ushered into Dr. Sandler's office.

A few minutes later Glenda's intercom buzzed, she picked up the phone, and after listening for a few seconds, replaced it. "Dr. Sandler will see you now Mr. Williams," she said briskly as she stood up to show him the way. He waved her off, saying, "Stay seated, I can find my way." She smiled in appreciation. As soon as he opened the door with one hand he clicked the on button with the other, both clicks happened at exactly the same time, just as planned.

Dr. Sandler was just standing up to come around his desk as Colin entered the room. "Mr. Williams, a pleasure to meet you. I'm Dr. Sandler." They shook hands for a brief instant, both men sizing up the other. "Won't you please be seated?" Dr. Sandler asked, indicating two chairs right in front of his desk. There was other furniture in the room in separate areas, but apparently this was to be the meet and greet area, Colin thought. He took the chair that was right in front of Dr. Sandler's crystal candy bowl.

"Got a sweet tooth, huh?" he asked as he watched Colin eye the bowl. "Yeah," Colin replied, "I'm a sucker for a sucker." He laughed. Dr. Sandler laughed with him and then told him to help himself. Colin took a cellophane-wrapped butterscotch and popped it into his mouth.

"Well, Mr. Williams what brings you to my office today? What can I help you with?" Dr. Sandler asked tentatively.

"I discovered my wife of seventeen years cheating on me several months ago and I haven't been able to get it out of my mind for a minute since. We're separated now," he added, "and the divorce will be final next week."

"What exactly are the problems this is causing for you?" Dr. Sandler asked.

"Well, I can't sleep. I try to eat, but sometimes I can't seem to swallow. I'm short with all my employees and friends and I don't really care a damn about anything anymore. I'm also probably drinking more than I should be."

"Got it bad, huh?" Dr. Sandler asked.

"Yeah, 'fraid so. She was everything to me. I'm still in love with her, even though now she's in love with somebody else."

"Any kids?"

"No," he lied. He didn't know why he lied, he just felt that was the best answer right now.

"Well, first things first," Dr. Sandler said, "We'll get you something so you can get a good night's sleep every night and then we'll figure this thing out together. That okay with you?"

"Sure," Colin replied. "I'm anxious to get back to normal, if that's possible."

"Oh, it's possible all right, in fact you can count on it. We'll have you back to your normal self before you know it." Dr. Sandler reached into his desk and took out a small folder. "I'd like to see you next week if you can fit it in and in the meantime would you try to fill out some of these questionnaires? If you can't, don't worry about it. It just helps me get to know you better a little sooner." He took out a prescription pad from his center desk drawer. "I'm going to write you out a prescription for a mild sedative. Take it at night just before bedtime and it should help you get to sleep. Don't take it on a night that you've been drinking," he admonished firmly.

"Thanks, Doc." Colin said. "Do you mind if I use your bathroom? Seems I dribbled some butterscotch on my tie."

"No. Help yourself," he said as he continued filling out the prescription form.

Colin went into the bathroom and closed the door behind him. Immediately he turned on the water faucet as he quickly scanned the room. There was only a cabinet under the sink and all it held were cleaning supplies and extra paper products. Colin dipped his tie in the sink and then turned off the water.

While he rubbed it with wet fingers he looked through the trash can. Nothing of any interest there. Except... what was that under the clear liner? He moved the trash at the bottom aside and through the clear plastic liner he saw a prescription bottle. He dropped the trash, gathered the liner from the top and lifted it. He picked up the bottle and put it into his pocket, replacing the liner with his other hand. Making sure things were as he found them he opened the door and walked out, still rubbing his tie as he looked down at it. "Ever notice how you can wear a junkie tie for years and not spill anything on it, but the first day you wear a $200 one you demolish it?" Colin asked with a lopsided grin.

Dr. Sandler laughed. "Yeah, but it can't be all that bad. I've got some club soda. Here, let me take a look." He reached into a credenza behind him and grabbed a bottle and a rag. He tilted the opened bottle over the corner of the rag and applied it to Colin's tie. After a few brisk rubs he said, "There you go," as he stepped back to admire the job he'd done. "Good as new."

Colin smiled. Now Dr. Sandler knew Mason was very wealthy. The tie had been evidence in a trial for a high class shoplifting ring. It showed obvious quality and he was sure Dr. Sandler noticed the Lord and Taylor signature on the inside tongue. That, along with all the other borrowed clothes he was wearing, should convince him he was worth the time and trouble to try to cash in on.

"Thanks, a man of many talents. Can't wait to see if you can fix my life as easily," Colin said as he took the folder and prescription the doctor was handing him.

"Set a date with Glenda and I guarantee you, we'll get you straightened out."

He put out his hand and Colin shook it. He was really a very likable guy, Colin commented to himself.

Colin went back out to the reception area to Glenda's desk to set up his next appointment. "That'll be $140 Mr. Williams," she said politely. He had to cover his choking sound with a cough. He had already informed her before his session that he wanted to settle his account after each appointment, saying he didn't want anyone at his office to know he was seeing a psychiatrist.

Colin reached into his pocket and took out his new Armani leather wallet. He extracted two crisp bills, one a hundred dollar bill and the other a fifty. He made sure it was obvious that there was more where they came from. He'd had to delve into his savings account to play the rich guy role. He placed them on her desk in front of her and never mentioned the change. An appointment was made for the following week and he left the office.

He waited until he was alone in the elevator before he loosened his tie and commented to himself about the fee. Geez, $140 for just a half hour consultation. Next week's session would be a full hour! For MaryAnn's sake I hope I nail this guy soon!

When Colin got into his car in the parking garage he took the confiscated prescription bottle out of his pocket. It was slightly sticky from having been in the bottom of the trash can up against a wet paper towel The ink on the label was badly smeared and all legible writing had been practically obliterated, except for the date and the pre-printed pharmacy information. The prescription had been filled over two months ago. The lab at his old office had made more out of less before so he drove over to beg another favor from a good friend. For some reason he couldn't explain, he didn't believe the bottle belonged to a patient. He had the feeling that this could be something important.

Colin had learned a long time ago that the best element you could hope for in any investigation was luck. He could only surmise that the reason the bottle was still in the trash can instead of having been emptied along with everything else long ago was due to the time-saving habit of cleaning crews to drop several empty liners in the bottom of each trash can at one time. So all they'd have to do is pull the next one up after removing the full one, instead of going for more supplies. After tonight this bottle would have been on its way to the dump since the next to the last liner was being used now. Yes, he'd take luck over intelligence any day.

After stopping at the lab and leaving the pill container he drove home to listen to the tape and to change into his work out clothes.

Jacqueline DeGroot

Chapter 85

Downtown Washington, D.C.

David left the office early the next day and drove downtown to Browne and Sons Jewelers. He had known one of the sons since his old college days at GW. Rather than waiting til November as they had agreed he had decided to get Jenny an engagement ring now. He had to do something to smooth things out with her. She'd only taken one of his calls and that had been to tell him that she was too busy to talk to him.

He'd just see if diamonds were a girl's best friend. The roses he'd sent that morning to her office might soften her up a bit but he was counting on the ring to remind her that she was his and what he'd done a few nights ago, although crude, was certainly understandable. How many men who were engaged these days didn't have sex with their fiancé? Leave it to him to fall in love with the one puritan in the lot.

He selected a high quality, 2-carat, brilliant cut diamond in a high-pronged platinum setting. He had it boxed and wrapped and hand delivered to Jenny at work.

When Jenny answered the summons to the showroom she was met by a very distinguished looking gentleman who identified himself as an employee of Browne and Sons. He had a package for her and it would require her signature of receipt after she opened it. She knew that Browne and Sons were ritzy Downtown jewelers so she had a hunch what was in the small box so she asked him to follow her to her office. She carefully unwrapped the box under the scrutiny of the man and Tammy who had been standing on the showroom floor watching her exchange with the man.

When she lifted the lid to the small blue velvet box she gasped in surprise. Nestled in the ridge in the middle of the box was a huge sparkling diamond, similar to the ones she'd seen over the years on the fingers of the wives of her wealthier clients. Tammy leaned closer in to see it and gasped as she flattened her hand against her chest. "Jenny, it's beautiful! David has such good taste," she chided as she lightly elbowed Jenny in the ribs, "and so much money!" she whispered.

The man handed her a filled out form asking for her signature. She read it quickly, put it down on her desk to sign it and handed it back to him, saying, "Thank you. Thank you very much." He nodded and left.

Jenny snapped the box shut and Tammy looked over at her. "Aren't you going to put it on?" she asked incredulously.

"No," Jenny said simply. Tammy knew about the doubts Jenny had about David, but she was sure that Jenny had told her that they were going to become engaged soon.

"Why?" Tammy asked.

"I don't know," Jenny said as she put the box in her suit jacket pocket. "I just don't know if I'm doing the right thing." Just then she was called to the Used Car Manager's office. "I don't want to think about it right now. C'mon we've got work to do, I know this is a payment close they need help on." She walked out of her office with Tammy right on her heels.

"Prince Charming asks you to marry him and you're hesitating, I don't get it. What more do you want?"

"I want love without doubts. Now please, Tammy. We'll talk later. There's too much going on right now. Toby needs this deal for bonus. We've got to find a way to get down to the customer's payment and close this deal for him."

All afternoon they worked on that deal, finally getting the bank approval they needed just minutes before the banks closed at 6 pm. These "last days" of the month were killers. Everything in the car business is done by the month. Unfortunately many years ago people got wind of this and stopped coming at the beginning, waiting until the last few days. Now the crush was hard to handle.

Of course, everybody wanted the best deal and of course, all the dealer owners wanted the monthly deal projections met, so everybody scrambled to get it all done in the last one or two days. On top of that you had the two, three and four year lease deals that were made on hectic "last days" of the month in previous years coming due at exactly the same time again, at the end of the month. When customers would complain to her that their salesman refused to put them out for a fourth test drive so they could go home and think about their car buying decision for a few weeks, she wanted to shake them and scream, "If you want to have individualized, one-on-one attention for hours of test driving, come on the first day of the month when all we're doing is twiddling our thumbs! Today's not the day!"

By ten that night she was sick of arguing with people over the value of their trade-ins, trying to convince supposedly intelligent people that you couldn't just take the amount to be financed, multiply it by the interest rate and divide it by the number of payments to get the monthly payment amount. That on top of repeatedly having to justify selling a car for a profit. Somehow people in this country had become convinced that car dealers are the only people in business that don't deserve to make a profit on the product they sell.

By 11:30, when the last deal was just going into a settlement office, Jenny turned off the showroom lights and kicked off her shoes. The night phone rang and thinking it was Mr. Royal asking about the end of the month totals, she punched in the code to be able to answer it from her desk since the switchboard had been closed for several hours.

"Hey, beautiful. I thought I'd hear something from you tonight about my little present," David breathed into the receiver.

On Jenny's many trips upstairs to the general offices she had seen at least three different messages that he had left earlier at the switchboard. "Hi." She sighed, more from exhaustion than from pleasure, but the way it came out certainly sounded kittenish even to her ears.

"It's a really late night for you tonight, huh? Did you find time to eat?"

"I don't remember to tell you the truth, everything's a blur from about four o'clock on," Jenny said.

416

"Are you wearing my ring?" he asked softly.

"Sort of," she answered honestly. "It's in my pocket."

"Why?"

"Because it would be kind of obvious on my finger now wouldn't it? And we did agree to wait til Thanksgiving." Recognizing how harsh that must have sounded she quickly added, "but it is beautiful. I love it. It's exactly what I would have picked out for myself, only larger. You spent too much."

"Nothing's too good for my future wife. You sound awfully tired. Do you want me to come pick you up and drive you home?"

"No, I'll be okay, we should be locking up in a few minutes. I'll drive with the windows open and the radio turned up."

"Okay, but be careful. This is not always a friendly city at night, you know."

"I know."

"I'll call you tomorrow. I love you. Good night."

"G'night." She reached over to cradle the receiver and missed, it clattered about on the desk top before falling on the floor, the only noise in the otherwise quiet showroom.

"Getting a little punchy are we?" Tammy asked from the doorway.

"Yeah, I guess so. All done?"

"Yup. Dan's in the service lane with his customers switching their stuff over from their trade in. From the look of all the junk piled in the trunk and on the back seat, we've got time for a nap." Tammy pulled out a chair and plopped into it, putting her feet on the seat of the one beside it.

"That David?"

"Yeah. Wanted to know if I was wearing his ring."

"And why aren't you?"

"You know, Tammy, some days I think marrying him is the best idea in the world but then there are days, days like today, when I feel that this isn't what I want. I keep thinking there's somebody else out there that I'm supposed to be with. Somebody who is my all-consuming love, the one I'm supposed to be paired

417

with. I know he's going to come into my life one day, and wouldn't it be awful if I wasn't available to go to him?"

"And you're sure David isn't him?"

"No. And that's another thing, shouldn't I be sure? If you love someone shouldn't you be overwhelmed and awed by the completeness of it? I think I am capable of more passion than I feel for David. And to tell you the truth sometimes all I feel for David is irritation. The physical yearnings aren't there either. At least not for me. I am not anxious to have sex with him. Now what kind of a marriage is that going to be?"

"You're lucky to have the attention, Jen. He's a wonderful man."

"Yeah, I know. That's been the problem."

"Well, when you're done with him, I'll take him!" Tammy said with a smile. "Looks like they're done out there. Let's go home."

Jenny grabbed her things and gave Tammy a hug. "Thanks for listening to me. At least I don't have to resolve anything tonight. I've got until the end of November before I said I'd wear his ring."

"November, huh? This guy who's supposed to step into your life had better hurry," Tammy said as she walked away heading for her demo.

Chapter 86

Fairfax, VA

The next week during Colin's appointment with Dr. Sandler they discussed Colin's marriage. The good and the bad. It was almost as if Dr. Sandler wanted him to relive each and every moment of their seventeen years together. All the events of their marriage down to the minutest detail. Colin had to be very careful not to mention his police work, and although he felt it would be safe to talk about Lynn and many of the ups and downs they'd been through, he'd already decided before that it would not be a good idea for him to talk about Adam. He didn't want the doctor to think that there was an heir waiting to contest his settlement money when he *died*. His police work having been such an important part of their marital decline he decided to substitute some of their major issues with in-law problems.

He and Lynn had never really had any in-law problems but he found himself embellishing details about his wife's parents with great enthusiasm. Lynn's sweet mother was turned into a nagging old hen and Lynn's hard-working father became an overbearing military tyrant. When Dr. Sandler's logical train of thought lead to questions about Lynn becoming a dominating, bitchy wife, he went with it.

He tried to remember all the times he and Lynn had really fought, which really hadn't been that many. They hadn't communicated enough to have anything to fight about. But for Dr. Sandler, he made them epic, painting a picture of marital disharmony going back for many years.

By the end of their first real session Dr. Sandler had read all the questionnaires Colin had returned and had asked him many questions about them. He had also listened to Colin enumerate all the negative and positive aspects of his marriage with all the emotion of a man blind sided by infidelity. And he'd learned part of the key he thought he could use to eradicate Colin's broken heart.

Before Colin left, almost as an aside, Dr. Sandler asked, "So tell me Mason, how are the pills working? Are you sleeping any better?"

"They're working fine. I sleep almost all the way through the night on the nights I take them. The other nights I just drink til I pass out," Colin replied laughing.

"And eating? Still no appetite?"

"It goes in spurts, some days I'm ravenous and on other days I don't eat a thing."

"Well, I think it's time we address this depression. Chemically first and then though therapy starting with your next session. I'm going to give you another prescription. This one is for a mild antidepressant. It's such a low dosage that it can be taken several times a day as needed. But no more than 4 in any given 24 hours, okay?" Not waiting for an answer, Dr. Sandler removed his prescription pad from his desk and started writing. "You'll find these more effective if you take them throughout the day as you find yourself feeling a little melancholy. So, keep them on you, in your jacket pocket or something, so they'll be handy when you need them. And don't take a sleeping pill within four hours of taking one of these, got it?"

"Yeah, I got it. With my blood pressure medicine and the two prescriptions from you I'm beginning to feel like I'm turning into a junkie."

"Now, Mason, don't think that way. Each medicine you're on is for a specific problem. Soon you won't need the sleeping pills or the Sinequan. And I'd be willing to venture that in six months you won't be needing the blood pressure medicine either."

Colin didn't like the sound of that. It had an ominous sound to it, whether Dr. Sandler had meant for it to or not. He frowned perplexedly at Dr. Sandler.

"You did know that some forms of high blood pressure can be treated with hypnosis, didn't you?" Dr. Sandler asked.

"No, I guess I didn't," Colin replied as he took the piece of paper Dr. Sandler was handing him.

"Well, one thing at a time. First we treat your emotional problems, then we'll move onto the physical ones. See you next week."

They shook hands and Colin left the office. The bill this time was $280. $70 for each quarter of an hour. And he still had the medicine to buy, and without a prescription card at that. This prescription, just like the last was in the name of Mason Williams. He hadn't bothered filling the last one, this one he would need to get. Dr. Sandler had made it pretty plain that he expected Mason to carry these around with him all day long. He would need to make sure he removed four a day from the container as if he was taking them. Sinequan. Just like he'd prescribed for Pete.

Colin went down the elevator to the parking level and eased himself into his car. It was even harder to do in an expensive suit, if that was possible. He was rotating three suits and the necessary accoutrements "borrowed" from the evidence warehouse. The shoes were a tad small so his feet were beginning to protest. He still had one more place to go before he could go home and change clothes so he kept his feet in the cramped shoes, knowing that if he took them off it would be hell to pay to get them back on.

He drove to McLean to the Metropolitan area's main office of First Union and went into the tomb-like quiet and coolness that only banks, churches and libraries seemed to have this time of the year. He took a seat in the reception area to wait his turn. After a few minutes he was introduced to a Mrs. Dorothy White. She looked far too prim for his way of thinking and he had a hunch he wasn't going to get very far without a search warrant. Time to switch tactics. He let his badge fall down into his deep jacket pocket.

He introduced himself as Dr. David Sandler. She smiled, shook his hand and proceeded him into her office. "Dr. Sandler, what may I do for you?"

"I seem to have lost my last two month's statements for my checking account. Well, actually I don't think I lost them, I think my accountant did," he said with a bright smile. She smiled back at him. Well, that was a start. "Is it possible to get copies of them?"

"Certainly. I can arrange to have duplicates mailed to you or I can run a print out for you on my computer. Which would you prefer?"

"The printouts would be fine."

"Then please, have a seat. I'll have them ready for you in just a few minutes."

"Do you happen to have the account number with you?"

"Yes," he said as he took out the piece of paper he had copied from the computer screen a few weeks ago in Debbie's office. He read the numbers to her.

She typed them on her keyboard. "Here it is. Current balance $496,874.00?"

"Oh, Damn! I brought the wrong account number, that's one of my business accounts. I need the statements on my personal account. Let me see if I have that number in my car." He started to stand up.

"Oh, that's okay," she said, "I can find it from here." She typed for a few minutes more and then said. "Here it is. Balance $1,208.23?"

"Yeah, that's it. Unfortunately I can't seem to keep that balance as high as the ones for my practice," he said with chagrin. She smiled back at him, "Don't worry, neither can I. It'll just take a few minutes for this to print in the other office." She got up to retrieve it.

Colin had no doubt that if this woman hadn't been so impressed with his attire as well as the healthy balance in *his* business account, that she never would be providing this information so readily without any identification. He smiled at his own cleverness.

When she returned to the office and handed him the printouts he quickly scanned them.

"Is that all you needed?" she asked.

"Well, actually I needed a copy of this check here," he said as he pointed to the list of checks, stopping at the one for $100,000 showing on the first statement. The lost statements had my canceled checks in them. Do you keep copies of them anywhere?"

"Well, yes, actually we do. For awhile at least anyway. They're on microfilm. That's a separate department. I can call them for you and you can go upstairs and pick it up if you'd like."

"Oh, that would be great," he said enthusiastically, smiling his appreciation to her.

She picked up her phone dialed an inside extension and spoke in an authoritative manner to the person who answered. After she hung up she turned back to him and said, "You can go on up. Fourth floor. Records department. Ask for Flo. She'll be happy to make a copy of it for you."

He shook her hand and thanked her very much for her time, praising her for her efficiency. She beamed and self-consciously patted the French twist behind her head, tucking in strands of coarse dark hair that didn't need to be tucked.

A half hour later when he left the bank, he had everything he'd been looking for. The last two month's statements on Dr. Sandler's personal accounts and miniature copies of all his checks for the past six months. He would definitely need a magnifying glass to read some of them, but the one for $100,000.00 was clearly legible. As he had suspected, proceeds from the David L. Sandler Foundation had been used to secure the lot and pay the up front money to the builder for Dr. Sandler's new mansion on the hill in Great Falls.

Colin removed his tie and suit jacket before inching into the hot leather seat of his Mustang. That was another thing he hated about this car. He had wanted cloth seats, but the souped up sports model didn't come that way. When had he started compromising on everything so easily? With great difficulty he reached down and removed his shoes and socks from his hot, cramped feet. Driving over to the Association Hall he made a mental note to take the time tonight to write down new goals for his future and to make a list of all the things he wanted to get and to accomplish for himself. Within the next few years he hoped things would be very different for him. Better write everything down, he said to himself or I'll get side-tracked again, thinking about the fog he had been moving through for the last six months.

His divorce was final now and all his friends had said he'd been lucky. No alimony, only three years of nominal child support and the house had been sold and the equity divided evenly. Somehow he didn't exactly feel lucky though. What he did feel was lonely. Maybe tonight would be a good night to hang out with the old gang from work. The thought of that cheered him a little as he pulled his little white convertible into an empty slot. He grabbed his gym bag from the trunk and walked up the sidewalk to the doors.

He made a pretty unusual sight. An extremely handsome man with his chiseled profile carrying an over stuffed leather work-out bag. He was the image of a successful business man, from the sleeves of his white oxford dress shirt rolled to his elbows, exposing a wrist draped with a gold link bracelet and one with a thin stylish gold watch, to his obviously expensive trousers ending with a sharp cuff before his bare feet stuck out. He moved confidently across the pavement toward the front doors of the Association Hall.

Chapter 87

Chantilly, VA

Later that evening, after Colin had showered and changed, he sat in his little living room in the one real chair that he owned. In front of it was a card table and in front of that was a small television sitting on a shelf made from two cinder blocks and a piece of wood shelving. The chairs for the card table were in his bedroom, open and up against the wall. They served as his dresser. Socks and underwear were stacked on one, T shirts on another, shorts on yet another and his junk *drawer* was the last one.

In front of him was the invitation to his high school reunion. Many months ago when he'd first received it, he entertained the idea of going. It would be a hoot seeing all his old buddies and squiring Lynn around on his arm. He'd always told them he wasn't going to marry a dog. And he hadn't. Lynn was still youthful and pretty. Now, he'd be just another middle-aged divorced man, one of those third wheels hanging on to every twosome, trying to fit in and be with someone.

He had to get used to the idea that Lynn wasn't coming back and now he had to get used to the idea of going to these things alone. He supposed he could ask somebody, but who, and why the heck would they even want to go? What a boring night it would be for them. He put the invitation aside telling himself that it was still two weeks away, he had plenty of time to decide.

Next he popped the audio tape into his tape recorder and listened to his session with Dr. Sandler. What a lot of rehashing he'd done today. No wonder he was so morose.

He jumped up, grabbed his car keys and drove to Tres Amigos, right in the heart of Fairfax City. There were always off duty and on duty officers hanging out there. As soon as he walked in he was hailed by several members of his old Criminal

Investigations Bureau team, including Judy. He took the seat they pulled out for him and ordered a beer.

Many beers and many hours later he left the restaurant feeling that at least he still had a connection somewhere. He was just about to open his car door when he heard his name being called from the outside eating area of the front porch just to his left. He turned to see who it was and had to squint against the bright lights on the veranda. It was Suzy, one of the deputy sheriffs he'd known for years.

She stood up and was on her way down the stairs to meet him. From the stuttering steps she was taking he figured that she'd had a few too many. She came over to him and gave him a big hug, making sure her big breasts moved back and forth across his chest.

"Coll-in, where ya goin'? It's too early to go home now," she wailed.

He unwrapped her arms from around his neck and said, "I gotta go. It's gettin' late. You should be goin', too. Don't you have to work tomorrow?"

When she nodded energetically, he asked, "Do you have someone to take you home?" It was obvious that she was in absolutely no condition to drive.

"Yeah," she said. "You. You'll take me home won't cha Coll-in?"

Great. Just what he needed. With any luck at all she'd throw up in his car and then he'd have yet another reason to hate it. "Yeah, sure," he said. "Hop in."

"Wait, I gotta get my purse." She made it back up the steps, grabbed her purse and told her companions she'd just gotten lucky.

Meanwhile Colin started the car and put the top down. This lady was going to get a lot of fresh air!

She slid in beside him and closed the door. He had to reach over her, reopen the door and shut it again as she hadn't shut it right the first time. "Sorry," she mumbled as she stroked the back of his arm.

A few minutes later it was nice to notice that she had sobered up a bit and was staring up at the stars in the sky, reciting the constellations and pointing them out to him. He had no idea how accurate she was, he'd never even been able to make out so much as the big dipper. A seaman, he could never be. "Where did you say to make the next turn?" he asked her.

"Two blocks down there on the right."

When he got to the second block he had his turn signal on, ready to turn when he noticed it was a little park. "This is a park, not where you live, quit playin' games!" he said testily. He pulled into the park to turn around. She shocked him with her next words.

"Colin, don't be so anxious to get rid of me, don't cha want ta fool around? How 'bout a head job?" She said as she reached over and grabbed at his crotch.

He had to apply the brake to keep from hitting a tree. "Suzy, cut it out, will ya?" he said as he put the car in park and tried to pry her hands away from his zipper.

"C'mon, Colin. Let's have a little fun." She reached up and pulled her sweater over her head and threw it into the back seat. Then she reached behind her and unhooked her bra. The bra quickly followed the sweater into the back seat. She gathered her huge breasts, one in each hand and shoved them together. "C'mon if I can't suck you off, then you can tittie-fuck me."

Colin just stared, his mouth having gone slack jawed. The vision of his fully erect penis delving into that warm fleshy cleft left him breathless.

Suzy took that opportunity to unbuckle his belt and zip down his zipper. Before Colin knew what was happening he was helping her to free himself.

As soon as he was released from his encumbrances she bent her head and began licking and sucking on him. Oh, God. It had been so long. And not just six months either. It had probably been years since a female mouth had touched him there. This was not something Lynn had been fond of doing. It usually required a special vacation trip and getting her drunk in the afternoon for him to inspire her to service him like this.

He knew he should stop her, if for no other reason than they were out here in the open in a park that was clearly posted with signs saying No Loitering after Dark. It would be embarrassing if they were caught because chances are they would know the officers. There wouldn't be any repercussions, they always excused their own, but it would be fodder for the mill for a long time. But he couldn't stop her. It felt too damn good. He stretched his arm out to caress her nipple as he laid his head back against the headrest. Had there ever been anything that felt this good he wondered?

Slowly and with languorous care she worked her magic and before he was ready to end the delightful pleasure she was giving him she brought him to a shattering release. As he pumped his load into her mouth, she gagged and moved off of him. The result was a sticky steering wheel, console and all his clothing.

"Oh, God! Colin, I'm sorry. I just couldn't take it all!" she moaned, wiping out her mouth with a Kleenex from her purse. She grabbed a few more and dabbed at his crotch.

"Never mind!" he said. "I'll get it." He took the tissues from her and wiped up the best he could.

Suzy quickly leaned back to grab her sweater and bra from the back seat, almost slapping him in the face with her breast. "Other than that mess at the end, was I all right?" she asked timidly.

"Yes, you were all right." She had been better than all right, but he wasn't going to tell her that. No sense encouraging her, this was not something he planned on repeating.

"Okay, tell me where you live, remember you've got to get up early and go to work tomorrow."

She mumbled an address that was in an apartment complex he was familiar with.

He did the best job he could with his clothes while she put her sweater back on. He watched as she just stuck the bra in her purse. He started the car and they drove the rest of the way to her apartment in silence, the wind ruffling their hair.

When he pulled up to her apartment entrance he said, "Forgive me if I don't see you to your door, but I'm not even sure how I'm going to get into mine without being seen," he said with a slight smile.

"Oh, that's okay. Will we be seeing each other again anytime soon? I can give you my number if you'd like to call me sometime."

She was almost begging and it bothered Colin a lot. What a cad he'd been. Hell, he hadn't even kissed her. But he wasn't the type to lead someone on and truth be told she didn't appeal to him in the slightest.

"I don't think so Suzy. This was nice, but I'm really not ready yet for a relationship. Heck, I'm still praying that my wife'll dump that jerk and come back to me. I'm not the kind of guy you want in your life now. I'm all take and no give. You deserve better."

"No, I don't Colin. I could take whatever you were able to give."

"No, I wouldn't do that to you. Good night." He gave her a quick peck on the lips and reached over and opened her door for her.

Driving home he had the emptiest feeling he'd ever had after an orgasm. Hell, this was worse than masturbating he told himself. At least then he hadn't hurt anybody. He knew then that the swinging singles life was not going to do it for him. He didn't want to have sex just for the sake of his body. He wanted it to mean something. He wanted to find somebody he could love again and he wanted to roll over and pull her into his arms after they were both spent. Where was she now he thought as he slowed for a traffic light and looked up at the stars.

Chapter 88

Tyson's Corner, VA

As she maneuvered the ancient hulking station wagon around the curb and reparked it in the place she had taken it out of ten minutes earlier, Jenny thought that this had to be the absolute worst part of a sales manager's job. Appraising cars usually fell to the hands of the used car manager and she normally didn't have to do this, but today was Dean's day off, so the chore fell to her. She climbed out of the 1976 Ford LTD station wagon and brushed off the back of her skirt with her hand.

Typically a prehistoric wreck like this didn't even require a test drive. After all, how much could a thirteen-year old car with 198,000 miles on it be worth? And this one had sure seen better days. Generally anything drivable was worth a hundred dollars wholesale. This one was drivable, but she really felt that she should be able to deduct a dollar for each chicken bone on the floor of the back seat from its value. Then the customers would owe her to take it off their hands. She had only driven this one because the customers had been standing outside looking at the new car they wanted to trade this on and she didn't want to hurt their feelings by making them think she didn't want to even get in it, which was exactly the case.

Over the years she had been in some pretty disgusting trade-ins. These cars were in essence people's living rooms, kitchens, dining rooms, bedrooms and more frequently than one would like to believe, their bathrooms—especially for the children. The smells of some of these older cars were so musty and smoke-filled that she had often wished she was wearing a bio technician's sterile suit. It had long ago become her practice to head directly to the ladies' room after depositing the keys and appraisal book on the salesman's desk after evaluating a car. She always made sure she washed her hands thoroughly after having had her hands on the steering wheel of some stranger's car. You just never knew what people did in their cars. When she watched people driving down the road they were usually either smoking, picking their noses or chewing on their nails. Yuck!

She also washed her hands every time she shook someone else's hand. She had always done this even before it had became popular as a way to avoid spreading germs. Being a student of human nature she was amazed at how many times people touched their mouths, noses, ears and even feet! There was a game she played while watching people at airports or in theaters when wiling away extra time, see how fast you could count fifty facial touches. Rarely did the game take more than seven or eight minutes.

Washing her hands after appraisals and hand-to-hand contact had become such a well-known, ingrained habit of hers that if anyone was looking for her and was told that she was appraising a car or she had just closed a deal, they would just go and wait at the door of the ladies' room for her to come out.

As she made a few notations on the salesman's appraisal pad that he could use to devaluate the car in the customer's mind during the negotiations part of the deal, she heard her name being paged in the showroom. She hurriedly wrote $100.00 on the pad, underlined it twice indicating that he could go two hundred more if he absolutely needed to and signed her name. On the way into the showroom she placed the pad and the customer's keys on the up desk so the salesman could find it when he needed it. Then she crossed the showroom to her office and picked up the phone. "Jenny Miller, May I help you?"

"Hi Jenny. It's Ron, I'm still here in Detroit at this Dealer meeting but I couldn't wait til I got back to tell you this. You've been chosen to do a series of Management Training videos for Pontiac. They just asked me about it today. They wanted to know if it would be all right with me for you to do them. I said, 'Hell Yes'. It would be an honor to have you do their National program. So what do you say? They're all right here waiting for an answer."

"Gee, Ron, this is really out of the blue. And you know how I feel about cameras and pictures and all. And I've done the Detroit thing once already, remember the Walk-Around Demonstration Competition?" He'd tried many times over the years to get her to do some print and television commercials for him, but she'd always declined. Public speaking just wasn't her thing.

"I know Jenny, but this will help so many others to become more professional, just like you. They'll treat you like a queen here in Detroit for two weeks. And they are also talking a nice chunk o' change, m'dear." He gave a deep sigh, "and it would really be a feather in my cap."

That was the only thing she heard that swayed her. He had done so much for her, how could she refuse? "Okay, I'll do it. When do I have to be there?"

"They'd like you to come in two or three weeks if you can."

"Okay, go ahead and arrange it with them, as long as it's okay with you, it's okay with me." They went over the day's totals so far and then said their goodbyes.

Jenny replaced the phone and took a deep breath.

Just then Tammy came into her office with a deal for her to check and sign. "Why so glum?" She asked.

"I gotta go play Hollywood in Detroit for the big wigs and you know how much that thrills me," she said as she took the deal from Tammy, read over the numbers and signed it on the bottom so it could get in line on the list to go into a settlement office.

"What for?" Tammy asked.

"Some training tapes. They're gonna be sorry. I am not photogenic and I'll be sooo nervous everybody will laugh." She mimicked in a sugary falsetto voice, "Yes of course Mr. and Mrs. Jones, I can certainly see why you feel your old used up piece of junk station wagon is worth $6,000. After all, each of your eight kids has thrown up in it at least three times on your ten trips to the Grand Canyon. And that big hole in the middle of the back seat where your dog clawed the upholstery to shreds? I don't think we'll have any problem finding a new owner that has a dog with the exact same color hair. And by the way, I think it's very adventurous of you to drive with those banana peels as tires. Must be how you got that big chrome bumper all bent out of shape. And, yes, it certainly would be worth more money if you didn't have to climb in from the passenger side to get to the driver's seat. And what was that on the steering wheel anyway? You just pulled the duct tape off today because you needed it to reattach the rearview mirror?"

Tammy chuckled as she took the folder back and left Jenny's office. Calling over her shoulder as she went, "With a performance like that maybe you'll win an award and go on to Hollywood after all."

"Yeah, right," Jenny said as she reached down to answer her phone that had just started ringing. "John, there's no more money on that car! Three hundred is more than generous, anyone else would've only put $50 on it! " She listened for a minute and then said, " Oh, all right, I'll come talk to them. I'll be right there."

She hung up the phone and left her office to see if she could close the deal on the trade-in she had just appraised a little while ago. They wanted a thousand dollars for it because they'd just spent $300 on the brakes and another $400 on new tires. Heck, the tires were worth more than the car. Why were people always spending money on a clunker just before trading it? Did they think that with new tires the rust wouldn't show up so badly?

She ended up closing the deal by offering to move the tires from their trade-in to their second car that was still back home at no charge. This way she'd have tires on the piece of iron she was just going to wholesale so it could get onto a carrier and the customers didn't have to feel like they'd just lost $400 on tires. And more importantly, they felt like they had won. Exactly as a customer should feel. These were the types of closes Jenny was known for. Find the key, then compromise.

Another busy day for Jenny and her sales force. And they were rapidly becoming her sales force. It was apparent to all the salesmen and sales managers how important each and every deal was to her. She fought like a mama cat for each one, not letting go until there wasn't a shred of hope. She had earned respect as a top-notch salesman years ago. Now she was earning their respect as a phenomenal closer. Cash buyers, trade-in buyers, finance or lease buyers, it didn't matter, she really knew her stuff and she wasn't afraid to keep pulling something out of her sleeve until she got the opportunity to shake hands over someone's desk. And then of course, she'd just have to go wash them again.

Chapter 89

Fairfax, VA

Colin pressed the button for the sixth floor and once the door closed he patted his pockets for the tape recorder and the pills. He had removed enough pills from the bottle to correspond with the number he should have taken by now and had carefully wiped the outside clean of his fingerprints. He then used his handkerchief to put the bottle in his right outside jacket pocket. The tape recorder was all set to turn on as soon as he stepped off the elevator. It was in his left front pants pocket, the microphone threaded through a hole in his pocket and taped down with flesh colored band aids just under his T-shirt, which was under his oxford cloth dress shirt.

As soon as the elevator doors opened he flipped the switch on the side of the mini recorder. He was excited about this session with Dr. Sandler. The clandestine nature of his sessions was one reason, but the other was his curiosity over the hypnosis part.

He had some trepidations about being completely out of control over what was going on around him but his overriding sense of adventure took over and quashed his fears. Chances are he probably wouldn't even be able to be hypnotized, he thought. He was sure that since he was so strong-willed that he would not be susceptible to carnival brain-washing techniques.

Dr. Sandler saw Colin within moments of his arrival. Colin was asked to get himself comfortable by removing his jacket and shoes. Then he was shown to a small alcove with hangers in it he could use to hang his jacket. Colin noticed that the hangers were really nice wooden ones, there were also a few scented satin-wrapped ones for the ladies. His were all wire or plastic, depending on what the dry cleaners gave him.

Next, he was instructed to lie down on the long sofa with his head against a cushion that had already been covered with a clean linen cloth. As soon as he laid down he saw a small projection screen suspended from the ceiling. It was the perfect height for viewing, he didn't need to duck or raise his chin to focus on the center of it.

"Now Mason," Dr. Sandler started, "let me explain what's going to happen so you can relax and concentrate for me. In a few minutes I'm going to turn on a special projection unit located behind you. I will ask you to focus on the scene being played out before you. You are to try to listen to what I'm saying as long as you can and then I will give you some suggestions on how you can deal with your grief over your divorce from Lynn. I may ask you some questions, but they will be rhetorical. You do not need to talk, just concentrate on what I am saying and the images you will see on the screen. Are you ready?

"I guess. What happens if it doesn't work, if you can't get me under?"

"Then we'll try something else. But don't think about that now. Concentrate on my words."

Dr. Sandler pressed a button on the small remote control box he held in his hand. An image started moving on the screen. To Colin it appeared to be something like a computer simulated car race, only there was no car. It was like he was driving on a stretch of gray road that ribboned out far ahead of him. He couldn't see anything of the car, he just felt like it could have been a car propelling him forward, slowly at first and then a little faster. There was a slight flashing sensation off to one side as if a shadow was crossing the road at very exact intervals. Like the passing of telephone poles, one right after the other all the way to the horizon.

"Mason, you are on a trip. It started the day you were born and it continues today as it will continue tomorrow and the day after that and so on and so on. Imagine this trip is your life. You are traveling on this highway heading towards your destiny. Along the way your life has taken a few wrong turns, but now you are on the right road again. Driving, driving, driving, always looking ahead and seeing where you are going. Sometimes you are excited about driving so you drive very fast, but right now you are tired of driving so you are starting to slow down, slow, slow, slow, just barely moving. Now, you close your eyes to rest."

"You went off the highway a few years ago at the wrong exit. It took you a long time to realize that you were lost. In fact, you didn't even know you were lost. Somebody had to tell you. You know who that was don't you? Yes of course, you do. It was Lynn. You thought she was the right course for you, so you married her. And after awhile you discovered you weren't having as much fun on this trip as you had planned. Lynn became cold and distant. Whenever you were having fun, she gave you a hard time about it. She didn't like your friends. She didn't like it when you watched TV, or played golf with the guys. She nagged and nagged about every little thing. You tried to find more reasons not to come home and then she'd nag about that too. Nothing ever made her happy, so you stopped trying."

"You weren't happy either, but you didn't know that. This was the course you had taken. You were supposed to stay the course. And you would have too, if Lynn hadn't chosen to take another road without you. Her journey is taking her a different way. She is tired of trying to change you to make her happy. She's going to start her trip again and make someone else unhappy. You should be grateful you are on the right road again. This time your destination will be true. It may take quite a bit more driving until you find what you're looking for on this journey. But it's a worthwhile trip."

"You are going to be so happy when you do finally find what you've been looking for. The woman that will make you forget Lynn ever existed. She's going to be just perfect for you. Sweet and kind, where Lynn was mean and nasty. She will be your true love. The one you will finish the journey with. Beautiful and kind and living only to please you, not herself. You should be happy that Lynn left you to try to train another for her pleasure. For if she had not, you would still be on the wrong road and you would miss finding the key to your destiny, the woman made especially for you. She has your heart already. You must continue on your drive to catch up with her and then your heart and her heart will beat as one. Do not try to drive faster to catch up with her. Just stay on the right road until you find yourself driving along side of her and then you can ask her to share your journey. And you will be happy again."

Dr. Sandler stood up very slowly and moved to the alcove. He felt Colin's pockets and a small smile crossed his face as he felt the small plastic pill bottle in the right front pocket. He slowly strolled back towards the seat he had just risen from.

"It's time to pull back onto the road, to get back in your lane and continue on your journey. Open your eyes and follow the road, keeping your eye out for your next exit, but don't worry, you won't miss it. She'll find you just as you'll find her. Put your hand up and put your car in park." Colin lifted his hand and put the imaginary gear shift into park. "Open your eyes."

Colin opened his eyes and blinked a few times. He had fallen asleep? Had he actually dozed off when he was on an assignment? He quickly put his feet on the floor and sat up. What had happened? He honestly couldn't recall anything after the screen flashed with the race game. He shook his head and asked, "What happened?"

"You were under," Dr. Sandler said with a smile. "Are you surprised?"

"Yes, I guess I am. I didn't cluck or anything did I?" Colin asked.

Dr. Sandler laughed, "No, you didn't cluck. But we can try that next time if you'd like."

"That's okay."

"So, how are you feeling?"

"Fine. How am I supposed to feel?"

"Think about your divorce. How do you feel about that?"

Colin thought for a moment. "I feel relieved. And I feel a tingling sense of anticipation about something about to happen. Where's all that coming from?"

"It's coming from you and your new attitude about the future is coming from you, too. I'm just there to steer the way for you. Your next driving lesson will be next week, we will need to reinforce these messages for awhile. And don't quit your medication just yet. Just because you're feeling all cheery right now, don't undo what we're working towards. Keep taking everything until I tell you to stop, okay?"

"Okay," Colin said as he slipped into his shoes. Grabbing his suit coat jacket he shrugged his shoulders into it and felt the weight of the pills still in the pocket where he'd left them. "Next week, then." He walked out and paid another $280 and then headed for the elevators.

He drove straight home so he could fingerprint the bottle and listen to the tape. He was dying to know what he'd been hypnotized to do or think. Imagine! He'd really gone under! This was getting a little scary.

Chapter 90

GW Parkway, VA

David was driving back from Georgetown. It was 4:30 am. He had been summoned by Congressman Tyler to his daughter's apartment. That's just the kind of person it would have taken to get his private home phone number at two o'clock in the morning. He was just getting back from a rare house call. When he'd arrived at her apartment it had been just past three. He was ushered into Jessica's bedroom, which not surprisingly, had a little girl quality to it. It was all white French provincial furniture with gilt edging and lacy white eyelet linens trimmed with lavender ribbons and there were small groupings of stuffed animals on the window seat.

Jessica was past the stage of just being inebriated or rip roaring drunk. Her body was starting to have trouble filtering the alcohol out of her system. She really should have been in a hospital but the Congressman didn't feel that his reelection campaign would deal well with yet another of Jessica's scandals. He'd tracked down Dr. Sandler in the middle of the night and asked him to come over. As soon as David saw her he filled out a prescription for Hydroxyzine Pamoate as an injectable and sent one of the congressman's aides out to an all night pharmacy.

He hoped that they had it in stock. Actually he secretly hoped that they didn't. If he didn't get some of that into her soon, they would probably lose her if she wasn't hospitalized. He wondered if the congressman knew how close to death his daughter was at this exact moment. The campaign had already been done with Jessica and he certainly couldn't be faulted if she expired right now. He had been waiting for just this sort of thing to happen to Jessica for weeks now.

Twenty minutes later when the aide returned with the syringes he used some vodka he found in Jessica's kitchen to swab her arm and then injected her with the medicine. This was only the second time in his career he'd ever used this particular drug. As a small pill it was used commonly as an antihistamine, as an injectable right into the blood stream it became a highly effective treatment for acute alcoholism in an adult psychiatric emergency. Soon the nausea, vomiting, anxiety and extreme agitation would subside. Then maybe, with some rest and no alcohol for awhile, her body would start to cleanse itself again. Maybe.

When she seemed somewhat settled he went to talk to her father. "Have someone keep checking on her through the night and into the morning. She's quiet now, but she could easily vomit in her sleep and choke. As soon as she's up and around, which probably won't be until the day after tomorrow at the earliest, have her come see me. We have to deal with this drinking problem right away. She's going to kill herself this way."

"Thank you for coming out like this doctor. I'll leave one of my aides with her until I can get a nurse tomorrow. And I will definitely get her out to see you as soon as she's feeling better, even if I have to drag her there myself. Doctor, do you have any idea what's causing this rebellious, self-destructive behavior?"

"Yes sir, I do." But he made no move to elaborate.

"I'm listening?"

"Yes, you're listening now, because she's being a problem. But you weren't listening before when she wanted to talk about her mother and how much she was missing her."

The Congressman just nodded, silently accepting the criticism due him.

Dr. Sandler left the luxurious condo with the magnificent view of the Potomac River out the living room windows. The aides were just starting to clean up the trashed apartment. Jessica had really been in quite a psychotic state, pieces of broken crystal were everywhere. Just as he turned to close the door behind him he saw why. He smiled. Someone had sent her flowers, he saw the card on the glass table by the door. The flowers were strewn all over the carpet, the water from the broken vase splashed all over the wall. He reached over and picked up the card and read it, then tucked it into his pocket. The short message said simply, "Love, Mommy."

Three days later when Jessica came to see him he was shocked at her appearance. Her hair was dry and brittle and her face was pasty white and bloated. The dark eye make up she had become accustomed to wearing accentuated the deep shadows under her eyes and gave her a ghoulish look. It hardly seemed that this could be the same woman who was a kittenish vixen only months ago.

During hypnosis David preyed on her vanity by strongly implying that all the alcohol she was drinking was causing her to gain weight. In actuality she was losing it quite noticeably. He explained to her that he would be giving her a new prescription for a medicine to help her with her alcoholism, that the instructions on the bottle would say not to take it if she had been drinking. Then he informed her that even though very few people knew it, it was really a wonderful diet pill if taken in conjunction with alcohol. Two or three pills with alcohol and she would be slim and trim in no time at all. Then he talked about her mother and all the wonderful things they would do together in heaven when Jessica arrived.

When he brought her out of her trance-like state, he handed her the prescription for Hydroxyzine Pamoate that he had already filled out. If she took two or three of the pills each time she went out drinking, it would only be a matter of time before she passed out driving on the GW parkway or went catatonic from the two interacting. Either way, it was only a matter of time before she killed herself. And he wouldn't be to blame, the instructions he had clearly written to be included on the instructions to the patient right on the bottle would say, "DO NOT TAKE WITH ALCOHOL." No one would ever know why she had chosen to disregard that warning. Maybe he could be faulted for prescribing such a medicine to a known alcoholic, but what was he supposed to do? There were very few treatments that would be effective at this point with such an uncooperative patient.

After Jessica left he grabbed his sport coat and left to go see how the house was progressing. It was almost time to make a second payment to the builder and he wanted to make sure that all the work was being done properly and to his exact specifications. On the way back he'd stop and talk to Jenny. He hadn't been thrilled to hear that she was going to be away by herself in Detroit for two weeks but he knew how loyal she was to Ron Royal and as long as he wanted her to go, he knew that there would be no stopping her. If he hadn't had such a full slate at work, he might have considered going with her, but then who would check on the house each day?

He went down to the parking garage, got into the Trans Am and pulled out onto Main Street. On the way over he thought a lot about Paisley. He wondered if Christmas would be a good time to buy her a pony. Maybe he should wait until her birthday in June, then the stables would be ready for sure.

Chapter 91

Chantilly, VA

Even though Colin was in a hurry, he'd put up with this sticky steering wheel long enough. He kept forgetting to bring down something to clean it with and he'd had to drive with just his fingertips on the lower portion of the wheel. What a grim reminder of his night out last week.

He opened the door and climbed back out just seconds after he had finally gotten in. He went back upstairs to his apartment and grabbed a handful of wet paper towels and a few dry ones. Damn, this was stuff teenagers did, not grown men!

He was on his way to his third appointment with Dr. Sandler. At almost $5 a minute he couldn't afford to be late. As it was he knew he was well over MaryAnn's budget for his fee and expenses. And he had nothing to show for it yet. A lot of circumstantial stuff but no solid incriminating evidence that he could use. Maybe today.

After last week's session he had listened to the tape twice. The second time he made the mistake of lying on his bed and before he knew it, he'd been hypnotized again, not to regain his normal awareness til the end of the tape when Dr. Sandler had awakened him. He'd also dusted the pill bottle for fingerprints and to his disappointment had found none. The bottle had been cleaned again, more pills removed and reinserted back into the same jacket pocket as before. The mini recorder had a new tape and fresh batteries. He was ready for his next hypnosis session.

When he arrived at Dr. Sandler's office exactly on time, he turned the recorder on and waited to be called. He was told that Dr. Sandler was running a few minutes behind due to an earlier session. After ten minutes he asked where the men's room was and went down the hallway to rewind the tape and start it over again. A few minutes after he returned he was ushered in to see the doctor.

"Sorry, to keep you waiting. It doesn't happen often but I was finally getting a break through with someone and I couldn't stop just then."

"Oh, that's okay, I understand. I don't have anywhere I have to be after this."

"Oh, yeah. I hear about those banker's hours all the time."

Colin chuckled, "Hey, it's nothing like psychiatrist's hours. At least we're open on Saturday."

"Well, I'll have you know, just last night I made a house call at three in the morning."

"Whoa, you got me there. I don't do any house calls."

Dr. Sandler laughed. "Ready for your session?" he asked Colin.

"Yup, I sure am. Can't tell you how much better I've been feeling all week. I don't wake up thinking about Lynn and I don't go to sleep thinking about Lynn. Do you think we can work on the in between times now?"

"You got it. Get comfortable. You know the program now, hang up your coat, take off your shoes and lie down."

As Colin situated himself on the leather sofa he thought to himself, this guy sure is likable, just a normal kind of guy you'd have a few drinks and shoot the breeze with. That was Colin's last thought before he was asked to focus on the screen again. This time the screen was like looking through a car windshield as rain drops continually pelted it while he drove. He was under in just a few seconds this time.

Dr. Sandler started by reinforcing negative feelings Mason should have for Lynn. He was much stronger this time in trying to build vehemence between him and Lynn. He used his notes to recollect things Mason had said earlier to him and then twisted them around to suit his purposes. Ultimately he would need for Mason to begin to hate Lynn with a passion in order for his campaign on Mason to work.

He brought up imaginary times for Mason to remember when Lynn had humiliated him in front of his friends. He tried to portray her as a spendthrift and a sloppy housekeeper. And then he left a nagging question in Mason's mind as to whether she had been faithful to him in the early stages of their seventeen years of marriage.

After David was pretty sure of the animosity he had created between Mason and Lynn, he started working on the campaign. "You know, Mason, it might not be a bad idea at this juncture in your life to get a new will written. Even though you're divorced, should anything happen to you now, your estate will go directly to her. You don't want that to happen now, do you? She's gotta be the last person you want to leave all your hard earned money to. Leave some to someone you really care about, then leave the rest to an organization you believe in, like your alma mater or maybe a foundation you admire. Put your money where you want it to go now, before it's too late and the old ex gets it. Just imagine it, Lynn and her new love living life on easy street because of you. Don't make it easy on her, she doesn't deserve it."

"This therapy has helped you a lot, you no longer have the pain you were living with on a daily basis. You can get on with your life again and what a wonderful life you still have before you. It's time you cut all the ties to the past and make new connections for the future. The David L. Sandler Foundation is in need of benefactors such as yourself, caring individuals who understand the commitment psychiatrists have for their patients. People who've felt first hand the healing in their lives. We can save others, too. With your help."

"When you wake up you will have confidence that a new love is on the horizon. Don't leave things undone. Be ready for her. Right now as we speak, she is getting ready for you. Picture her in your mind. She is beautiful with long blonde hair, emerald green eyes and a petite curvaceous body just waiting to join with yours." David stopped as he realized he was describing Jenny. Oh, what the heck, he thought, Mason would never run into Jenny, and besides, there were lots of women that could be described like that. "She is sweet and nice and caring, she's your idea of the perfect woman. You already love her, so don't give up on finding her."

"Now, you've driven enough in the pouring down rain. Let's take a break and pull over to the side of the road, just ease off the gas pedal and steer the car to the right."

Colin did exactly as he was asked. He raised his hands and made as if he were steering a car off to the right.

"Now put it in Park," Dr. Sandler said.

Again, Colin reached up and put the imaginary gear shift in place.

"Now, open your eyes. Your journey is done for the day."

Colin opened his eyes, blinked several times and sat up. He really felt groggy and at the same time very light hearted.

"Well, how are you feeling?" Dr. Sandler asked.

"Terrific. I feel great."

"Good. Remember to keep taking your medicine. I think in another month we can wean you off of it. Then we'll start working on the other medicines you're taking."

"Thanks, Doc," Colin said as he put his shoes on and stood up to get his jacket.

"You're welcome, Mason. See you next week."

Colin put his jacket over his arm, subtly feeling for the pills as he folded it over. He went out to the reception area, paid his $280 and went down to his car. He was anxious to get home to check out the tape and to fingerprint the bottle again.

As soon as he went through the door he started peeling his clothes off. The band aids had been pulling on his chest hairs every time he breathed deeply and he couldn't wait to get the microphone off his chest. The shirt stuck to his back it was so wet from his perspiration. This was not the time of the year to have to wear a suit, tie and T-shirt. A shower would feel really good right now, but he was too anxious to hear the tape. First he checked the pills. They hadn't been touched. He felt deflated, he'd thought for sure that today would've been the day until he remembered that he hadn't even left his money to the benevolent doctor yet. That of course would be the doctor's first priority.

Then he rewound the tape and pushed the play button. To keep what had happened before from happening this time he stood up and paced while he listened. Man, this doctor's voice was so soft and soothing! No wonder he was so good at what he did. Three quarters of the way through the tape he knew he had Pete's murderer. And what was even better, he had the motive, all on tape. Dr. Sandler had made his move!

After he finished listening to it all he tried to analyze his feelings. Had all the things the doctor had said about Lynn affected the way he was now thinking of her? It was very hard to be objective about this. He knew his feelings for her had changed since he started seeing Dr. Sandler, but was that necessarily bad? If he could never be with her again, if she was to be out of his life forever, wasn't it better this way? That he'd been talked out of loving her bothered him a little. But he'd known all along that sooner or later he would have stopped loving her anyway. Sooner was better, wasn't it? He was no longer miserable without her. He supposed it did bother him a little that this wasn't the normal course of events and that he'd let someone else have control of not only his thoughts, but his emotions, too.

He didn't hate Lynn the way he thought the doctor wanted him to though. He could see that was the direction the doctor was headed in, but he didn't think of her as he used to either. He had to admit that now he did have tendencies to believe that she was bitchy, mean, sloppy and unfaithful. Boy, this hypnotism was pretty strong stuff. And he had no doubt in his mind that he'd be on his way to an attorney's office right now to sign a new will if he'd really had any money or assets to leave anybody.

And of course, all this talk about a new love was nothing but hokum, but even though he kept telling his mind that, a part of him was hoping that it would be true.

He walked over to the refrigerator and took out a beer. He had enough to go to the magistrate's office to get David Sandler indicted on a murder charge, but he didn't think he had enough to get the conviction. He needed Dr. Sandler to mess with his pills and to leave his fingerprints on the bottle as evidence that it was him, the good doctor, who was killing people for the money they would be leaving to him. And he needed him to do this quickly before more people were killed. Could he chance waiting one more week?

Maybe the doctor wouldn't touch them even given one more week. He had no idea what Dr. Sandler's time frame was. He knew that it was almost eight weeks to the day that he had started seeing Pete before Pete died. Colin had only been seeing him for four. He would have to make Dr. Sandler move faster. Another month would be too long to keep this kind of thing to himself.

He was probably waiting for some type of confirmation that the will had been changed and then a decent interval between that and the actual death so no one would become suspicious. But that hadn't happened with Pete. To Colin's way of thinking anything less than a year would look suspicious to him as it had with Pete's recently amended will.

Had he done the same to others already? How many others? There was an awful lot of money in that foundation's bank account. If so, he was apparently getting away with it, maybe he was getting brazen, knowing there was no way to connect a random death to him. Maybe he was getting desperate for the money. God! He threw up his hands. Too many questions! He needed a few minutes away from this. He went into the bathroom and took a long cool shower.

Then he got his note pad out and called his friend at the lab where he had dropped off the pill bottle. He finally tracked his friend down and was told they'd have the results the following Friday. Today was Wednesday. Okay, he'd give it one more week. But first he had to get some help getting a phoney will drawn up. Maybe if Dr. Sandler was convinced Mason had already heeded his advice he would play the game out a little faster. He called a lady attorney that he knew who had always had a slight crush on him. For the price of a good dinner maybe he could get her to draw something up for him. He rang her office number and was put through right away.

"Sandra! How are you? Yes, Yes, I know, it's been a tough few months. But I'm ready to tackle dating again. Are you game for dinner? Tomorrow would be fine. I'll pick you up at seven. Is that okay? Okay, just give me your address." He wrote down the address she gave him and said goodbye. What a cad he was. Well at least with this one he wouldn't have to clean the interior of his car. He would tell her right up front that he didn't believe in kissing on the first date. After the other night, he needed to go back to the basics of dating again.

Chapter 92

Chantilly, VA

Colin spent most of the next day reviewing his notes and trying to figure out a way he could get Dr. Sandler's patient list. Then he called a friend of his to see about getting a list of all the people who had died in the last year from drug related problems. It would require a three jurisdiction search since the metropolitan area consisted of the State of Virginia, the State of Maryland and the District of Columbia. The District of Columbia, having such a high rate of illegal drug use, would constitute a large chunk of the list, most having died because they were junkies. It was estimated that the list could easily top a thousand. If he could get it though, he could cross reference it against lists of wills that had been probated.

But that created another problem. The court houses where these would be filed were County courthouses. There must be at least a hundred counties between Maryland and Virginia combined. It would take him months to compile a list to work from.

No, the only way to approach this was from patient files, if Dr. Sandler hadn't destroyed them. He wondered how chummy he could get with Glenda, Dr. Sandler's receptionist. That idea didn't hang around for too long. Then he considered breaking into the office late at night, but that might tip him off and of course, it was against the law to do that. How many times had he been faced with breaking the law trying to preserve it? He didn't want to count, or to think about the times he'd succumbed.

He'd just have to wait until after his next session on Wednesday and after he received the report back on the pill bottle he had found in Dr. Sandler's bathroom. Then he would go from there.

He finally left his apartment in the late afternoon to go work out. Afterwards, he drove around for awhile trying to decide what restaurant to take Sandra to.

She was a pretty sophisticated lady, graduated magna cum laude from Wesley and then Harvard School of Law. She had been a prosecuting attorney when he'd first met her over ten years ago. Scuttlebutt now was that she was up for a judgeship. Her career was everything to her and she'd sacrificed the idea of marriage and family to dedicate herself to it.

She was hard nosed and dogged in her pursuits and had earned herself the nickname Mad Dog among her peers. At least that's what she always attributed her nick name too. Nobody was going to tell her that she sort of resembled a Bassett hound because of the way she wore her hair parted in the middle with large loopy braids hanging above each ear and drooping almost to her shoulders.

At seven o'clock Colin pulled into the driveway of her townhouse in a very nice neighborhood near downtown Fairfax. When he rang the door bell he heard the sound of several little dogs barking. She opened the door while she held onto the collars of two of them, calling to the third, "Pepper, pipe down, it's okay. C'mon in."

He stepped into the foyer and smiled at her, "Got a handful there." He noticed she had done her hair a little differently, it was in a bun secured behind her head at the nape of her neck. And it was the first time he'd ever seen her without her thick glasses. She could pass for cute he thought, in a bookish kind of way. She was a bit heavier than he last remembered her and it was obvious that she was trying to camouflage it by wearing all black, either that or she was rehearsing dressing as a judge.

"Yeah, they can be, but they're sweet, too," she said as she kissed them both on the mouth as they licked her face. The issue of the first date kiss was completely resolved in his mind.

"Ready to go?" he prompted.

"Sure," she said, "just let me put them in their little houses." He watched as she took each one in its turn and put in its own little crate, complete with blanket, water and food.

"What kind of dogs are they?" he asked.

"Yorkies," she said. "That one's Mitzi," she pointed to one that had a pink ribbon in its top knot. "That's Molly," she pointed with her elbow as she put on her black jacket. "And that's Pepper," she said, waving to the little black one. "You be good and maybe I'll bring you home a doggie bag with some goodies in it."

"Do you always pen them up?"

"Got to, they have the worst separation anxiety you've ever seen. The house would be torn apart."

"What do you think about Italian? I thought we could go to the Olive Garden, if that's alright?"

"That would be fine," she said as they walked to his car.

He opened her car door for her and then she watched him as he maneuvered himself into the driver's seat.

"You don't really fit in this car so well do you?" she said as she laughed.

He grinned at her, "So you noticed. This was a spur of the moment decision I made just after my separation. I have since decided that I need to allow myself at least several days before making any big decisions."

They had a good time talking and laughing, recalling funny things about the cases they had worked on together while they enjoyed a bottle of wine and a nice dinner.

He was truly enjoying her company and told her so. She blushed. Over dinner he told her about the will he needed. She listened intently to everything he said and then asked if there was any such person named Mason Williams at that address with those assets. When he replied, "No," she said she'd do it as long as it didn't have to be notarized. He thought he could get away with that, she nodded and said he could pick it up at her office the next day.

They ate their tiramasu with coffee while they finished the last of the wine. He'd given her the lion's share and she was beginning to get a little tipsy.

All the way back to her townhouse she talked about her *babies* as she cradled the Styrofoam container holding their promised dinner in her lap.

Contrary to what he'd told himself earlier, when he walked her to the door he kissed her lightly on the lips as he said good night. He told her he'd had a really good time. And he meant it.

Chapter 93

Chantilly, VA

As Colin prepared for his session with Dr. Sandler he was especially careful to wipe off the new bottle of pills he'd had to get refilled. He had "used" up all the pills from the initial prescription and he wanted to make sure the new label reflected that it was a refill with no more refills available. For all he knew Dr. Sandler could be calling the pharmacies to check on his patients, to make sure they'd refilled their medications. He'd come too far to screw up on a tiny little detail. He was trying to do things exactly as the new attitude-adjusted Mason Williams would. He'd better remember to bad mouth Lynn a bit when he saw the doctor.

He checked to make sure he had the will Sandra had drawn up for him. He was only planning on flashing it to show Dr. Sandler that he'd taken care of everything as instructed. Sandra had enclosed it in a special folder that had "Last Will and Testament" embossed in gold. Unless someone sat down and read it line by line, it looked like the real thing all the way down to the paragraph where it read he was leaving The David L. Sandler Foundation $250,000.

The recorder was in his pocket ready to go and his note pad with all his meticulous notes detailing everything he knew about the case was on his kitchen counter. Just in case something happened, he wanted to make sure this investigation didn't end. Last night he had met with MaryAnn and filled her in on what was happening. He told her today's session would be pivotal if they were to get a conviction.

On his way to Dr. Sandler's office he said a few prayers as he had done many times in the past when he was getting uptight about a case and its outcome. He pulled into the parking garage and headed for the elevators. Just before he reached the sixth floor he switched the recorder on.

As he sat in an arm chair off to the side in the reception area he kept glancing at Glenda while she was working. He wondered if she was involved in any way. He quickly decided against it. What would be Dr. Sandler's reason for involving her? Besides, other than scheduling appointments and doing some light book work, what could she contribute? Did she wonder about all the money and the new Foundation? Maybe she didn't even know about it.

He glanced around her work area. Other than an appointment book, a receipt book and a phone message pad there really wasn't much on her desk other than the phone. There were no files out here but he had noticed a tall mahogany file cabinet in the corner behind Dr. Sandler's desk. The patient files must be in there. He was hoping there would be a rolodex with the patient names around Glenda's work station somewhere that he could "borrow" for awhile. Either it was in one of her drawers, or all the information was on the computer on the credenza behind her.

Glenda's phone rang and she picked it by just answering "Yes?" followed by, "Yes, doctor." She looked over at him and said, "The doctor will see you now."

He stood up, smiled at her and went into the doctor's office. Didn't that woman ever smile? She apparently was only there because of her efficiency, not her personality.

Colin took a deep breath, "Here we go," he thought. Feeling the same old surge of adrenaline he'd always felt when he was undercover and trying to get the proof he needed for a case.

"Hello, Mason," Dr. Sandler called out from behind his desk as he stood to come over to shake his hand.

"Hi, Doc," Colin said as he shook his hand. "Look here," he said as he opened his sport coat with his left hand to reveal the inside pocket where a tall jacket-type folder was sticking out. Clearly embossed on the top front were the letters declaring it an envelope for a Last Will and Testament. Colin tapped it with the forefinger on his right hand. "Just came from my attorney's office. I've written that woman completely out of my life, and out of my death!" he said with a chuckle. "Your treatments have made a new man out of me. Now I feel like a man with a future instead of one with just a rotten past."

"Mason," Dr. Sandler said as he eyed the folder Colin was pointing to, "I'm so glad to hear you say that. Now we can get on with the next part of your treatment. Are you up for some relaxation imagery? Maybe we can bring that blood pressure under control."

"Sure. Just tell me what I have to do."

"Well, first you have to do what we always do."

Colin gave him a confused look. Dr. Sandler gave a pointed looked at Colin's coat and then his shoes.

"Oh, yeah. Almost forgot. Jacket and shoes." He quickly went to hang up his coat and then shucked off his shoes over by the sofa. "Do I lie down for this one?"

"You don't have to, but that probably would be better."

Colin positioned himself on the sofa as he had all the other times, being careful not to pull the microphone wire out of the recorder.

"Mason, in Therapeutic Imagery we find out all we can about a patient, his likes and dislikes and then tailor a relaxation exercise especially for them. It is so important that you are able to imagine something so strongly that you can convince your brain it's real. So, the greater amount of information you can feed to it to make it seem more real, the stronger the messages will be to the nervous system to effect the change we want. This is not a passive experience, you must be involved and directed towards the goal. I will be here just to show you how and to get you started. Then you will go into another room and practice on your own. Ready?"

"Yes," Colin said and closed his eyes.

Dr. Sandler came over and sat on the sofa by Colin's hip. Colin's eyes opened wide and Dr. Sandler chuckled. "These exercises require me to monitor your pulse so we can see what works best for you." Colin relaxed and Dr. Sandler wrapped his fingers around Colin's wrist.

"Close your eyes and try to picture tunnels. Lots and lots of tunnels, all intersecting going off in all directions. Now, fill these tunnels with little stick people. Give them small heads and small bodies but fill their arms with lots of things. Briefcases, grocery bags, knapsacks, packages of all kinds, books, clothing—just fill up everybody's arms. Now imagine them moving so fast that they keep bumping off of each other, like bumper cars, continually struggling to get by each other. Now imagine that these tunnels are your blood vessels and all these stick people are the components of your blood. They are moving quickly through the tunnels, in a chaotic cycle of everyone bumping into the walls and into each other as they hurry, hurry, hurry to get through the tunnels. Now, blow a whistle." Dr. Sandler put a small child's plastic whistle up to Colin's lips. He obeyed and blew it softly.

"That whistle is the signal for all the stick people to slow down. Slow them down. Slower. And slower again. Make them go so slow that it seems their feet are coming up out of molasses with each step. Have them look at each other and laugh as they exaggerate their movements. Now have them all toss up whatever they are carrying and have them turn to each other and begin to waltz. They are all waltzing now, ever so slowly and smiling as they move slowly through the tunnels. Laughing and waltzing, not a care in the world."

Dr. Sandler removed his fingers from Colin's wrist. Then he stood up and walked over to his desk. "Okay Colin, open your eyes."

Colin opened his eyes and looked around.

"Hey, did it work?" he asked.

Dr. Sandler smiled. "Yes, it worked. Quite well in fact. Now let's see what you can do by yourself. I have a small room right over here that was designed just for this type of relaxation therapy. I want you to go in there by yourself and try one of these three exercises I've outlined specifically for you."

Colin took the paper Dr. Sandler was handing him. He saw three short paragraphs. He stood and followed Dr. Sandler as he crossed the room and went over to a door.

Dr. Sandler opened the door to a room that was quiet and dark. The walls and ceiling were covered with dark flocked wall paper. There was a small covered light in the corner, giving off just barely enough light to see with when the door was closed, like a very intimate restaurant. There was a black leather chaise in the center and Colin was instructed to lie down on it. Handing him a small flashlight he asked Colin to read the three paragraphs and pick the one he wanted to try. One reminded Colin of Pac man, one had him as the drummer in a symphony orchestra, and one had him meandering around in a kayak in a mountain river. He chose the kayak and Dr. Sandler went over to a bank of stereos up against the wall. He pushed a button and the room filled with the sound of rushing water.

Dr. Sandler turned around and smiled at him. "Now, I'm going to leave you alone for about five minutes and then I'll come back and check on you. In the meantime you will be hooked up to this bio feedback machine so I can get an idea of how successful you are at bringing your heart rate down by yourself. While I hook you up, reread the scenario you're supposed to act out in your mind." Dr. Sandler pulled a small table on wheels over from the corner. He attached a blood pressure cuff around Colin's arm and turned on the machine. "Ready?"

"No chance of drowning now, right?" Colin asked.

Dr. Sandler chuckled. "The idea is to slow the water down, not fall out of the boat." He turned off the flashlight and left the room, closing the door behind him.

Colin stared at the ceiling trying to concentrate on the noises outside of the room, but it was no use, the sound of the water rushing all around him was too loud. His hunch was that Dr. Sandler was checking out the will and possibly tampering with the pills. Well, he'd know soon enough. Both had been wiped clean of fingerprints and both would be checked as soon as he left here.

He tried to lift his hand to his head and was reminded about the cuff that was around his arm monitoring his blood pressure. He'd better get busy doing this exercise or when the doctor read the bio feedback tape he would wonder what he'd been doing all this time that was increasing his heart rate.

He closed his eyes and quickly got into his kayak and pushed off from the shore. Using the oars he pushed off against the rocks trying to keep from capsizing. Then he visualized the hot sun beating down and the water beginning to dry up until the rushing river became little more than a gentle flowing stream. By the time the doctor opened the door to check on him, the stream had become little more than a trickle and he was mired in the mud. He'd gone a little too far in imagining the water evaporating.

Dr. Sandler was pleased with his recollection of his kayaking experience and with the read out and told him he was going to give him a few more exercises to try at home. He gave him a CD and a small booklet. "After you do these exercises twice a day for two weeks, we'll meet again and if your blood pressure stays consistently lower, we'll talk to your other doctor about discontinuing some of your medication. Any questions?"

"How long should these relaxation sessions last?"

"Try for 20-25 minutes if you can, but chances are 15-20 minutes each time will do the trick. Just make sure to do them twice each and every day. If you have any questions or if you get stuck in the mud again, just call me," he said with a chuckle.

Colin left the small room and went to get his shoes and jacket.

"And please make sure you keep taking your medicine until I say it's okay to stop, all right?"

"Okay," Colin said and called after him, "see you when I get down river. You said that'll be in two weeks, right?"

"Right." Dr. Sandler turned back to his desk and called for his next patient.

As Colin left Dr. Sandler's office a woman in her thirties was being ushered in to see the doctor. She was tall and slinky looking with a pale, heavily made up face. She looked a little familiar, but he just couldn't quite place her. Boy! That bugged him when that happened. It would probably be days or weeks before his brain processed it all and came up with who she was.

He paid Glenda the $280 plus another $25 for the CD and $10 for the booklet. Why this guy needed more money was beyond him. At these prices he should be doing just fine without other people's money.

He drove straight home and immediately got his fingerprinting kit out of the closet. He wasn't at all interested in the tape anymore, unless it had a full-blown confession, it probably didn't have anything useful on it.

He used a pair of hot dog tongs to remove the bottle from his jacket. After just one swipe with the dust brush he saw a print. Hallelujah! He got him! He was absolutely jubilant as he put the bottle in a baggie. He made one quick swipe over the front of the will and saw two distinctive sets of prints. He put that in a separate bag. He would have the lab do the rest. He would have no idea what to look for inside the bottle, but parts of fingerprints would probably be on the pills too. Then it hit him. That low-down, sneaky sleazeball was trying to kill him! And he'd thought he was such a nice guy.

Just then the phone rang. It caused him to jump because he wasn't used to that sound here, he doubted if the phone had rung more than twice the whole time he'd been living here.

"Yeah?" he answered as he put it to his ear. "Okay, I understand. What is it? Hey, thanks a lot man, I really mean it." He hung up and reached for a pen. He scribbled something on a sheet of note paper by the phone. His friend from the lab. They couldn't get anything except a first name—Michael, and the last letter of the last name—h. But they were able to get the prescription number just to the right of the heading.

Colin had a hunch what this was, but he couldn't be sure until he checked it out. He removed all his dress clothes and

461

pulled the band aids off of his chest. With any luck maybe this was the last time he would have to pull out any more chest hairs on this case. He took a quick shower and dressed in an old pair of jeans and a T-shirt. Grabbing his badge off of his *junk drawer* he went out the door and down to his car.

On the way over to the pharmacy in the York Towne shopping center he thought about what his next step should be. Who was he going to go to with all this? The hierarchy in the Department dictated he go to the homicide division Lieutenant first, who would then go to the Captain in charge of the Criminal Investigations Bureau, who would in turn finally alert the Major who was head of the Major Crimes Section. He knew all of them. They were all his friends and he didn't want to step on anybody's toes, but this was just too important. He had to go to the one who could authorize him to stay on the case. Chances were that unless he went to the Major himself, a detective on the force would be assigned to replace him.

As he pulled into an empty parking space in front of the store he saw a sharp looking black Pontiac Trans Am. Now that's the car he probably should have gotten he said to himself as he lifted himself out of the Mustang by holding on to the top of the door. He was still looking over his shoulder admiring the car when the automatic doors opened. He turned to go into the store and found his way to the back of the store where the pharmacy was.

He asked to speak to the pharmacist on duty and was led to a consultation counter a few feet from where the register was. The pharmacist came over to see him. He was an older gentleman, totally bald except for the slightest fringe around his head going from the back of one ear to the back of the other. He had a wide grin and twinkling eyes and Colin immediately liked him. His name tag said Harold Beeker.

Colin reached into his jeans pocket and produced his badge case. He flipped it open so the man could see his ID and his badge. No one ever looked at the date.They just looked at his picture and the impressive shield attached to the other side of the case. He flipped it closed and replaced it in his pocket. Then he handed the man a small slip of paper with the prescription number he had gotten from his friend at the lab.

The man nodded his head and went back behind the tall counter in the back and within a few minutes he came back out with another piece of paper. Colin pulled out his note pad from his back pocket and wrote down the information, turning to look up at the man several times as he pointed to the paper and asked questions. Then he handed the paper back to the man, nodded his head and reached out to shake his hand. Weaving through the same aisles he left the store and got back into his car.

He never noticed the man several aisles over who had been watching the whole exchange.

Chapter 94

Fairfax, VA

October 23, 1989

David stood transfixed as his eyes followed Mason until he was out the front door. A chill had coursed down his spine when he had seen Mason flash what appeared to be some sort of badge to the pharmacist. He had stood there in the toy aisle watching the whole thing, wondering what it could mean. A feeling of foreboding was giving him a cold, crawly feeling all over his skin, just as if he'd come in to a chilly air conditioned room with wet clothes on.

He picked out the coloring books and puzzles he wanted to buy for Paisley and took them to the back counter to pay for them. When he caught the pharmacist's eye he called over to him. "Wasn't that Mason Williams you were just talking to? I thought I recognized him from college." The pharmacist walked over to him and said, "No, his name was Colin. Colin Scott. I remember seeing it printed on his police ID."

When David's eyebrows shot up in shock, the pharmacist quickly added, "There's nothing to worry about, he was just asking about a prescription we filled about two months ago."

David mumbled, "Could've sworn I knew him in college." He took back his charge card the cashier was handing to him, grabbed the bag of toys and left the counter.

Two months ago, he'd come here to get a prescription filled for "Michael Smith", the Sinequan that he'd used for Pete. It was while he had been waiting for that prescription to be filled that he had seen these Sesame Street puzzles and coloring books. Paisley just loved Bert, Ernie and Oscar. When he found out that Jenny was going to be in Detroit for two weeks he'd arranged with Jenny's mother to come over to their house to watch the kids for a few hours on Saturday so she could have a break. He had come back to this store tonight to get those very same toys for Paisley.

And now, it seemed he'd chanced upon discovering that *Mason*, the banker was really *Colin*, the policeman. What reason could he have to give him a false name and occupation? None, unless he was the one Colin was investigating. The complete realization of what this meant caused his knees to buckle and he had to grab for a shelf to keep from falling.

Boxes of laxatives fell to the floor and he knelt to replace them. People use these so they can shit he thought numbly. And that's where he was, in deep shit. Telling himself to calm down and stop overreacting he purposefully strode through the store and out to his car. He noticed his hand was shaking as he tried to insert the key into the ignition.

After he started the car he sat slumped over the wheel trying to piece things together. He knew. David wasn't sure how he knew but he was absolutely certain that Colin knew. What other reason could there be for him to be a patient with a false identity. He'd been undercover all this time. All this time he'd been there to watch and listen. And listen. Oh, sure, he thought. He'd listened. And how many others had, too? He'd probably been wired the whole time. He tried to think back, to remember all that had been said. Hell! He'd done the campaign! And just today he'd switched out the pills.

For the first time in his life he felt defeated. Absolutely defeated. He'd weathered abandonment, foster homes, being a ward of the state until he'd practically finished medical school and then a hopeless, loveless marriage. Now that things were finally starting to get better for him, they were going to put him in jail. Once again, the state would get him.

Well, that was something he just couldn't face. He'd rather die than go to prison. Oh, Jenny, Jenny. His sweet Jenny. The anguish that was in him was welling over. The thoughts kept coming at him as he realized one horrible thought after another. He'd never be Paisley's father. He'd never have Jenny wrapped in his arms with his legs between hers. He'd never enjoy the first game of pool in his billiard room in his new mansion in Great Falls and he'd never watch Paisley in her riding outfit prancing up to him on her very own Chestnut mare.

Tears streamed down his face as he sat there in the car, oblivious to the curious stares. After awhile he slowly backed the car out of the parking space and drove home. When he got there he mechanically parked and locked his car, walked over to the elevator and pushed the button for his floor. All these things were done without him even being aware of them.

He removed his jacket and threw it into a chair with Paisley's toys. Ironically he realized that if it hadn't been for Paisley's toys he wouldn't have had an inkling about what was going on until they came to get him.

That was the question. When would they make their move? And how much did they really know, anyway? What had tipped them? Did they know about Betsy? Jeremy? Leroy? Henry? Pete? "What do they know?" he screamed to the walls.

Reviewing each case in his mind, he went over and over every detail. Regardless of what they already knew, soon they would know that there was no Michael Smith and that he'd bought the Sinequan for himself. They would make the connection that Pete died from an overdose of Sinequan. If they knew about Pete, how had they found out? Was that measley $15,000 bequest the one that led them to him? He slammed his fist against the back of a chair hard enough to topple it forward. How ironic that would be. How had they discovered he'd written that prescription? How long had they been watching him, anyway? He was going nuts. He recognized the fear of his own paranoia clouding everything over.

Forget what they knew. Undoubtably they knew enough, or Mr. Colin Scott would not have been playing the grieving patient. He wondered how much of his story had even been true. At a minimum they had his *campaign* on tape and "Mason's" medicine doctored to lethal proportions. They had motive, opportunity and *weapon*. It wouldn't take long to get the big picture. They might not uncover all his misdeeds, but it would only take one to put him in one of those hell holes they called prison cells.

Okay, so what was he going to do now? Pacing back and forth he went over all his options. Every one gloomier than the last.

First, he would take care of his daughter. He would make sure she was set for life. That she would be able to choose to go to any college anywhere in the world, not just the one the State decreed she could go to if she kept her grades in the top ten percent of her class.

Next, he would see to it that Jenny remained faithful to him forever. His mind whirred as an idea came to him. The idea of it fueled him and gave him renewed courage. He would allow her to live and to take care of Paisley as long as nobody else was having her. As soon as somebody else took her, he would take her to be with him. As long as she was good, she could raise Paisley, but if she allowed another man to pleasure her, to take what was rightfully his, she would die and her parents would raise Paisley for him.

Yes, this was perfect.

He reached for the phone and pressed the speed dial button on his phone. It dialed her number at the dealership. When he asked for her, he was told that she was with a customer. He left a message for her to call him at home as soon as possible.

Twenty minutes later his phone rang and he jumped to get to it, afraid she'd hang up if he didn't get to it right away.

"Jenny?"

"Yes, David, what is it? You sound strange."

"Just a little upset, I need to talk to you tonight. Can you meet me at my office when you get off from work?"

"David, I may not get out of here until eleven and I still have to go home and finish packing. Can't we talk when you take me to the airport tomorrow?"

"No. I have to see you tonight. Jenny, I wouldn't ask if it wasn't extremely important. Please. I won't keep you long."

"Okay," she said with a sigh. "You know, I've never really been there before so meet me at the Mobil gas station down the street."

"Okay. Call me when you're leaving."

Two and a half hours later Jenny called to say she was leaving. David grabbed his car keys and went down to his car. He had at least a half hour on her so he went straight to his office to make sure everything was ready. Then he drove to the gas station to wait for her. When he saw the lights of her Bonneville pull onto the lot he honked his horn and led the way to his office.

They parked side by side in the parking garage and he came over to help her out of her car.

"David, what is all this? Why did I have to come here, tonight of all nights?" She sounded tired and she certainly was irritable.

"You'll see. There's something we have to do tonight and this is the best place for me to do it."

He pushed the button for the elevator and while they were waiting he took her in his arms and gave her a very passionate kiss. The elevator doors opened and he was not quite willing to let her go yet. She pulled away, "David, the elevator."

They rode in silence to the sixth floor and then walked down the quiet, carpeted hallway. When they reached the door to his office he used his key to unlock it. After he closed the door behind them, he locked it. He switched on the lights and led Jenny through the reception area to his office which was also locked. He unlocked it and flipped the light switch. As soon as she was on the other side of the door he closed it behind them. Jenny was beginning to feel a little uneasy when he took her hand and led her to a black leather sofa. He sat down and pulled her down beside him.

Suddenly she thought she knew what he wanted. "David, you know I'm not ready for this yet," she stated.

He put his finger on her lips. "Shh, it's not what you think. I brought you here because I need to tell you something, but you can't know it yet, so I need to hypnotize you."

"What?" She asked.

"I can't explain, you'll just have to trust me on this."

"David, I don't even know if I can be hypnotized."

"Trust me, you can. I'm the best there is."

"Why can't you just tell me?" She said with impatience.

"That won't work."

"If you're trying to make sure I'm not going to make it with somebody while I'm up in Detroit, you ought to know, I'm not an easy lay!"

"Yes, darling," he said as he smoothed her hair away from her face. "Believe me, I know that. It's nothing like that. I need to tell you where you can find something if I'm not around later to get it for you."

"What?"

"Never mind now, you're asking too many questions. You'll find out when the time is right. Now just lay back, put your head right here." He cradled her head with his hands and eased her down until her head was in the slight indentation. He lifted her ankles and removed her shoes, letting them fall onto the carpet.

He sat in a leather arm chair behind her and using a remote, dimmed the lights. Pressing another button he lowered a screen. Suddenly the screen lit up and there was a long pointed crystal prism with a myriad of rainbow colors bouncing off the different facets. The prism was suspended by a silver thread that was moving back and forth in some white sand. The point was making perfect circles over and over again, each one slightly overlapping the last.

"Keep your eye on the tip of the prism. Follow it around and around. Don't let it out of your sight. Around and around it goes and goes, making circle upon circle upon circle, around and around, never ending, never stopping, just like my love for you." He pressed another button and the prism sent out shards of color in a wild Technicolor pattern, mesmerizing Jenny as she focused on it. Seconds later she was under.

"Jenny, everything I tell you tonight you will forget. It will go to the very back of your mind and it will stay there until it's time to surface. I will be taken from you soon even though I don't want to go. It's the only choice I have. A man will kill me. It will seem like an accident, but it is not. His name is Colin Scott. If you are missing me, blame him. Go to John Marshall's office in Fairfax. He is my attorney. He will have a key for you. Use this key to find a letter of explanation and to learn about Paisley's legacy. You will only remember these words after a certain trigger occurs. That will happen when you achieve an orgasm with another man. As soon as any man causes you to climax you will remember everything I've told you tonight, instantly. When I count back from five to one, you will wake up. Five, four, three, two, one.

"When is something going to happen? I've got to get home to pack." Jenny wailed.

"It's already happened honey," David said as he sat beside her on the couch. "C'mere and let me hold you for awhile. It may be a long time before I get to hold you again." He pulled her into his arms and kissed her deeply. The way he had worded the trigger precluded him from making love to her tonight, unless of course, he showed no concern for her pleasure. But that wasn't how he wanted her to remember him. Keeping his kisses soft and gentle he held her in his arms, savoring the feel of her and the essence of everything that was his Jenny. When she looked up into his face and said she had to go now, he smiled down at her. "I know." He pulled her up off the sofa and walked her through his office, down the hallways to the elevator and put her into her car.

"Aren't you going home, too?" She asked.

"Not just yet, I've still got a few things I have to do. I'll see you tomorrow."

"Don't forget, you're driving me to the airport."

"I won't forget. See you at the dealership tomorrow night around six. That should give us plenty of time to get to the airport and get you through security before your flight." He gave her a kiss on the cheek and closed her car door. He watched her pull out of the parking garage and then hung his head down.

After all the plans he'd made, he could hardly believe that all his dreams had disappeared with the advent of one Colin Scott. His hands, hanging down from his sides began to turn into hard fists. Hatred was not a new emotion for him, but it had been several years since he'd felt it like this. Not since his school days when they'd taunted him about being Mr. Nobody's son had he had his blood boil like this.

He went back up to his office, sat at his desk and started making a list of things he had to do. After a few minutes of the eerie silence of the empty building, he grabbed his note pad, locked up and drove home.

As soon as he got home he walked into his darkened study, not even bothering to turn the lights on. He slumped down into his chair as he tossed the note pad on the desk blotter in front of him. It was late, he was tired but he had a lot of thinking and planning to do. God! Just when had everything he'd ever dreamed about started slipping through his fingers?

Chapter 95

Chantilly, VA

October 23, 1989

He just knew it. There was no Michael Smith at the address given with the prescription order. He'd even driven over to the address in Fairfax City and checked it out. A Mr. and Mrs. Gervase lived there with their two kids and four cats. The phone number was also phoney. It connected to a 7-11 on Route 123. The prescription had been for 15 Sinequan capsules, 150 milligrams each. And the prescription had been written by Dr. David L. Sandler. Needless to say, Michael Smith had not had a prescription card.

He was ready to go to the Major. It was after nine o'clock on a Wednesday night. No sense trying to track him down now, he'd call on him first thing tomorrow morning.

The phone rang and he distractedly went to answer it. "Hello?" He said into the receiver.

A female voice said,"Colin? Colin Scott?"

"Yes." He answered a bit hesitantly.

"This is Barbara! Remember me?"

Barbara? He thought? Who was Barbara? And then it dawned on him who she was. "Of course I remember you. Who could forget you?" Who could forget the first woman he'd made it all the way with? He thought to himself.

"How the heck are you?" he asked and "How'd you track me down?"

"I just called your mother. She was happy to give me your number. And I'm just fine, how about you?"

"Okay, I guess. I just got divorced this month and I retired from the Department a few months ago. I'm trying to figure out where I want to go from here."

"Yeah, I got divorced, too. Bummer, huh?"

"Yeah."

"Say, are you planning on going to the reunion party Saturday night?"

"I hadn't really decided yet. Why? Are you going?"

"Yeah, I think it'll be a gas, seeing the old gang. Hey, why don't we go together, just like old times?" she asked. Then added seductively, "I'm just dying to see you again."

"Yeah, okay. I guess we could do that. You want me to pick you up somewhere or just hook up there?"

"How about coming to my mother's house? She still lives in that same house down the street from your parents. I live a couple of hours away from here now, in Richmond, but I always stay with Mom when I come to visit."

"Okay, around seven?" he asked.

"Yeah, that'll be good."

"Okay, see you then."

"Colin?"

"Yeah?"

"We had some good times, huh?"

"Yes, we sure did. See ya Saturday."

"Bye," she said wistfully.

He hung up the phone and walked over to the chair in front of the TV. As he grabbed for the remote he thought, Geez, Barbara! Wonder what she looks like. Gads! It had been years since he'd thought about her. At one time, they'd been very close, going steady almost their entire senior year. That was until he'd met Lynn and taken her to the prom instead. He and Barbara hadn't spoken since. He hoped she wasn't planning on doing a "Carrie" thing at the reunion. He laughed out loud at the thought and flicked on the TV. As he switched through the channels looking for an adventure movie he thought, if anybody wanted to kill him, it would be Dr. Sandler after he found out who he really was.

He fell asleep in his chair watching Steven Segal pulverize his enemies and woke when he heard apartment doors closing as people headed off to work. He rubbed his neck where it had gotten kinked from the chair and went to take a shower.

After he dressed and wolfed down a bowl of Life cereal he gathered all his notes together, as well as the tapes and the two baggies and left the apartment. He drove straight to his old office and even used the familiar parking space he'd often thought of as *his*.

He called out "Hi" to a few people as he made his way to the Major's office. When he approached the desk of the Major's secretary, he winked at her. "Hi, Gloria. The Major in?"

She smiled back at him. "Well, well, look who's here. Are you still coming back to get your monthly dressing down from the Major?"

"No, this time I need to talk to him about a case I've been working on."

"Well, let me see if he can make the time to see you. You don't have an appointment, you know," she said with a smile.

"If I promise to buy you lunch do you think you can squeeze me in?"

"Oh, I can squeeze you in alright," she said in a sultry voice. "Don't you ever worry about that." She picked up the phone and pressed a button.

"Major, C.G. Scott is here to see you, just like old times. You got a minute to see him or should I ask him to come back?"

Colin could hear the booming voice on the other end. "Send him in, send him in!"

Colin winked at Gloria and said, "I'll call you about lunch."

Gloria smiled back, "Call me about dinner, so I won't have to come back to work afterwards."

He chuckled as he walked into the Major's office.

Colin and Major Ryan went back a long, long way. They had been golfing buddies long before Neal Ryan's career track had put him in a supervisory position. The Major stood up to meet Colin as he entered his office. They shook hands, good friends that they were. The few times the Major had reined Colin in during the past years were for his over zealousness on a few cases. It had caused some tension once or twice, but that was all forgotten now.

"Colin, What brings you back to the Zoo?" referring fondly to the nickname everyone used when talking about the building that currently housed the Major Crimes Division.

"Got something I need you to take a look at. You got time?"

"Sure." He motioned for Colin to have a seat in one of the chairs in front of his desk as he reseated himself in his.

Colin started with meeting MaryAnn Riddel. He explained the intricate schedule found under the bed, the dry cleaning found later, Pete's demise on the day of his anniversary, all the interviews he'd had with Pete's friends and the discovery of the amendment to Pete's will. Then he explained everything he'd been doing for the last month or so, culminating with the description of what was on the tapes and displaying the baggies containing the will and the pill bottle. After he had filled the Major in on all he knew and what he additionally suspected, he ended with: "So, I think I may have stumbled onto a serial killer, but I can't go any further without a list of his patients, current and expired."

The Major sat back in his chair and quietly thought things through for a few minutes. Finally he said, "If we pick him up tonight after 5, that will give us all day today to get these pills checked out and then we'll have twenty-four hours to charge him, so that'll put us past 7 or so on a Friday night. With any luck he won't be able to get his attorney over the weekend and we'll have two days to try to get him to talk. In the meantime that will give you, AND a detective from homicide time to check out those files. Who do you know in homicide that you can get along with?" The Major asked.

Rather than answer the insult implied by that question, he rambled off three names.

"Good, I think Lawrence is available. I'll have him brought in." He picked up the phone and told Gloria to get Richard Lawrence down here as soon as possible, as well as the Lieutenant in charge of homicide and the Captain of the Criminal

Investigations Bureau. He also wanted to meet with the prosecuting attorney before lunch and what was the new number for the police lab?" When he hung up the phone, he said to Colin, "I was going to leave early today to play some golf." Pointing at the baggies on the desk he said, "Get that stuff over to the lab."

Colin jumped up to do as he was told. The Major shook his head as the door slammed behind him. This could be nothing, or it could be huge. He'd better make sure everything was handled by the book and that everybody was informed every step of the way or he'd have a lot of questions to answer later.

Chapter 96

Fairfax, VA

October 24, 1989

By 4:30 they were ready. The lab confirmed what Colin already knew. There were fingerprints on the pills as well as on the bottle and the pills were not the same as the 50 milligram pills that they compared them to from a pharmacy. They appeared to have more powder in them so they were being sent away for further testing. They would wait until David Sandler was arrested to compare the fingerprints rather than chance having the prints they'd lifted being lost or bogged down in the National Registry at the FBI headquarters. A plain clothes detective was waiting in his unmarked car to follow the doctor home from work.

Once they were sure he was in his apartment, six officers would enter the building and make the arrest. There were four undercover detectives and two uniformed officers. Colin was to be permitted to accompany them as a ride-along. There would be two squad cars circling the block as back-ups, should he manage to elude them somehow.

David left the office and went down to the parking garage. He'd had a hectic day today trying to get things done. First thing this morning he had asked Glenda to cancel all his appointments for today and for tomorrow. Then he'd gone to his bank and from there to his attorney's office. He'd called the builder in Great Falls and told him he'd changed his mind. He instructed him to sell the home after it was finished and to settle up any overages from the sale with his attorney. He bought a casket and a funeral plot in a local cemetery and left the papers on his desk before he left the office. Then he filled out the papers to buy a gun. He would be able to pick it up on Monday.

Now he was driving home to get a quick shower and to change before it was time to pick up Jenny and take her to the airport. He'd had this awful melancholy cloud hanging over his head from the moment he woke up this morning and remembered that Colin Scott was on to him. How long did he have before Colin and his friends would make their move? He was very grateful that Jenny would be in Detroit when all this was likely to be happening. She wouldn't have to deal with any of this. He'd seen to that. Saturday he'd go spend some time with Paisley.That would cheer him up. That thought buoyed him a little as he took the elevator to his apartment. Once inside he hurriedly showered and dressed.

It was almost 5:00. He'd told Jenny that he would be at the dealership by 6:00. Traffic being what it was at rush hour, he had just about enough time if he left now. He grabbed his keys and went down to the parking garage.

Just as the elevator doors opened he saw them. He tried to push the button to close them but an officer threw his body between the doors to stop them from closing. As the door connected with the officer's body, temporarily immobilizing him when it crushed up against him, David grabbed the officer's gun. The snap had already been undone in anticipation of their confrontation, so it was easy pickings. David had the gun in his hand pointed at the officer just as the doors reacted to the pressure against them and released his entrapped body.

"No, you can't take me now!" he hollered, pushing the officer away. "I have to take my fiancé to the airport. Get out of my way!" The officer fell back against the elevator door opening, landing on the floor, preventing the doors from closing. He put his hands on top of his head and sat there wild-eyed.

Just outside the elevator the whole contingency stopped as they realized what had just happened. One by one, they started to back away, giving David, the man with the gun, a little space.

David was frantic. He wasn't ready! They had come for him too soon. He looked down at the gun he held in his hand. This

478

wasn't the gun he had planned on using, but it would certainly do. He looked at all the officers as they fell back, seeking cover.

Suddenly David spotted Colin. He instantly felt a surge of rage that he could not control. He stepped forward. "You!" he spat out as he pointed the gun at Colin. His hand shook with his anger. "This is all your fault! I've lost everything because of you!" He flexed his finger over the trigger for one split second before squeezing it.

Colin, in anticipation of his action jumped behind a cement pillar just as a bullet sliced the air beside his ear. Coming out on the other side of the pillar, his weapon drawn, he took aim and fired before David could fire again. Several other bullets pierced the doctor's skin simultaneously, but Colin's was the one that killed him, leaving a small brownish hole just above his left eyebrow.

David fell back to the pavement never knowing whether he'd shot Colin or not. As the blood poured from the back of his head onto the garage floor, the officer in the elevator slumped down, dropping his head into his hands.

The crime scene guys were called, as well as a contingent of sergeants, lieutenants and one Major who had been sitting at his desk awaiting word of the arrest.

It would be days before things got sorted out and many more months of investigating before Colin could identify some of Dr. Sandler's other victims. But it would be years before he knew the complete scope of David Sandler's powers.

At 6:30, after many attempted phone calls to David's apartment and to his car phone, Jenny gave up waiting for him and had one of the Service porters drive her to the airport. It would be almost a week before she found out why David hadn't picked her up and taken her to the airport that Thursday night.

Chapter 97

Fairfax, VA

October 24, 1989

The ambulance came and took David's body to the coroner's office while Colin and all the officers who'd been there at the shooting were interviewed one by one in separate rooms. By eleven that night Colin and the others had been completely exonerated of any charges relating to the shooting, pending a formal IAD investigation. All of the officers testified that the doctor had fired first using one of the officer's guns.

Colin was asked to assist in the follow up investigation and was hired on as an outside temporary consultant by the Department. It would be as if he was back on the force, just dedicated to one particular case. They would start the following morning by getting all the patient files and thoroughly going through David's office and apartment. The search warrants were arranged for that night before everyone left to go home.

As Colin drove home he remembered MaryAnn. So far he hadn't seen or heard any reporters nosing around, but he knew they had connections in the department and there would be something in the paper or on the TV news by tomorrow. He decided that even though it was late he would stop by and see her. She was probably wondering what was going on since he hadn't called her after his last session with the doctor.

When he pulled into the driveway all the lights were off in the house. He hesitated for a few minutes trying to decide whether he should disturb her or not when he noticed the outside front door light go on. Somebody was up after all.

He got out of his car and walked up the driveway just as the door opened. MaryAnn stood in her bath robe holding the door for him. "I thought you were my daughter returning from her date. I was wondering why she was still sitting in the car after the engine was turned off. I'm relieved to see it's you."

"Hi," he said in a tired voice. "Well, it's all over. We went to arrest him tonight and he grabbed an officer's gun and tried to kill me. Luckily, my instincts had me tensed for something and I was ready. I got him first. He's dead."

"Oh, Colin," was all she said as they wrapped their arms around each other and hugged. MaryAnn was sobbing and wiping her cheeks when they pulled apart.

"I knew Pete wouldn't leave us," she said softly.

"Well, turns out you were right. He didn't leave you. Someone took him from you, and now he's gone, too."

"Colin, thank you so much for all you've done for me and the kids. We'll never forget this."

"Funny, my whole police career, I never shot anybody. I'm retired less than six months and look what happens."

"You look beat, Colin. Go home and get some sleep. Then get a bill together for me."

"That won't be necessary, the Department's going to handle everything. They feel they should have given Pete's death a little more attention than they did. Now they want me to see if there were any others. I'll be back on the force for a few months trying to piece everything together."

Another car pulled in beside his on the driveway. "Well good night, Colin. Looks like I can go to sleep now, too. The kids will do a lot better now, knowing how Pete really died. Thanks, again."

He hugged her again and then ran down the steps, anxious to get home to his own thoughts and to try to get some sleep.

On the drive home he started trembling a little. He realized that he needed to eat something. All the adrenaline he'd used up tonight was now causing him to crash. He drove through a drive-in Taco Bell and bought a couple of soft tacos to take home. That and a couple of beers and he should be able to sleep after he wound down.

Man, he thought, I could've been killed tonight! He'd still had some doubt in his mind as to whether David Sandler was really a murderer as the evidence indicated, until he'd seen the look in his eyes just before he'd fired that shot.

That was the look of a man angry at the world, a man trying to find love and acceptance. He recognized that look because lately he'd seen something like it in the mirror. He never doubted that Dr. Sandler had done what he'd done because of love. Who was the woman he loved so much? He'd heard the doctor scream that he had to take his fiancé to the airport, just before he'd noticed that the doctor had the officer's gun in his hand. He wondered who she was and how she would handle hearing about his death.

Chapter 98

En route to Detroit, MI

Jenny sat in her first-class seat sipping a glass of champagne as she caught up on some crossword puzzles and some newspaper articles that she'd been meaning to read. Pontiac, in their very generous way was taking very good care of her, as they always did. Being a woman GSM she was a novelty. Being beautiful and single made her hard to forget. During her whole career she had graciously deferred the preferential treatment that they always wanted to give her, but now she was enjoying the lavishness of somebody's expense account.

As much as she loved doing these puzzles, she was going to have to give them up. Every day she cut the puzzle out and slipped it under her pile of puzzles from the previous days. Now there really wasn't much pleasure in it. It had become a chore as every day she struggled to get two or three done, trying to catch up. It was the same with the newspapers. They were piled on her coffee table, jammed into her briefcase and articles were cut out and saved in paper-clipped stacks for her to read whenever she had a spare moment. The problem was there were no spare moments anymore, and the papers and puzzles kept mounting. She decided that as soon as she got home she would cancel her subscription to the newspaper. Maybe if she wasn't paying for them she wouldn't feel they were being wasted if she didn't read them. Who needed to know all this stuff anyway?

She had always prided herself on the fact that she stayed abreast of everything going on in the world, her state, her county and her city. But she was now beginning to realize the folly of it all. I mean, really, when was the last time someone asked her about the goings on in Bosnia, or in Richmond, nevertheless Fairfax County's Courthouse or Herndon's Town Hall. Never. The talk was all of Washington and the latest scandals and you didn't need to get anywhere near a newspaper to hear all about those. She wondered if David could help her get over her obsession with newspapers and the daily crossword puzzle.

She wondered where he was. It was so unlike him not to show up when he said he would. Tammy said she'd try to track him down and let her know what had happened. Maybe after she got to Detroit and was checked into her hotel room he would call. She had already told him the name of the hotel she would be staying in, but she hadn't known the phone number. He said he'd call information to get it and that she could expect a call every night while she was away.

She was really looking forward to this trip. As much as she loved her children, it was really going to be nice to get away. Children were a lot of work. Just getting them ready for school or playtime each day before going off to work herself sometimes left her frazzled. She did feel bad for her mother though. Now she'd have to do it all by herself for two weeks. Well, at least she'd have David to help her on the weekends. She took another sip of champagne and went back to the puzzle.

When the plane landed in Detroit she was met by a Pontiac representative who ushered her and her luggage to a waiting car and drove her to her hotel, which was almost an hour away from the airport, but close to the Pontiac headquarters. She checked into the hotel and asked if there were any messages. There were none, so she called her parents to let them know she had arrived safely. It was too late to talk to the kids as they were asleep and too late to call Tammy at the dealership as it would have been closed for at least an hour by now.

She called the front desk and left a message for a wake-up call then hung up all her business suits and unpacked all her cosmetics. Finding the key to the mini-bar she took out a soda and a candy bar and sat propped up against the headrest on the king-sized bed reading the newspapers she'd brought with her. An hour later she was sound asleep in the dark, quiet room.

The next day was Friday and she was given the grand tour of the Pontiac headquarters, Tech Center and some of the testing sites. She had a picture taken of herself standing in the huge wind tunnel to show the kids. In the afternoon, after a scrumptious lunch, she was met by the video crew who would be taping the training series. They tried a few sequences with her to try to ease her nervousness and then they all had dinner together at the hotel. Saturday they would get to work in earnest and Sunday would be a day for sight seeing.

Getting ready for bed that night she realized that she still hadn't heard from David. Well, he was supposed to help her mom tomorrow with the kids. She'd call there sometime in the early afternoon to check on them. Surely David would have surfaced by then.

Chapter 99

Chantilly, VA

Colin was so anxious to get started on the patient files that he woke up almost every hour thinking he'd over slept. By 5:30 am, he realized he would not be able to get back to sleep again so he got up, shaved and showered and then sat in his easy chair in his underwear in front of the TV eating a bowl of cereal watching the six o'clock news.

There were usually a handful of shootings every night around the beltway, but apparently the media hadn't gotten wind of this one yet. He listened to the weather segment. He didn't know why. It wasn't likely he'd be playing any golf today so he switched off the TV and went into the bedroom to get dressed.

He drove to the CIB offices and waited for Dick Lawrence to arrive. They had agreed to meet at eight, pick up the search warrants and go to the doctor's office to wait for his secretary to arrive. Dick showed up at ten 'til eight and they left to go to the magistrates office.

They arrived at Dr. Sandler's office a few minutes before nine and waited until 9:30 for Glenda to show up. When she didn't show they started looking for the rental management office. They finally found someone who had a key but it took a few minutes to explain the search warrant and convince him that they really were police detectives before he agreed to let them in.

One of the first things they found were the papers David had left in the center of his desk, just before locking up last evening, the deed to a cemetery plot and the ownership papers and receipts for a casket he'd bought just the day before. Colin sat down hard in David's chair as he stared at the papers in stunned silence.

He'd known! Somehow he'd known he was onto him! This gave a whole new meaning to the shooting that had occurred last night. Dr. Sandler had known he was going to die. He'd apparently accepted that fact rather than consider going to prison. He'd meant for one of the policemen to shoot him, but he'd meant to take Colin with him first. The significance of Dr. Sandler's last words had a different significance to him now than they had last night, "You!" he'd said. "This is all your fault! I've lost everything because of you!" The words rang in his ears just as the sound from the gun kept reverberating in his ears along with them. This was a cop-assisted suicide! The doctor had planned on being taken out, maybe even by Colin.

He reached over to the phone and lifted the receiver to call the Major when he noticed the redial and speed button. He punched the redial button. It was answered by a feminine voice proclaiming this to be the office of John Marshall. Colin had heard of John Marshall, he was an attorney in the city of Fairfax.

"Is Mr. Marshall in?" he asked.

"No, sir, he's in court today. May I take a message?"

"No, I'll call him back on Monday. Thanks." He disconnected the call and pressed the speed button.

"Royal Pontiac and GMC," a sugary voice replied.

"Does anybody there know a Dr. David Sandler?" Colin asked.

"Hold on. I'll ask," she said.

She came back on the line a minute or so later and said. "The title clerk says he's bought a few cars here. Would you like to speak to the Service Manager?"

"Yes, please," he replied.

"One moment. please."

"Dave Stroud. May I help you?"

"Yes, I'm with the Fairfax County Police Department, and I'm wondering if you're familiar with a Dr. David Sandler."

"Yes, Sir, I am. He's one of our best customers, buys a new car almost every six months, and he's real particular about how he keeps 'em."

"What kind of car is he driving now?" Colin asked.

"Unless he's traded within the last few weeks, it's a loaded up black Trans Am with all the trimmings in gold."

Colin sat bolt upright. He'd parked right next to one the night he'd gone to check on that prescription number. There was silence on the line for a moment and then the Service Manager spoke.

"Would you like to speak to his salesman, sir?"

"No, that's alright. Thank You."

"Sir, would you mind telling me what all this is about?"

"He died last night and you're on his speed dial for his office phone."

"He died?" the service manager asked incredulously.

"Yes, sir. Thanks for your help." Colin hung up.

Colin punched in the number for the Major's direct line. After relaying everything about the papers he'd found and telling him about the last call Dr. Sandler had made yesterday from his office phone, he asked the Major to send over a couple of guys in uniform with a van. They needed to get this stuff moved into a secured office in the CIB building so they could go over it.

As they were stacking things up preparing to move them, Glenda walked in. "Hey! What's going on here? Did the doctor tell you to do this?" She spun around and saw Colin. "Mr. Williams! What are you doing here?"

"Glenda, please come in here and sit down. I need to talk to you," Colin said as he gently took her elbow and led her over to the leather sofa.

"First, I am not Mason Williams. I'm an undercover investigator. My name is Colin Scott." He showed her his badge and then went to sit on the corner of the desk. He decided she didn't need to know more than the absolute basics unless she had some information to share with him. "We suspected Dr. Sandler of taking money from his patients. I was trying to get proof. When we went to arrest him last night he shot at us and we had to shoot back. He was killed last night." He wasn't ready to tell the world that he had been the one to kill him, they'd find that out soon enough.

"Oh, no!" she gasped, clutching her handbag to her chest with both arms. "I knew something was wrong yesterday when he had me cancel all his appointments. I just came in today to get my pay check."

"Do you know what he spent the day doing yesterday?"

"No, he sent me home as soon as I had contacted everyone."

"Glenda, did you know about him stealing from his patients?"

"Oh, heavens, no! I can't believe he was doing that!" she cried out.

"Glenda, did you have anything to do with keeping track of the medications the doctor prescribed to his patients?"

"No. Only he knew that kind of stuff. I never knew what they were being treated for. Dr. Sandler was very careful to protect his patients' privacy. Those files are confidential you know. You just can't take them and read them."

"I know. We're taking them to a special place that stores confidential medical files." He lied, because he knew she'd raise a stink if she knew where they were really going.

"Oh, okay."

"Glenda, are there patient files on the computer?" he asked nodding towards the door that led back to her reception area.

"No, just the appointment calendar, the billing information and some games for me to play to pass the time. I guess I'll have a lot of time to play games now. It looks like I'm out of a job," she said dejectedly.

"Sorry. Can I get any passwords needed to access the computer records before you leave? And your full name, address and phone number in case we have any further questions. We found the checkbook over there. I think I saw a check already made out to you as the last entry."

She walked over and opened it. There on the last page past the stubs was a check already written and signed by Dr. Sandler made payable to Glenda Jameson in the amount of $5,000. That's when she started crying. She held the check to her heaving bosom with one hand while wiping her eyes with a tissue with the other. "I can't believe he's gone," she said between sobs as she put the check in her purse and left the key to the office door on top of her old desk. She found a small box and put her personal items in it and then left the office, sniffling.

Ten minutes after she left, Linda Sandler showed up. She was all indignant and proprietoral. "Just what is the meaning of all this? Who said you could take anything? Everything here belongs to me now. What are you some kind of scavengers or what? First you kill him and then you rob him. Is that the kind of law enforcement our money's buying us now?" Clearly this was Colin's least favorite type of person, judging by her Cruella Deville demeanor and apparent greediness over her ex-husband's estate.

Colin waived the search and seizure warrant under her nose as he tried to explain to her that they were only taking things having to do with their investigation, nothing with any monetary value. Then he slapped the cemetery plot and casket papers into her hand. "Maybe you should take care of burying him before you spend all his money, if in fact he left it to you. We have reason to believe he saw his attorney just yesterday. YOU'D better make sure before you take anything out of here that it belongs to you. I wouldn't want to have to track you down and accuse YOU of "scavenging".

"Ohhh," she screamed as she shook so hard her Louis Vitton shoulder bag fell off her shoulder. "We'll just see about this! I know exactly what's in here and nothing had better be missing when I get back!"

Dick Lawrence stood up from the floor where he had been stacking boxes. "Good Lord, you can't fault him for divorcing that one! What say we get these last things loaded and lock up and be outta here before she gets back?"

"I'm with you one hundred percent," Colin said as he bent down and grabbed two cartons. He was anxious to get to work on these files and they still had his apartment to go over. Colin had found some audio tapes in the back of David's desk drawer and he couldn't wait to see what they revealed. They finished loading up, rechecked the office and therapy room then locked the office door. Grabbing Glenda's key from the reception desk he checked her drawers, unhooked her computer and, carrying it under one arm, he locked the main door behind them.

Returning the key to the rental management office he advised them that no one was allowed to remove anything else from the office until the court said so. If they needed the offices they could store the contents and the estate would reimburse them for any expenses they incurred. If they didn't hear anything from anybody within a few months they should contact John Marshall. Colin had found several legal documents in Dr. Sandler's office that had been prepared by him, so it was safe to assume that he was the doctor's attorney, at least for business purposes.

Colin had put the key Glenda had left on the desk in his pocket, just in case it turned out that they'd forgotten something.

Colin and Dick, along with the two uniformed officers, unloaded everything into a prepared office at CIB. Then they grabbed a quick bite to eat before tackling Dr. Sandler's apartment.

First they started with the car. It was immaculately clean. It was indeed the same car Colin had seen the other night. Dr. Sandler must have been in the store watching him as he talked with the pharmacist. That must have been how he had known they would be coming for him. He'd go back there later with a picture to see if anybody remembered him just to confirm his suspicions.

It was a little harder getting into the apartment than it had been the parking garage. They'd been in the garage just last night and he'd remembered the access code for the gate. The superintendent in charge was very skeptical and insisted on staying with them the whole time they were in the apartment. Surely he must know that the doctor was dead, Colin thought. It had happened right here in the parking garage just last night, for Pete's sake. He wondered if the ex-Mrs. Sandler had already alerted them.

Dr. Sandler had a very nice apartment. It was very tastefully decorated. Colin cringed when he thought about the sharp contrast there was between his "bachelor pad" and this one.

In Dr. Sandler's home office he found a patient rolodex which would come in very handy. He also found an odd assortment of pills in assorted baggies with little notes inside them. Colin thumbed through the books that were on a burled mahogany book shelf behind the desk that matched it. The first row of books contained two that the doctor had written and several other psychiatric reference books. The next shelf had collections of periodicals in leather bound cases and the third had a Physician's Desk Reference as well as several other books on prescription drugs. At the end of that shelf were three little books on erotica. That was a little odd, he thought.

The kitchen yielded two bottles of champagne, some cheeses, a box of crackers and some ice cream. Apparently he ate out quite a bit, just like Colin.

The bathroom had one of the most expensive razors Colin had ever seen as well as a customized chrome shower head that could be turned to almost any angle. The towels were quite obviously the best money could buy. They were the thickest and softest he'd ever felt.

The bedroom was surprisingly sparse compared to the rest of the house. As if he hadn't quite decided what style to furnish it in. In the center was a massive platform bed with a built-in head board containing built-in night stands on the ends. The comforter on the made-up bed was bold black and white spirals with thin red lines dissecting them. The lamp bases on each night stand were like smooth onyx, the shades were white with small red pleats all around. This was definitely a man's bedroom, except that it was clean.

There were no dressers. When he opened the closet he saw why. Colin had never seen a closet the likes of this one. On one side the sport coats were hung, very evenly spaced exactly above the rack that held the matching pants. Next were shirts neatly pressed and ready to wear, sorted by color. Sweaters were in clear plastic bags on a shelf along the top. Beyond that was a tilted shelf holding at least thirty different pairs of shoes. Socks were rolled up and sticking out of little cubbyholes and on the other wall were at least forty little drawers filled with underwear, rolled up ties, cummerbunds, cufflinks, handkerchiefs, belts and suspenders. Across the top of that shelf were some hats. At the very back of the closet was a bag full of toys. The man certainly knew how to dress, but what were the toys for?

Having found nothing more that would help with the investigation, they thanked the supervisor and signed a receipt he had already filled out listing the items they were taking. On the way down to the parking garage in the elevator Colin asked Dick, "Did you see anything that would make you think the man had a fiancé? I saw nothing, no pictures, no photo albums, no cutesy memorabilia."

"I didn't see anything either. It's like he sterilized the place as if he knew we were coming," Dick said.

"He did," Colin replied.

As an after thought he said, "Let's take a look a what's at the end of the trash chute."

"Oh, Colin, do we have to?" Dick said with a grimace on his face, "that stuff smells so bad, there's always dirty diapers and rotten food."

"C'mon, if he cleaned up, that's probably where he tossed everything."

"Yeah, and everybody else."

As it turned out the incinerator had been fired up that morning so it was too late to find anything useful. They did find a few metal picture frames with cracked and charred glass, the pictures completely obliterated by the intense heat. Colin had his doubts as to whether they could be from the doctor's apartment until he realized that the frames were sterling silver. Who threw away picture frames that were sterling silver? They had to have been his. What or who was he hiding?

They went back to the office and Colin started going through everything. It was after midnight before he left to go home. He took the box of cassettes with him, figuring that he could listen better, undisturbed, at home.

He walked into his apartment a half hour later with two hoagie subs in a bag and the box of tapes under his arm, a six pack of Coors dangling from the other hand.

Time to eat and have a few brews while he worked. He knew there was no way he'd get a good night sleep until he was sure nobody else was in jeopardy. Right this very minute somebody could be taking some kind of pills the doctor had "doctored".

Six 90-minute tapes later he knew the story of Liesel. In fact he felt like he knew Liesel. It was almost noon on Saturday and he was getting tired. He drove over to the office to find the file on Liesel Palmer, hoping that she hadn't already been one of his victims. He found the folder and opened it. Written in red ink on the inside jacket was a hastily written note: Relocated to Washington State. Account paid in full.

He sat at his new desk and dialed the number that gives officers access to phone and address information. In a few minutes he was connected to a corresponding service for the Washington State Police. He had a phone number within minutes. He punched in the numbers. The phone rang several times before it was answered. A groggy man's voice said, "Hello?"

Damn! He'd forgotten about the time change. He should have probably waited at least another hour before calling.

"Is Liesel Palmer there?"

"It's Liesel Hoffman and she's asleep! Who wants to know?"

She's alive, he thought somewhat relieved. "I'm an investigator from Fairfax County, Virginia. My name is Colin Scott. I'm sorry to be calling you so early, I forgot about the time change. I'll call back later."

Daniel, wide awake now said, "No, it's okay, what's up?"

Colin sketchily explained what he knew and what he suspected. Then he asked if Liesel was taking any medication prescribed by the doctor.

"Well, she was many, many months ago. She moved back here almost eight months ago. She's married to me now and as far as I know the only thing she's taking is prenatal vitamins. We've only got another month to go in our pregnancy."

"When she wakes up could you ask her if she's ever changed her will to include the David L. Sandler Foundation?" Colin asked.

"Hold on she's awake now." A few minutes later Daniel came back on the line. "Yeah, she says she did."

"Would you mind if I flew out to see you early next week? Maybe you could clear a few things up for me and I know I can clear a few things up for you."

"Sure, just let us know when you get here."

"Meanwhile, don't let her take any pills until we check them out. Okay?"

"Okay."

Colin went back home to take a nap. Tonight was the Reunion party. With everything that had been going on, he'd almost forgotten about it. He hoped he could get a little rest before he had to perk up for all his old school chums, and Barbara.

Chapter 100

Chantilly, VA

When the alarm went off at 6:00 pm Colin was still groggy and if it hadn't been for his date with Barbara he would have just turned it off and rolled back over. He dragged himself out of bed and went into the bathroom to take a shower. Maybe that would help.

Thirty-five minutes later he was freshly showered and shaved and wearing one of the new suits he had "borrowed" from the property room. One more wearing before turning them in on Monday wouldn't make a difference to the Department, but it sure would show his former classmates that he had style and that he could afford very expensive suits. The shoes would be a problem later, as experience had shown him that in three or four hours tops, he wouldn't be able to feel his toes. Dancing would be out of the question after that.

He drove to his old stomping grounds, past his mother's house to the small house down the street that Barbara had grown up in. It hadn't changed a bit. Well, maybe the trees were a little bit bigger but the same lawn ornaments were still stuck in the flower beds. A shiny blue aluminum ball rested atop a cement triangular base and a painted wooden fat lady with red and black polka dotted underwear was bending over tending to the mums. It was nice that some things never changed.

He'd felt a pang of guilt as he'd driven by his parents' house. He really needed to stop by and visit with them. He used to do that all the time. The odd thing was that now he was almost ashamed to go home. He felt that he'd somehow let them down by failing at his marriage. When he stayed away too long, it was always hard to make contact again. He had to get over the guilt of not visiting or he'd only have more guilt to worry about come Thanksgiving when he'd have to surface.

He parked his car in the bluestone driveway remembering all the nights he'd done just the same thing in a blue Chevelle Super Sport. That car had fit him like it had been made for him. He wished he still had it. The time he'd taken Barbara's virginity in the back seat seemed just like yesterday. He looked to the back seat of the Mustang, he doubted that he could even get back there with or without Barbara.

Just as he put his hand up to open the outside screen door the inside white wooden one with the three small glass diamond windows opened. There stood Barbara all decked out as if she was going to the prom. He'd have recognized her broad grinning smile anywhere but she had changed a lot. The years had not been as kind to her as they had been to him. She was at least thirty pounds heavier and her beautiful blue-black hair was now a dull gray with streaks of silver in it. Her complexion looked as smooth as ever but she had caked on so much makeup that it was hard to tell. He didn't remember her eyebrows being quite so heavy but those magnificent sparkling blue eyes under them were as welcoming as they'd always been.

"Hi!" she called out as he opened the screen door. "Come in, come in," she said as she motioned with her hand.

"Hello, Barbara," he said softly as his eyes assessed the rest of her. Her low cut, spaghetti strapped gown revealed a nice cleavage he didn't remember her ever having and although her waist was thicker than it had been it did taper in before the gown flared out at her hips again. It was a tawny peach color and her peau de soie covered pumps matched the shade perfectly. He would've bet a hundred dollars that somewhere down the line that dress had been a bridesmaid's gown.

While Barbara looked him up and down with a very approving eye he was reintroduced to her mother. "Colin, how nice it is to see you again. Your mother speaks of you often, always telling me about the wonderful awards you're always getting at work. We were all so sorry to hear about you and Lynn. How is Adam doing in school this year?"

He was ashamed to admit that he had no idea. He'd talked to him two weeks ago on the phone but Adam had been anxious to get back to the TV show he'd been watching, so they hadn't talked long. "Oh, fine." He supposed he was or Lynn would have told him so. "Mother said you lost your brother. I was so sorry to hear that. We all liked Uncle Charlie."

"Yes, I miss him dearly," she said with a slight tremor to her lips. "Well you two go and have a good time, and remember as long as she's living in my house she still has a curfew!"

"Mother!" Barbara wailed. "Why do you always have to embarrass me so?"

Colin helped Barbara on with her coat. It was a red cloth coat. "I know it doesn't go with my outfit, but it's the only coat I brought. Maybe I'll leave it in the car when we get there."

"Fine by me." He really didn't care. He was anxious to get there, shake a few hands and leave. He didn't know if it was because he was still tired or if he was all keyed up about the case, or because Barbara was not at all what he had expected. You really can't go back, he told himself. Nothing's ever the same.

Falls Church High School was just down the road so they didn't have much opportunity to talk, but he did find out that she had three kids, ages 17, 13, and 10. They were all with their father this weekend.

He told her a little bit about what he'd been doing since they'd last seen each other and then they were at the school. He parked the car and went around to her side to help her out, the bucket seats were so low slung that you almost needed to lift yourself out of them.

The party was in the gym and it appeared to have been decorated exactly the same as it had been for the prom. When he read the banner across the front he realized that there had been a theme to this reunion that he had not been aware of. It said, "Welcome Class of 1965 to your 1990 Prom night". Even though it was still 1989, they were celebrating their reunion year in October '89 instead of later during the summer of '90 when a lot of people would be on vacations. No wonder Barbara had called and no wonder she was dressed as she was. They'd broken up just before the prom and she had been devastated. Most of the women had corsages pinned to their dresses and Colin felt like a heel that he hadn't known to get one for Barbara.

She didn't seem to mind though as they moved from one couple to the next reminiscing, laughing about old times and asking the same three questions; "So what do you do now?" "Do you have any children?" and "Where do you live?"

The way Barbara was holding on to him he was sure that most people assumed they were married, so he had to keep finding a way to let everyone know he was recently divorced. He didn't want anyone to think that she was his wife.

He was forced to dance two slow dances with Barbara and two with other girls he had dated at one time. Then he found a quiet table for them to sit at while they ate chicken wings and Swedish meatballs with vegetables and ranch dip. They weren't allowed to have any alcohol because they were using the school building but someone had managed to spike the fruit punch with a fair amount of vodka.

After about two hours of socializing and "Do you remember?" questions he was ready to go home and told Barbara so. She was not anxious to leave but she agreed anyway.

As soon as they were in the car, Barbara turned to him and said, "Let's go to your place, so we can talk for awhile." He didn't feel like talking or anything else for that matter but he didn't know how to turn her down without hurting her feelings so he said okay. They stopped at a 7-11 on the way to pick up a bottle of wine for her and some hot dogs for Colin. He was still hungry, the buffet hadn't even begun to fill him.

There was no place in his apartment for them to sit so they sat on his little balcony with its view of the closed pool in two webbed lawn chairs, Barbara guzzling the wine and Colin wolfing down the hot dogs with some beer. It was an unusually warm night for early autumn.

Barbara kept up a constant banter about her ex-husband, her job and her kids, intermingled with thoughts about how their lives would have been so different if they'd only stayed together.

When she suggested they go skinny-dipping in the pool he suggested they call it a night and went inside. She followed him and put her arms around his neck. "We were always pretty good together. Don't you want to see if we still have that old magic between us?" she said as she stood on her tiptoes and kissed him on the lips. He had to bite his lips to keep from saying, "Barbara, I was 18, it would have been magical with anybody."

He was trying to pull away when her tongue breached his mouth and her thigh started rubbing against his groin. She sensed his resistance, "C'mon, for old times sake. Let's go one more round."

"Barbara, things have changed. You can't just have sex with anybody anymore, no matter how close we used to be. It's not the same. And the precautions you have to take now, I'm afraid, I'm not prepared."

"Oh, don't worry about that, I don't have any diseases and I can't get pregnant anymore. I had all that stuff fixed years ago." She unzipped the back of her gown and pulled the straps off her shoulders. "Besides, if you're really concerned I've got some condoms in my purse over there on the counter," she said inclining her head toward the kitchen. She pulled the straps off her shoulders and pushed her gown down past her hips and to the floor. He saw the combination bra and girdle that was apparently responsible for her full uplifted cleavage.

"Barbara, please," he said before she silenced him with another kiss. She put her hand between his legs and cupped his balls. "Remember how good I was at sucking on these?" she asked as she kissed his throat. She knelt in front of him and put her mouth over his manhood over top of the pants, breathing hot air through the material as she massaged his balls with her hand. When the bulge of his erection was visible through his clothes she reached up, undid his belt buckle and zipper and let the pants fall to his ankles. She pulled his underwear down past his knees and took him into her mouth. He groaned as the waves of pleasure overtook him and his common sense.

He reached down and unhooked the back of her tight foundation garment trying to get her breasts freed. Keeping him still in her mouth she reached back with both hands and helped him with all the eye hooks that went down past her waist.

When he had pulled her breasts out of the cups they'd been in, he was surprised to feel that they didn't have the form he'd expected. They weren't firm and heavy as he thought they'd be, they were loose and floppy and very soft. The nipples were massive though, and hard, and that pleased him. He pulled on them and rubbed them between his fingers listening to her soft groans.

He reached down and grabbed her by the elbows and pulled her up. "C'mon," he said, "let's go to the bedroom." There was something so cold and unfeeling about this but now he was fully aroused and looking for some form of release. He stepped out of his pants and removed his socks and was unbuttoning his shirt as they walked to his bedroom. He made it to the hallway before he remembered the condoms, he walked back to get her purse. She had removed that one article of clothing she'd been wearing, unhooking her stockings from it before shimmying out of it. He followed her into the bedroom noticing her saggy butt cheeks and flabby thighs. No you can't go back, he thought again.

When she turned to get into the bed he saw her breasts for the first time and was shocked by the way they drooped against her chest. What had appeared to be luscious, full, uplifted breasts all evening were actually ugly, white-veined, low-hanging ones.

He was feeling the edge of his arousal waning. She reached up and pulled him down on her, rubbing his shoulders and sucking on his nipples as she placed her knee between his thighs. "You don't have to do anything to get me ready, I've been ready and waiting for you for twenty-five years. Here, feel." She took his hand and put it between her thighs, mechanically he moved it around and instinctively he inserted a finger. She gasped with pleasure and wrapped her hand around his cock. Jerking it up and down until it became rock hard again.

"Colin, take me now, please," she begged as she arched her body up to his. She helped him put the condom on and then he placed the tip of his penis against her and pushed. He hardly felt anything. He knew he was inside her, but he couldn't feel her closing around him. He withdrew and thrust again thinking he wasn't all the way in. But he was. She was so loose he couldn't get any friction and the condom wasn't helping matters. He pushed up against her harder and harder trying to get enough sensation to stay hard and to please her. But apparently she was used to this because he felt her hand rubbing between their bodies down where he had entered her as he continually thrust into her. She cried out and spasmed and for the life of him he couldn't tell if it was something he'd done or something she'd done. He continued with his thrusting making sure she was satisfied and then he just stopped.

"Oh, Colin, that was wonderful! Just like it used to be," she had no clue that he hadn't even come, or that he didn't even want to. All he wanted to do was to take her home and come back and go to sleep. He lifted off of her, discarded the condom in the waste basket and walked out to the living room for his clothes. He carried hers back to the bedroom for her and waited in the living room for her to come out of the bedroom.

"Remember your curfew," he said. "She's probably already sent the cops out looking for us."

"You are the cops. Say, you wanna get together tomorrow? I don't have to go home until Monday."

"Sorry, Barbara. I gotta work. I'm on a special assignment." Then he threw in, "I'm afraid it's going to be bell to bell, seven days a week for awhile. It's a pretty important case," just in case she wanted to come up next weekend.

"You didn't have a good time, did you?" she asked.

"Barbara, it's not that. My divorce is just too new. You've had awhile to adjust to yours. I really loved my wife and I guess I'm not really looking to love somebody else just yet." Which was not true. He was ready, she just wasn't the one he was looking for. He thought about the woman Dr. Sandler had spoken about. That was the woman he was waiting for. "C'mon, I'll take you home." He helped her into her coat and ushered her out the door.

After dropping her off he drove back home, berating himself for his behavior tonight. No more casual sex he told himself. No more, unless it meant something. He was beginning to feel like a slut. What was the male counterpart to that word, he asked himself. He felt cheap and used and dirty. Geez, is this the way women felt when they put out for the wrong reasons?

He went back up to his apartment and went to bed. Ten minutes later he was stripping the sheets from the bed. Barbara's perfume had permeated them and it was nauseating him. He didn't have another set, so after throwing them out into the living room he laid back down on the bare mattress and fell asleep.

Chapter 101

Chantilly, VA

As soon as Colin woke up he threw on an old sweat suit and went to the Association Hall to work out. Then he stopped at his favorite breakfast place, Le Peep and had their Omni omelet with some freshly squeezed orange juice. He bought a newspaper to read while he ate and he scanned it for any news item on the shooting. Page 2 of the local section had the paragraph he was looking for.

"Dr. David L. Sandler was shot and killed by former Fairfax County Master Police Officer C.G.Scott as he and five Fairfax County Police officers were trying to arrest him for questioning in connection with the death of Mr. Pete Riddel, a former patient of his. The shooting occurred Thursday evening in the parking garage of Dr. Sandler's apartment complex. Dr. Sandler wrestled a gun from a uniformed police officer and fired at the officers. Scott returned the fire along with several of the other officers. Dr. Sandler was pronounced dead at the scene. Dr. Sandler was a prominent psychiatrist practicing in the City of Fairfax. Scott has been cleared of any wrong doing in the shooting and has been contracted back to the County to help on the case. Since his retirement from the County, Scott has been working undercover on this case as a private investigator. Pete Riddel died over two months ago in what was originally believed to have been a suicide."

Colin turned to the obituaries and found a small paragraph there also. Sandler's ex sure wasn't wasting any time or money posting the announcement. There wasn't even a picture. "Dr. David L. Sandler, noted psychiatrist and author died Thursday October 24, 1989. He is survived by his former wife Linda Sandler. Memorial services will be at the Money and King Funeral Home in Vienna, Virginia with interment immediately following at Fairhaven Memorial Gardens in Fairfax."

Colin closed the paper, threw some money on the table and left to go to the office.

By four o'clock he had a list of all the patients that had died within the last two years and a list of all the current patients. Seven had died, 258 were still alive. They would need to contact each patient to ask them several pertinent questions and then they would need to research each death. Tomorrow Colin would need to go to Dr. Sandler's bank and to see John Marshall, his attorney. Tuesday he would fly out to Seattle to see Liesel Palmer Hoffman.

Since Friday, when he had requested an up-to-date list of all the recorded deaths in the Metropolitan area, he had received new computer printouts almost hourly. None of the most recent names matched the patient list and so far that was a relief. The list he had requested last week from a friend in the department had also finally made its way to his desk. This was the list of all the drug-related deaths. There were two names on that list that matched the dead patient list: Henry Blocker and Pete Riddel.

Monday he would send Dick to find a copy of Henry Blocker's autopsy report and death certificate as well as a copy of his probated will, if there was one. He strongly suspected that there was one after having read Mr. Blocker's file folder. He was very wealthy at the time of his death if Dr. Sandler's notes could be believed. Written in red pen and underlined on the inside folder were the words, "settled lawsuit with insurance company, no longer pro bono, new millionaire." Looking further through the file he found numerous mentions of different drugs that had been prescribed. Colin was probably going to have to hire some medical help to understand all this stuff. He thought of the pharmacist that had been so instrumental in opening his eyes on this case, the man who had filled Pete Riddel's prescriptions. What was his name? He reached for his note pad. He knew he had it written in there somewhere. Maybe he would be willing to put in a few hours for Colin at the County's expense. There it was, Robert Jones, or in Colin's mind the man who had reminded him of Dennis the Menace's father.

He grabbed his jacket and car keys and went to see if Robert Jones was working today, taking Blocker's folder with him to study later at home.

Robert Jones was off that day so Colin left a message asking him to call him the next day at his office number. Colin went down the card aisle and grabbed two cards, one studio card for his son to let him know he was thinking about him and one mushy one for his mother just to say "hi". Then he drove home to read Henry Blocker's file and to order a pizza. After last night he just wanted to stay home and chill out. This coming week was going to be very hectic.

When he arrived at his office early Monday morning he had already made many phone calls and had an outline of the things he needed to do and the things he needed Dick to help him with. He met with the Major for a few minutes and then started calling patients and trying to track down information on the seven deceased ones. When Dick showed up he gave him his assignments and sent him on his way, asking him to check in every few hours with him or the Major.

Then Colin sat back down in front of the phone. Just before he called each patient he pulled their file, skimmed through the notes and checked the date of the last prescription. If it was over four months ago and there hadn't been a refill ordered he was less concerned but still he asked the same questions. "Did they have a will leaving any property or assets to Dr. Sandler or his Foundation?" If the answer to that question was "no," he continued with, "are you currently taking any medications that were prescribed by him or any other doctor?" If that answer was "no," he asked when their last appointment was. If it was more than six months ago, he informed them that Dr. Sandler had died and that their medical file would be destroyed unless they requested it to be forwarded to another doctor.

He had called ten patients by ten o'clock and all had said "no" to the will question, so he decided to take a break and go to David Sandler's bank. Just as he had suspected after finding out David had seen him Wednesday night at the drug store, the

Foundation account had no money in it. His personal account had less than a hundred dollars and his business operating account had enough to handle the incoming checks that had been written against it.

He had all the ledgers now since he had taken them from the doctor's office and his home study so he knew the checks that had been written and what they were for. Thursday he had written one to Glenda on the business account and two for the casket and cemetery plot on his personal account. The Foundation checkbook had a check taken out of it but nothing had been noted in the ledger as to how much had been removed from the account. But the bank confirmed his suspicions. Dr. Sandler had taken out $497,865 as cash Thursday morning at eleven o'clock. Somehow Colin knew he'd never find the money, but he certainly had to try. He didn't doubt that Linda would be trying to find it also if she ever found out about it. Her name wasn't on anything so if she was entitled to anything it would have to be through the settlement of his estate.

Colin had found out that the estate wasn't all it seemed to be. In reviewing Dr. Sandler's financial files that he'd found in his study he discovered that the Trans Am was financed and there was probably more owed on it than it was worth at this time and would probably be repossessed eventually. The condo was leased not owned, so there was no equity. He owed money in the form of installments to the decorating firm that had furnished his apartment and he had credit card bills totaling over $60,000 to Visa, Mastercard and American Express. He was already late for this month's $10,000 alimony payment and there were insurance notices demanding payments to keep coverage. All in all Linda was not going to fare well with David's death, even if she was the beneficiary unless the money from the Foundation appeared somewhere.

Colin suspected David had transferred his assets to his fiancé, but so far he could not find anyone who knew about her. Glenda hadn't even known he was engaged when he called her to ask.

The builder David had hired in Great Falls told Colin that the doctor had called him Thursday and canceled the deal. He was to finish the house any way he wanted and sell it, if there was any money left from his $100,000 first payment he was to send it to John Marshall's office in Fairfax. But the builder assured him that there probably wouldn't be anything substantial left. He would have to discount it heavily to sell it since it was customized to the doctor's unusual tastes.

When he asked the builder about David's fiancé he said he'd only met her twice and he didn't remember her name or anything else about her except that she was very pretty and surprisingly undemanding. He had thought that very odd, as most soon-to-be wives would be pretty much running the whole show for a new house being built. Colin had to agree with him there.

The personal checkbook had shown a check written a few weeks ago to a jeweler in Washington, the notation beside the amount had said engagement ring. Colin called Browne and Sons and talked to the owner. The owner explained that Dr. Sandler knew one of his sons from his college days so he'd come into D.C. to get a good deal on the ring. But again, nobody knew her name, nobody had even met her. He hadn't known that his son had arranged for a special courier to deliver it to her at her office in Tyson's Corner.

The more Colin dug the less he found out about Dr. Sandler, but the more he knew about the man. He was a loner, he had no friends except business acquaintances. He had no family, but he wanted one. He'd been married to a real bitch, but now he'd found a beautiful angel that he'd been afraid to share with anyone. And somewhere there was a child that he'd bought some toys for.

He grabbed the yellow pages for Northern Virginia and went in search of a rookie cop he could commandeer to call all the department store bridal registries. At least he knew the groom's name, maybe somewhere there was a bride's name to go with it.

Shortly after 2:00 pm he went to meet with John Marshall at his office in Fairfax. Mr. Marshall was very nice but not very

508

helpful. Yes, he'd met with Dr. Sandler on Thursday, and yes, he had written Dr. Sandler's will for him several years ago. But he honestly hadn't known he'd died until Linda had called on Friday afternoon. The appointment on Thursday? He could not remember what it had been about. He remembered sitting in his chair talking to his old college buddy and then he remembered shaking his hand and saying goodbye. The really strange part was that Colin believed every word Mr. Marshall said. This was too bizarre for anybody to make up and Colin had a good recollection of Dr. Sandler's hypnotic abilities.

The final disposition of Dr. Sandler's estate was as his three year old will decreed. All proceeds were to go to Linda Sandler. As the executor she would also have the added responsibility of liquidating his assets and paying his debts. Just wait 'til she figured all this out. She'd be livid when she discovered that he owed much more than he was worth and to top it all off, he had no life insurance and she had lost her $10,000 a month income from him.

It nagged at him as he left John Marshall's office. What had the doctor come here to see him about? Did it have anything to do with the Foundation's money? That money was cash now and it was hidden somewhere. John Marshall hadn't known about a fiancé either.

The mystery *angel* was probably on a yacht in the Mediterranean sipping champagne right now.

Jacqueline DeGroot

Chapter 102

Pontiac, MI

Jenny was sipping champagne from a very tall champagne flute at a very posh restaurant on top of a large building. She was being entertained by several Pontiac reps who were knocking themselves out trying to impress her. One in particular, Michael Kuyper, was working even harder to seduce her. She laughed at their jokes and oohed and ahhed over the elaborate desserts they had ordered for her to sample. In the back of her mind she was calculating the money this dinner was costing for the six of them. These certainly were fat times for the car business.

After she sampled a taste of all the desserts, she reached for the baked Alaska and finished that one off. It was scrumptious and her favorite of all desserts. She thought of her full tummy. Tomorrow she would have to visit the exercise room in the hotel's mezzanine section. She'd already discovered the pool and the sauna. Now she was mentally scheduling a time to use the treadmill and stair stepper.

After drinking a cup of rich, fragrant coffee she asked to be taken back to her hotel. Even though everyone protested her turning in so early, especially Michael, she was very firm. It wouldn't do to be on video tape tomorrow doing a training film on professionalism with a bloated face and red eyes from staying out too late and partying.

Since they'd all come to the restaurant in the same car after the afternoon's video taping session they all drove her to her hotel but Michael finagled a way to be alone with her by insisting on seeing her to her room. In the elevator he made his move by suggesting that they have a nightcap together in her room from the mini-bar. She politely declined saying that she really was tired and needed to get some rest. At her door he pressured her again, and had she been anywhere else she would have laughed at his pathetic, begging and cajoling, but she still had a week left to work with this guy on the taping.

"I'm sorry, Michael. Please understand, it's not you. I am ready to drop. Maybe tomorrow after the taping we can go out for a drink together." Placated by the promise of another opportunity to woo her, he leaned in to give her a kiss. She side stepped him and using her key she opened the door just enough to pass through it, said good night and closed the door behind her. Leaning back against the door she surveyed her little home away from home. Her eye was drawn to the flashing red light on the phone next to the bed.

Her first thought was that something was wrong at home. Hurriedly she crossed the room and punched in the codes to receive the message. It was from Tammy and she said it was very important that she call her at home no matter what time she got in. It was just barely nine o'clock, maybe she'd heard from David. So far no one had been able to locate him. He hadn't even shown up at her parent's house on Saturday as promised. And no one answered his office or home phone. Everybody was worried, it was so unlike David to just disappear.

Tammy answered on the second ring. "Jenny," she said in a hushed serious voice. "I found out what happened to David. It's not good. He's in Fairhaven. He died."

"What!" Jenny shouted.

"He was shot Thursday night, leaving his apartment to come get you."

"Tammy, I can't believe what you're saying. Are you sure?"

"Yes, Jenny, I'm sure. I just found out today, quite by accident. I had to go back to the service department today to check on a customer's car and I ran into Dave Stroud. He said, 'It sure is a shame about Dr. Sandler,' and I said, 'What about Dr. Sandler?' And he said, 'He died last week, shot by the cops. It was in Sunday's paper. Some cop even called me last Friday to find out why our number was on the doctor's speed dial. I told him he was one of our very best service customers, called us at least once or twice a week.' I didn't bother to correct him about

511

why Royal's number was on David's speed dial. Jenny, I finally found a copy of Sunday's paper. I had to go over to my folk's house and dig through the recycling, but I found the article Dave was talking about. Hold on and I'll get it and read it to you."

Jenny listened to the silence on the other end of the phone and then the rustling of a newspaper as she slumped down onto the bed to listen, her mind already reeling from the shock.

Tammy read: "Dr. David L. Sandler was shot and killed by former Fairfax County Master Police Officer C.G. Scott as he and five Fairfax County police officers were trying to arrest him for questioning in connection with the death of Mr. Pete Riddel, a former patient of his. The shooting occurred Thursday evening in the parking garage of Dr. Sandler's apartment complex. Dr. Sandler wrestled a gun from a uniformed police officer and fired at the officers. Scott returned the fire along with several of the other officers. Dr. Sandler was pronounced dead at the scene. Dr. Sandler was a prominent psychiatrist practicing in the City of Fairfax. Scott has been cleared of any wrong doing in the shooting and has been contracted back to the County to help on the case. Since his retirement from the County, Scott has been working undercover on this case as a private investigator. Pete Riddel died over two months ago in what was originally believed to have been a suicide."

"Then I found his obituary." Jenny heard more rustling of newspaper then Tammy continued. "It's just a very small paragraph. There's not even a picture. 'Dr. David L. Sandler, noted psychiatrist and author died Thursday, October 24, 1989. He is survived by his former wife, Linda Sandler. Memorial services will be at the Money and King Funeral Home in Vienna, Virginia with interment immediately following at Fairhaven Memorial Gardens in Fairfax.' That's it. He was buried yesterday, and we didn't even know about it."

Jenny started to cry. "God! He's gone and buried and I didn't even get to say goodbye. I was engaged to him!"

"Yeah, but nobody knew. He had no family so nobody even knew you existed." Tammy said with a sigh, "I'm sorry, Jenny, even though you weren't madly in love with him, I know he meant a lot to you and the kids."

"I guess his ex-wife must have taken care of everything. We weren't married yet, so I guess it's her job to see to things. Why would David have shot at the police? Surely he couldn't have anything to do with anybody's death. Why didn't he just go with them and answer their questions?"

"I don't know, Jenny. Nobody seems to know the answer to that question. Maybe when you get back you can go talk to the police and find out more. Is there anything I can do for you?"

"Yeah, you can call my parents tomorrow and tell them what happened. They've been pretty worried since Saturday when he didn't show up to watch the kids."

"I already called them. They were shocked, too. In fact, they've been trying to call you all night You should have more messages on your phone."

"I didn't even check after I heard yours. I'll call them now. Let me know if you hear anything else, okay?"

"Okay. I wish I was there to give you a hug right now."

"I wish you were, too," Jenny sniffed.

"G'night."

"Bye."

Why did people say that? "Good night." Now how could it possibly be a good night? Boy, we sure say a lot of things without thinking about what they mean. She dialed her parent's number.

As always, whenever something really bad happened in her life, as soon as she heard her mother or her father's voice, she broke up. This time it was no different.

"Oh, Baby, I'm so sorry," her mother said. "I know you two were very close. We were very fond of him, too. Rusty and Paisley are too young to know what's going on, but I'm sure they'll miss him."

"Mom? Did you know we were planning on getting married?"

513

"Yes, honey, he told me about it a few weeks ago. I guess he was so happy he just had to tell somebody. I never did understand why you didn't tell us though."

"I was still having doubts, Mom. He loved me a whole lot more than I loved him. But I did love him, just not the way he loved me. God, how he loved Paisley though! I'm kind of glad that she's so young now, she probably won't even remember him in a few months."

"Well, don't you worry about the kids, we're all fine here. You just take care of yourself and you call us if you need anything, okay?"

"Okay. The taping's coming along real well, I'll probably be done by next Monday."

"Good night, honey."

There, now even her Mom had said it. I guess "good night" just means "I'm hanging up now, tell me if it's all right by saying the same thing." She hung up the receiver, wiped her eyes and started taking off her clothes.

David—dead. The thought kept revolving around and around in her head. It was so hard to believe. They had made so many plans. They were building a house. David's dream house. She wondered what would ever become of it now. Without any further funds coming from David, the builder would have no choice but to stop the construction on it. Well, all that was Linda's problem now. Jenny and David hadn't been financially enmeshed yet and now the marriage she was so reluctant to agree to was no longer in her future. She felt a sense of relief mixed in with all her grief. She put on her pajamas and fuzzy socks and went to bed.

She woke up many times throughout the night feeling lonely and unsettled about her future.

When she woke up the next morning and went into the bathroom she groaned out loud when she saw her puffy face and swollen eye lids. One did not need to drink, party and stay out late to look like they were suffering from a hangover. All you had to do was lose one of your best friends and then lose sleep worrying over what the future would hold for you and your children. She pulled on her bathrobe and went down the hall to get some ice to bathe her face in. Like Michigan wasn't cold enough for her this time of the year. She just wanted to go home.

Chapter 103

Fairfax, VA

Colin was looking over the papers that Dick had brought back from Washington the day before. Henry Blocker's will, his death certificate and his autopsy report. The will showed Mr. Blocker as philanthropic, practically all of his money had been left to charity with a whopping $300,000 left to the David L. Sandler Foundation. The death certificate indicated a death caused by drug interactions, specifically a combination of Dilantin, tricyclic antidepressants, monoamine oxidase inhibitors and over the counter phenylproprandamine.

The autopsy report and police report were more detailed and listed the drug combinations again, along with mentioning that several packages of Dexatrim were found on the kitchen counter by the sink and a nasal decongestant spray was in the pants pocket of the deceased. The conclusion was that these over the counter drugs would certainly have contributed to the hypertensive crisis that ultimately killed him. The police report stated that in the vicinity of the badly decomposed body were several prescription bottles all referring to a Dr. Wilson as the prescribing doctor. None of the pills had been examined as far as he could tell by the report. He wondered if they had been kept.

He called the Dr. Wilson that was listed on the police report and learned from him that he had prescribed the medications that Dr. Sandler had recommended and had agreed with Dr. Sandler's suggestion that Henry have only one prescribing doctor since he was on so many different medications including Dilantin for the epileptic seizure problems that had caused his slight retardation. Dr. Sandler had even recommended that the Dilantin dosage be lowered to compensate for the Sinequan. He thanked the doctor and hung up. Sinequan, again. Boy, Dr. Sandler sure did like that drug.

He picked up the phone when it rang and spoke to Robert Jones who was returning his call. Robert was very excited to be asked to help in a murder case and even though he didn't say it, he was relieved to hear that Pete Riddel's death had not been a suicide. Robert agreed to keep everything confidential and to act as a consultant for the County on the case and Colin agreed to have the County pay him a fair amount for his efforts. He asked him a few questions about all the drugs on Henry's autopsy report and said he'd come visit him at the end of the week with some more questions from the patient files he was working on.

Colin was starting to put things away so he could prepare for his trip to Seattle when Dick called over to him from the corner where he was working on the last box from Dr. Sandler's office that they had to go through. "Hey Boss," he called over to him, "what about this bag of pills, you want it to go to the lab or somethin'?" He held up a bag of pills that Colin had found in Dr. Sandler's study in his apartment. Inside were several individual baggies with pills in them accompanied by pieces of small square note paper indicating what each one contained.

"Let me see that," he said reaching his hand out to take the bag. He dumped all the little baggies on his desk and turned each one over so he could read the note papers through the baggies. Parnate, Nardil, Hydroxyzine Pamoate, Tavist, Sinequan and one marked simply "Vitamins." Wasn't that what Daniel had said Liesel was taking? Yes, it was. Prenatal vitamins. Thank God, he had told Daniel to make sure she wasn't taking anything. He decided to call and make double sure and also to let them know he would be arriving on a flight sometime in the middle of the night and that he'd like to see them tomorrow afternoon if that could be arranged.

After his quick call to Daniel he asked Dick, who had assumed Colin's role in calling Dr. Sandler's current patients, if he would mind running over to the County's travel agent to pick up his plane tickets while he went in to see the Major and brief him on all they'd learned about Henry Blocker in the last two days. Dick jumped up and smiled, "Heck, I'd sure rather go pick up some tickets than go talk to the Major." He was gone and back again while Colin was still in the Major's office filling him in and answering all his questions.

Dick agreed to continue calling patients and to follow up on the officers he'd sent to Sandler's funeral services while Colin was away in Washington State. Colin grabbed a few folders to read on the plane, his note pad and the tapes Dr. Sandler had recorded of Liesel's sessions. It was a bit curious, her sessions were the only ones he had taped unless he had destroyed or hidden some others. Secretly he couldn't wait to meet her, she had a very sexy voice.

He went home to grab the suitcase he had already packed and to park his car in front of his apartment building. Then Dick drove him to the airport.

Chapter 104

Seattle, WA

Colin stepped off the plane carrying his duffel bag just after 10:30 in the evening. There was only one car rental place open and he stood in line waiting his turn to be served while he looked around at the mostly deserted airport. Everything looked so squeaky clean and the corridors on either side seemed to go on forever. Like square tiled tunnels with little people disappearing toward the edge with each step they took. It reminded him of the relaxation therapy technique Dr. Sandler had taught him, the one where the stick people were moving so fast and bumping into each other until he had slowed them down and they were barely lifting their feet.

He stepped up to the counter when it was his turn and smiled at the rental clerk, "I'd like the biggest car you've got and if the only car you've got is a mustang, I'll sleep here on the floor until one of the other agencies opens up."

"We have a Lincoln Town Car available, sir. Will that be all right?"

"Just peachy, I'll take it. Probably be returning it tomorrow."

"Okay, sir. If you'll just fill out this form and I'll need a charge card please."

Colin dropped his duffel bag, took his wallet out of his inside jacket pocket and pushed a credit card across the counter to her. He grabbed the paper and pen she had placed before him and filled out the form.

"How long will it take to get to Alder Lake?" he asked.

"It's about a two hour drive this time of night, could be three or more if you wait until morning." She handed him a set of keys and a small fold out map of the area, courtesy of the car rental company. "The car is right out the door there and to your right. You'll see a parking lot just for the rental cars. Your Lincoln should be in the first row. It's already gassed up and ready to go." She flashed him a big smile and he winked at her as he called back, "See you tomorrow."

He found the car with no problem and sat playing with the power seat control, ecstatic that he would be able to drive without the steering wheel rubbing up against his chest. How wonderful it was to be able to have his legs stretched out in front of him instead of bent in half on each side of the steering wheel.

His original plan was to fly in, get a hotel room for the rest of the night and drive out to Liesel and Daniel's place in the morning. But, as he wasn't the slightest bit tired right now, he decided to drive until he felt like stopping or at least until he was beyond the immediate Seattle suburbs so he wouldn't have to worry about the morning rush hour. He headed south on Route 5 enjoying the big car feel the Lincoln Town Car afforded him. This was nice. As soon as it was financially feasible he vowed he would trade the mustang in on a more man-sized car.

Just past Tacoma he pulled into the parking lot of a motel figuring that this was a good place to stop as it left him just about an hour's drive in the morning, and according to the map, he would be taking a secondary route soon and he didn't know what type of accommodations he'd find further away from the city.

After registering he bought a few juice drinks from a vending machine, got some ice and went to his room. He fell asleep almost as soon as he laid down and he awoke just past eight to the sounds of doors slamming and big rigs being started. He grabbed one of the juice cans from the ice bucket and headed for the shower.

When he was ready to leave the room he called Daniel and told him he was on his way and asked for last minute directions to their cabin on the lake. He and Daniel had had a few conversations in the last couple of days and Colin was finding him to be a fairly friendly guy. They had invited Colin to come out to their cabin for lunch, and since he hadn't had any breakfast yet, he was eager to get on the road and grab a bite to eat so he wouldn't show up at around eleven completely ravenous.

The scenery in some places was absolutely breathtaking. The ruggedness of the mountainous area blended with the charming little towns he drove through and he found himself relaxing and enjoying the drive despite the seriousness of the reason he was here.

He found the cutoff that Daniel described, just past the abandoned summer fruit stand and right where three large boulders were grouped together just before a gravel road. He turned right and followed the road as it meandered around a virtual forest on each side of him. He didn't know what he had expected but he hadn't expected this.

He came upon a large open area and there, set back from the road, was a magnificent rustic cabin with a porch that appeared to go all the way around the house. Yes, it was a log cabin, but yes, it had also easily cost a good half a million dollars to build. It was situated all by itself. The only other signs of habitation were the backs of the houses you could see on the opposite side of the lake. There were large picture windows along the front and three dormer windows on the second floor. There was an attached three car garage and a beautiful stone chimney off to one side.

He remembered the log cabin Liesel had been rescued from and he smiled. Apparently Daniel had convinced her that they could build a cabin in the woods that would make her forget all about the other one.

He pulled up in front of one of the open garage doors. One held a Jeep of some kind, one held a sleek Jaguar sedan and one held a beat up old pickup truck. As he stepped out of the car a man Colin figured to be Daniel came out of the front door and bounded down the stone steps. "Colin?" he asked as he put his hand out to welcome him.

"Daniel?" They shook hands and then started talking about the incredible view and the new house that Daniel was so proud of. Daniel led the way up the steps and called up the stairs to Liesel. "Liesel, Colin's here. Didn't you find those papers yet?"

"Yes, I found them, Daniel," she called out. "I'm just taking another bathroom break because of your son. I'll be right down."

Colin gave Daniel a quizzical look, "She had the baby, already?"

"No! But we know it's a boy. We asked to know because that was the deciding factor as to whether we were going to live in the city or in the country. If it was a girl we were going to build a more contemporary house a little closer to the city for her and Liesel to be close to dance & music lessons and shopping malls and all that girly stuff. If it was a boy, I wanted him to learn how to fish and sail and go hunting in the woods. As you can see, I won."

Daniel took Colin through the large country kitchen and huge family room, with the stone fireplace taking up almost one whole wall, to the back of the house and the rear deck facing the lake. The view was incredible. Everything looked so pristine and true to its color. The greens were vibrant, the blue of the sky was like it had been painted with soft water colors and the sparkling water in the lake was mirroring everything so you could enjoy it twice.

They sat down at a round patio table with a whimsical yellow and black polka dotted umbrella. It looked a little out of place. As Colin took a seat he looked up at it.

"I know, it doesn't quite go with the surroundings, but when you live on a lake you have to be able to tell people how to get to your house by boat. We just tell them to look for the yellow and black polka dotted umbrella. Works like a charm!" He laughed.

Colin looked down at the dock and imagined the groups of people that would be coming here for parties in the years to come. Just like any place in the country that was peaceful and serene, people were flocking to them. Ten years from now they'd probably have neighbors on each side.

Liesel came out on the deck to join them. Both Colin and Daniel stood up as she approached. Even eight months pregnant you could tell she walked with class. She was tall with short, cropped curly hair framing a beautiful classic face. When she smiled her nose wrinkled just a bit and she had two perfectly matched deep set dimples. Her sparkling eyes were the color of warm cocoa with just a touch of light green in them.

Daniel bent to kiss her on the cheek as he helped her into a chair and Colin could see that he absolutely adored her.

"Hello, Colin," she said in that same sultry voice he was so used to now. "I'm very happy to meet you, even though I'm still not sure what all this is about. It was wonderful of you to fly out here to see us personally."

"Well, let me start from the beginning so you can understand things better," Colin said as he smiled at her. He started by explaining about MaryAnn and Pete and then about the discovery of Pete's amended will. Then he explained about going undercover and what he had discovered. He recalled and related everything about the shooting and the subsequent searches. Ending with, "And that's how I found out about you."

"I took home some audio tapes I found in a box in Dr. Sandler's drawer. One of them was of your session with him where he *suggested* that you change your will." He took it out of his coat pocket along with his mini-recorder. He had already fast forwarded it to the exact spot in the tape. He inserted it and pressed play. They listened as Dr. Sandler coached Liesel and convinced her to equalize her guilt by providing down-the-road relief to battered women. As Liesel listened she recalled the session. It continued until you heard Liesel say she had to hurry home for Daniel's call as she got up and exited the office. Then they heard Dr. Sandler say, "Campaign accomplished," followed by a loud click as the recorder shut off.

Daniel grabbed Liesel's hand and smiled, "Anxious to get home for my phone call, huh?" He joked as he took her hand to his lips and gently kissed it. Liesel blushed from her throat to the tops of her cheeks.

Colin waited 'til the exchange was over and then cleared his throat. "So we know you were being targeted as a victim. Now, what can you tell me about the pills he prescribed for you."

"Well, I can tell you that if he hadn't prescribed Prozac for me, I wouldn't be pregnant today!" Liesel said with a delightful laugh.

Colin smiled back at her and at Daniel who was also laughing, "Okay, spill it, what does that mean?"

They both explained between howls of laughter what had happened the morning in St. Croix when Daniel had flushed Liesel's birth control pills by mistake. They all had a good laugh and Colin actually had to wipe the tears from his eyes before they could get serious again.

"Okay, so what happened to the Prozac?"

"He flushed them too," Liesel said.

"So, maybe those were the pills he'd tampered with. Were they ever in your pocket or purse when you went to see him?" Colin asked.

Liesel thought for a moment. "No, I always kept them in my bathroom in my apartment."

"Was he ever in your apartment?"

"Not that I was ever aware of."

"Hmm," Colin said as he thought out loud, "I wonder what he had planned for you?"

Just then Daniel spoke up, "Hey, remember when we got back from St. Croix you called him and told him about not taking the Prozac and he said you had to come in right away to get some other kind of pill?" he asked as he looked at Liesel.

"Yeah, I remember. He scared me so badly about having to take some other medicine because I had stopped the Prozac almost ten days earlier that I had to call a doctor as soon as we landed here to make sure I wouldn't become so depressed I'd be suicidal coming off the pills."

"What did the doctor here say?" Colin asked.

"He was the father of one of my college sorority sisters so I just called him up at home and asked him if there was another pill I should be taking since I was almost ten days off of Prozac. He said he didn't know what Dr. Sandler was talking about and offered to call him for me, but because of the time difference, I knew the doctor wouldn't be in, so I just forgot about it. I had just become engaged to the man I loved and I couldn't imagine being depressed about anything ever again."

"Do you have a phone I can borrow?" Colin asked.

Daniel got up and brought him a portable one. Colin flipped through his note pad and found Robert Jones' phone number at home. Colin knew it would be his day off today. He punched in the numbers and waited for Robert to answer.

Meanwhile Daniel and Liesel went to the kitchen to start carrying the lunch out to the table. After Colin spoke for a few minutes to Robert he hung up the phone and walked over to place it back in the cradle Daniel had taken it out of on the kitchen counter.

Daniel called over his shoulder to Colin, "You want a beer or lemonade?" Colin saw Daniel take a beer for himself from a refrigerator by the bar that contained only beer.

"What kind of choice is that?" Colin asked, winking at Liesel, "Off course, I'll take the beer."

"Well then you'd better go choose one, he must have fifty brands in that thing," Liesel said, winking back at him.

Colin walked over to the refrigerator and chose a Coors Light. "You leaving Washington as you did, probably saved your life," Colin said as the three of them sat down at the table again.

Both Liesel and Daniel stared at Colin. "According to the pharmacist I hired to help me on this case, and please excuse me if I have to read from my notes, I have a hard time remembering all this drug stuff. If someone is taking a selective serotonin reuptake inhibitor, for example, Prozac, and if they discontinue using it and replace it with another anti-depressant that is a monoamine oxidase inhibitor such as Parnate or any other tranylcypromine within ten days of discontinuing the Prozac, there will be severe adverse effects, usually death. We found Parnate in the drugs we took from Dr. Sandler's office. So, when you called him, he was trying to get you to come by so he could give you those pills to take before the ten days were up. If you hadn't flushed the Prozac then he was probably planning on taking you off of it soon and slipping you some Parnate somehow."

They all sat silently for a few minutes not even bothering to touch the food Liesel had prepared.

Liesel reached for the white envelope she had put on the empty chair beside her. She took out some folded papers and scanned over them. Colin saw that it was her Last Will and Testament.

"So, he was after this $200,000 I was leaving to the David L. Sandler Foundation, because he'd more or less asked me to. I feel so stupid."

Daniel stood up and knelt beside her and wrapped his arms around her waist. "Not stupid, just trusting." He tried to make light of the somber mood she was suddenly in, "Hey, you were smart enough to get out of town before he *parnated* you."

She laughed through the tears that had just started to fall off her cheeks. "I could have died."

"Yes, but you didn't. So now we will have another thing to be grateful for come Thanksgiving. This year if I don't start calling them all out right after breakfast, I won't be able to eat turkey until midnight." She laughed again and reached out to hug him around the neck. "I love you so much."

"And I you. Now c'mon let's eat lunch. Colin looks like he could use some sustenance, and I know he's going to just love your potato salad."

The guys quickly changed the subject to anything except the reason Colin had come here, until Liesel left to take a nap.

There were still questions they both needed to ask but they could wait until Liesel wasn't around. Neither of them wanted to upset her again. They became fast friends over several beers and many stories about fire fighting in Baltimore City and crime fighting around the city of Washington. There was usually a special kind of camaraderie between policemen and firemen. The boys were hitting it off well together. Daniel took Colin out on his boat and they did a little fishing on the lake.

That was when Colin told Daniel about the vitamins he'd found in Dr. Sandler's home study.

Daniel thought for a minute before saying, "I know the doctor who prescribed these, I go with her on all her visits to the OB/GYN, the prescription was filled here in Tacoma, but just the same, I'm not going to let her take anymore. This Dr. Sandler is really spooky. The sad thing is, that I'm the one who recommended she see him. A friend of mine in Baltimore touted him very highly."

"Would you mind if I had a copy of that will as evidence? I'll trade you the cassettes I brought with me of all Liesel's sessions," Colin said hesitantly, looking over at Daniel.

"You listened to them?" Daniel asked in a quiet voice, one eyebrow arched.

"Yeah. I know I shouldn't have, but once I got started listening to her story, I couldn't stop. I stayed up all night. At 4 am I found the one about the will. She needs to change that by the way."

"Yeah, I guess so," Daniel said. Then he asked, "Anybody else hear them?"

"No, and there aren't any copies anywhere, as far as I can tell. I brought them with me because I thought they were private and that she should have them. It doesn't appear that he recorded anybody else's sessions other than hers. Or if he did, he destroyed them."

"Liesel's family is pretty prominent around Seattle, it would kill her if she found out that her story was public knowledge."

"It isn't. You can have her paper files, too. I brought them also. No one will ever need to know why she was seeing the doctor. It's not relevant to the case at all. But the will is the motive, and even though Dr. Sandler is dead, I really want to connect all these loose ends."

"Okay, I'll get you a copy tomorrow before you leave. Liesel and I would like for you to stay the night with us if you can. We're having a few friends over for a barbecue later. I think she wants to hook you up with one of her girlfriends."

"Is that good or bad?" Colin asked with a grimace.

Daniel laughed, "Who knows? You never know when you're gonna meet the woman of your dreams."

They both looked at each other and laughed. Daniel threw another beer to Colin and said, "You got a bite."

Sure enough his line was jumping up and down in the holder. They went to reel in their first catch of the day.

After cleaning the fish they had caught that afternoon, Daniel showed Colin where the guest room was upstairs so he could shower and rest up for the BBQ party later that evening.

The guest room was cozy, with dark planked wooden floors and braided hooked rugs scattered about. The queen-sized bed was high off the floor with a big brass headboard and baseboard. There was a beautiful patchwork quilt on it and another draped on a rack at the foot of the bed. Colin carefully pulled back the quilt and laid down naked between the sheets, listening to the birds singing outside his open window.

The sounds of car doors opening and closing woke him an hour later. He felt refreshed and peaceful. Ahh, this was the life. As he dressed he looked out the window and saw couples getting out of 4x4 pickups and Jeeps with dishes in their hands. He noticed all the vehicles had red lights sitting on the dashes. These must be Daniel's friends that he worked with at the Tacoma Fire Department. With all the trees in this area of the country it would be crucial to get to fires very quickly. He went downstairs to join the party and to meet Daniel and Liesel's friends.

He was introduced as a friend of Daniel's visiting from Virginia. It pleased him to be considered a friend of Daniel's. He knew he was a friend of Liesel's too, but he also knew that avenue would have raised a few eyebrows and led to more questions.

A few single sorority friends of Liesel's were there and Liesel introduced him to all of them. They seemed nice and they were certainly interested in him but he found them to be a little too uppity for his tastes and besides, they were way too young for him. They were all in their twenties and they were all looking for a well-to-do husband. Colin could almost feel them fighting over him as first one took his arm and tried to say something amusing and then the next one did the same until he'd been handed around the little circle like a puppet. He hadn't understood anything any of them had said as they laughed and smiled and patted his arm.

Daniel came over and rescued him by handing him a can of beer and asking him to come help him cook the fish they'd caught that afternoon on the rear deck. Almost all the men had ended up on the back deck, standing around the grill and a large cooler filled with beer.

Colin whispered a "Thanks" to Daniel when he reached the grilling area and saw that Daniel needed no help whatsoever. The fish fillets were already on the grill basted with a lemon butter sauce. A few boats pulled up at the dock below them and Colin saw that the polka dot umbrella now had a spot light on it since it was becoming dark outside. He smiled.

It didn't take long for him to fit in with all the guys. Football, and raunchy jokes being universal just about anywhere you went. He was having a really nice time with Daniel and Liesel and their friends. He even danced a few dances with some of Liesel's girlfriends on the lower patio when he was asked to. The fish was delicious along with the steaks and chicken they had set out. Everyone had brought some kind of salad or side dish and pretty soon he was overfull from eating so much.

Groaning and holding his hands over his stomach he begged off eating any of the desserts each time one of the women brought him one. When it appeared that the women were getting serious about their quest by asking him to accompany them for walks or boat rides, he begged off, saying he had to go upstairs and pack for his late morning flight tomorrow. He was met with over-glossed pouting lips each time, but still he excused himself and went upstairs to his bedroom. He met Liesel at the top of the stairs.

"Calling it a night, huh?" he asked.

Jacqueline DeGroot

"Yeah, I can't seem to stay up much later than ten o'clock these days. But I can't complain, I've had a wonderful pregnancy so far, other than being tired so much, it's been a breeze."

"Well, you don't have too much longer to go and then I'll venture you'll be up all hours of the night!"

She laughed. And then she got serious. "Colin, thanks for coming all this way to make sure I was safe. It means a lot to Daniel and I."

"Ach! Don't even think about it. I've had a great time. You guys are wonderful hosts."

"Well, you'll have to come back sometime and plan on staying a bit longer. Bring your wife when you come."

"You know I don't have a wife."

"You will. A man like you will be snapped up pretty soon, count on it."

"Well, I hope when I find her that's she just like you." He bent down to kiss her on the cheek. "Good night."

"Good night, Colin."

As he closed the bedroom door behind him he thought to himself that if there was a petite blonde version of Liesel somewhere out there, he'd find her, he just knew it.

He woke up early the next morning, said his goodbyes and drove back to Seattle. He had left the tapes and files of Liesel on the guest room dresser and took the copy of Liesel's will that Daniel had pushed under his door sometime last night or early this morning. He returned the rental car and went to catch his plane. He had a lot of work left to do on this case and he was anxious to get back to it.

530

Chapter 105

Tyson's Corner, VA

Jenny threw herself into her job with even more vigor after she returned from her Detroit trip. More than ever she was determined to make Royal the number one dealer in sales on the east coast. She was trying to forget about her problems and get over the pain of losing a best friend. She tried not to think about him or what they had planned. Only once, in a moment of weakness, did she drive over to the house still being built. She didn't even pull over. She saw that there was a for sale sign out front and she drove right past it.

Every once in awhile she took out the ring David had given her and just looked at it, wondering what to do with it. She had never bothered to contact the police when she got back to find out what had really gone on. She almost didn't want to know.The less she knew, the less involved she would be. And she was trying to pretend that David hadn't even existed for her.

Thanksgiving came and went without the fanfare she and David had planned. Her life was settling into a new routine. Working and being with her kids were her two priorities. Everything else was extraneous and she didn't allow the time for it. Her diversions right now were Christmas shopping, baking and sending out cards.

She had stopped reading the newspapers and doing the crosswords just as she'd promised herself she would on the plane to Detroit. Now she read all of Rusty's school papers and praised him for his neat, thoughtful papers and admonished him for his sloppy, lazy ones. She watched Sesame Street with Paisley and Transformer cartoons with Rusty as her television entertainment.

When Christmas came she made the prerequisite appearances at the round of parties going stag or with Tammy. She enjoyed her family and friends and just being home, baking and wrapping presents with the kids.

On New Years she rented a few romantic videos and stayed up late watching them by herself. It was a very lonely time, but it was also a good time. A time to be introspective and to plan her future, a time to get to know herself and to dream about the future. Over the holiday she watched her favorite movie, "Ladyhawke" three times. She watched Paisley's favorite movie, "The Little Mermaid", five times. She cleaned out her closets and dressers and got her financial papers for the previous year filed properly and started new files for the next year that was already here.

When she went back to work and discovered that David's Trans Am had been towed in by a repossession company, she finally cried. When Tammy found her in the restroom she hugged her and said, "Well, it's about time." After that she was much better and her cheery outlook surfaced again.

The next two years were full of accomplishing goals and making money. The car business was booming and Royal was becoming more successful than ever before. They were the number one Pontiac-GMC dealership in their district, region and zone. And they had a sales force that was the envy of all. Jenny had achieved the level of professionalism with them that she had always wanted.

The automobile industry was actually in itself becoming more respectable in nice little noticeable ways. People were actually keeping the appointments they made, they were calling if they couldn't make one, they stopped insinuating that car salesmen would lie to make a deal, and they started to understand that the dealers needed to make a little profit selling cars.

It was then that Jenny started thinking about getting out of the business and retiring. Managing was beginning to take its toll. She was thirty-seven and she'd been selling cars since she was eighteen. Almost twenty years. Twenty years in the car business was like forty in any other. The retail hours in a city like Washington were bad enough, but the stress of the competition added a lot to that equation. Averaging 60 to 65

hours a week was not worth the money anymore, at least not to
Jenny.

And Ron Royal's kids were growing up now. They were
being groomed to take over. The girls were starting to marry and
their husbands were being trained to join in the family business,
also. She got along with everybody just fine and she even helped
train some of them, but their ideas and hers were different and
she didn't see the future of the car business the same way that
they did. It was time to start phasing out and she knew it.

She had looked at some property in North Carolina the last
time she and her parents had vacationed at Carolina Beach.
She'd always wanted to relocate to North Carolina, maybe now
was the time. After every vacation it was so depressing to pack
up the car and head north again. The last few years the pull of
Carolina calling her to stay was getting even stronger.

She left the kids with her parents one weekend and drove
down by herself to look around. She fell in love with Sunset
Beach and bought a lot in Sea Trail Plantation from Hazel Boyd.
She was one of the most sincere salespersons she'd ever met and
it was a pleasure buying property from such an upbeat, happy
sales rep who truly thought she lived in the nicest part of the
world. Jenny had to agree with her. The Brunswick County
beaches are as nice as they come. Jenny drove home, happy to
finally have her own little piece of paradise.

The hard part was telling her parents and sister about her
plans to move herself and the kids to North Carolina. It wasn't as
bad as she'd thought it would be, but it wasn't the best news
she'd ever told them either. They were supportive of her desire
to quit working so hard so she could spend more time watching
the kids grow up and being there for them, especially as Rusty
approached adolescence. They didn't understand why she had to
move so far away though. That they would miss them like crazy,
everybody knew, but they would be able to visit whenever they
wanted Jenny had assured them all, over and over again.

The next one to tell was Ron Royal. And even though he
understood, he didn't like it one bit and managed to talk her into

staying one more year rather than the six months Jenny had planned on.

The hardest of all was going to be telling Tammy. Telling her was going to be like deliberately breaking someone's heart. They had become so close over the years. Jenny made several stabs at trying to tell her, but got nowhere. So she finally just invited her to come over to her house for dinner one night, knowing that the for sale sign in the front yard would start the conversation for her.

The only buffer for Tammy's hurt was that they both had a year to get used to the idea. Tammy kept telling her that she wasn't just losing her best friend, but that she was losing her best boss.

The year went quickly as Jenny's house sold practically right away and she had to move herself and the kids in with her parents while working long distance with a builder at Sunset Beach. Even with most of her stuff in storage, they still filled her parents' house to full capacity. But it was nice to be home again for awhile before leaving again for good.

Every few weeks Jenny would take a quick trip down to see the progress on her house and every time she drove back she felt the tug trying to keep her there. She usually stayed in a rental condo right behind where her house was being built, right there on the Plantation. But one time she decided to check out the surrounding area and arranged to stay at Goose Creek Bed and Breakfast at the next beach up the coast, Ocean Isle Beach. The large beach style home was right on Goose Creek, which led right out to the Intracoastal Waterway. It felt to her like she was sleeping in the tree tops, it sure was peaceful. The owners, Peggy and Jim were the nicest people and they would later become best friends, Jenny just knew it.

By July of 1993 all the going away parties and retirement parties had been given and everything had been packed up. They were ready to go. Jenny had to buy a car since she'd had one provided for so long, so there she was pulling out of the driveway in an old used '84 Pontiac Parisienne she'd taken in as a trade a few weeks earlier. It would do until she could sort out her finances and see what she could afford and figure out what she wanted to drive. It was hard to figure out what she should drive for three or four years in a row after being used to having something different every couple of months.

Then they were on their way, just Jenny, Rusty and Paisley, to their new home and their new life in North Carolina.

Chapter 106

Fairfax, VA

After returning from Seattle, Colin finished writing his report and then grabbed the patient list that Dick had been working on. Today Dick was in Arlington trying to find Betsy Drayton's death certificate and autopsy report. He was getting some kind of run around because she was a Virginia resident who had died in the District. So far they hadn't tracked down the paperwork. They had managed to track down her attorney though, through her old housekeeper. She'd left $100,000 to the David L. Sandler Foundation. Because of the time frame, Colin figured that was the money he'd given to the builder to start his house with.

Colin scanned the list. There weren't too many more to call. A name jumped out at him from the bottom of the page. Shawn Vanscoy. Everybody knew who Shawn Vanscoy was. And everybody knew about his drug problems, so it probably wasn't that much of a secret what the doctor had been treating him for. He went over to the box that had the patient files in it. He thumbed through them until he found the one he was looking for.

Then he sat back in his chair and looked through it. In the very back were some folded up pieces of paper. Colin opened them. It was a copy of Shawn Vanscoy's will. How did he ever get that? He quickly scanned it looking for the Foundation's name and the amount. There it was—$350,000; not to the Foundation though, to the doctor personally. Something was nagging at him, way back in a corner of his mind, but it just wouldn't come. He put the folder down and picked up his car keys.

He drove down the street to the Giant Food Store. He didn't feel like fast food today. Sometimes he just grabbed a whole roasted chicken and picked at it at his desk as he worked. Today was one of those days. He made a salad at the salad bar, too. Whatever was leftover would be dinner.

When he got in the express line he stood waiting his turn, looking around to see if he "needed" any of the impulse items stacked above the conveyor belt. That's when he saw the tabloids and that's when it hit him.

Vanscoy's gay lover had died in their apartment from a drug overdose. He tried to remember when that had been. A year ago maybe? He wasn't sure. He'd noticed Dick's scribblings beside Shawn's name on the list. He had apparently tried to get in touch with him but Shawn no longer lived in that apartment anymore and there wasn't a forwarding address or number. Colin had seen some numbers written in Dr. Sandler's handwriting on the back inside flap of the folder. The notes indicated that those numbers belonged to Shawn's father. He would know how Colin could track him down. He paid for his food and went back to the office.

After trying several different numbers he finally got someone to answer. After identifying himself he asked to speak to Mr. Vanscoy. The woman who had answered the phone sighed impatiently, "I'm sorry, sir. I have to know what this is in reference to."

"It's about his son, Shawn."

"What about his son, sir?"

"He could be in danger, I have to speak to his father, I'm a police officer for crying out loud!"

"Sir, do you have any idea how many people want to talk with Mr. Vanscoy, saying they're policemen, or doctors or presidents? I answer at least ten a day myself and I'm not even his secretary!"

"Fine! Give him this number, tell him to check it out! If I don't hear from him today, I'll get six patrol cars and we'll come to his house! Then maybe he'll talk to me!" He hung up after giving her the number. A few minutes later Mr. Vanscoy's secretary was on the line saying, "Please hold for Mr. Vanscoy," as soon as he picked up the phone.

Colin sketchily explained about Dr. Sandler, the fact that he was dead and why. He told Mr. Vanscoy that he believed that there were still several patients who could possibly die due to their medication and that it was imperative that he talk with Shawn as soon as possible. He was given a phone number and an address in Pennsylvania. Colin thanked Mr. Vanscoy for returning his call so promptly, then Mr. Vanscoy promptly hung up.

Colin dialed the number and let it ring twenty-five times. No one home, or no one answering, which one? He looked at the address. He could probably get there in two or three hours if he beat the Baltimore rush hour. He went to go sign out a cruiser. He was not going to drive that mustang on any long road trips unless he had to.

Before he left he called the Metropolitan Police Department. He asked if they would fax him a copy of the autopsy and police report on Jeremy Spragg, Shawn Vanscoy's roommate. He waited by the fax machine until they came over the wire. He grabbed them and then headed for the County motor pool. He was halfway around the Washington beltway before he remembered his uneaten lunch still sitting in the middle of his desk. This was why cops were always grabbing donuts, no time for the good stuff.

He pulled up in front of an apartment building just before five o'clock. He got out of the unmarked cruiser and went to the apartment indicated on the piece of paper. He didn't hear any sounds from within when he put his ear to the door and there was no answer to his knock. He went to his cruiser to sit and wait.

Twenty minutes later he saw him walking down the sidewalk a briefcase by his side. It was definitely Shawn Vanscoy, but it was a clean cut version of the famous actor's son. He stepped out of the car in front of Shawn and Shawn instinctively put his briefcase in front of his face.

"I'm not the press. I'm the police," Colin said as he took out his badge case and flipped the shield out for him to see. "I came from Virginia to talk to you about Dr. Sandler."

"What about Dr. Sandler?" Shawn said, a slight tic telling Colin that he was a little leery of him.

"Did you know that he died?" Colin asked.

"He died?" Shawn asked incredulously.

"Yes, I shot him. Can we go in and talk?"

"After that you expect me to say yes? You kill my doctor and you want to talk to me?"

"I only killed him because he was trying to kill me, he was trying to kill you, too. In fact I think he might have killed Jeremy."

"Oh. Well, in that case, C'mon in," he said sarcastically. "It's not much, we'll have to sit in lawn chairs."

"Sounds like my place," Colin said with a smile.

When they sat down Colin asked Shawn if he had a will. Colin's days of interrogating had taught him that when you were questioning someone who was hostile, start off by asking a few questions that you already knew the answer to. It was very intimidating if they answered them wrong.

"Yeah."

"And how much did you leave to Dr. Sandler?"

"Who says I left anything to Dr. Sandler?"

"I do. How much?"

"I don't remember."

"Does the figure $350,000 mean anything to you?"

"Why are you here if you know all the answers to the questions you're asking?"

"I'm here to see that you don't kill your self by accident as so many of Dr. Sandler's patients have been doing lately."

"Okay, I'm ready to listen."

Colin explained how Dr. Sandler got patients to change their wills and then found a way to tamper with their medication so they would die. Shawn listened very intently until he was done.

"I was never hypnotized. He never asked me to change my will. I offered to do it," Shawn said defiantly.

"Why?" Colin asked.

Shawn didn't answer.

"Why?" Colin repeated.

"I promised him I wouldn't get him into any trouble."

"He's dead! It would be hard for you to hurt him any more that that!"

It was beginning to sink in. Shawn slumped in his seat.

"I wanted to get straight. My Dad was pulling out, taking away all my funds. I knew I had to get straight and get a job if Jeremy and I were ever going to have a chance together. I couldn't take the Methadone treatments at a clinic. For one thing I couldn't get there, I didn't have a car and I had to be at work when they were open. And, I didn't want to go there, everybody knows my face. Pretty soon the tabloids would be printing a weekly picture of 'See Shawn shoot up, Legally.' Dr. Sandler understood but he didn't believe I was serious. So I bet him my insurance policy proceeds. If he helped me and I got straight, I won. If he helped me and I didn't get straight, eventually he'd win. He was supposed to buy a Lamborghini when I punched out."

"So, he gave you a prescription for the Methadone?"

"No, I don't think you can get it unless you're a doctor. Somehow he'd get a box of pre-filled syringes and then give them to me. I took them home and used them there."

"Were you sharing them with Jeremy?"

"I wanted to, but he wasn't ready to do the program yet."

"I think he decided he was one day while you were at work. I think he took a Methadone syringe and shot up, only it wasn't Methadone, it was Morphine. And it was meant for you."

"He died from a Heroin overdose. That's what the cops told me."

"According to a report I read, it was Morphine and when they called to tell you that, your phone had been disconnected and they had no idea where to find you."

"Oh, Sweet Jesus! You mean Jeremy was really killed by an injection that was meant for me?" Shawn exclaimed.

"Yes, that's exactly it. And Dr. Sandler couldn't afford to try again to get you, it would have been too obvious. At least right away."

"You don't have any more of them, right? The police took them all, according to the report," Colin asked.

"No, I don't have anything anymore, I don't even take aspirin now. Seeing Jeremy die that way cured me for good, but I was already on my way to being straight when he died."

"I'm sorry. I wish I could have prevented his death," Colin said softly.

"Well, it looks like he prevented mine," Shawn said just as softly.

"C'mon, I'll take you out to dinner before I head back to Virginia. You can tell me a little more about the man who hung up on me today."

"My father?"

"Yeah."

"He doesn't mean anything by it, he just doesn't ever say good-bye."

Chapter 107

Fairfax, VA

A week later Colin and Dick sat down to review the things they were working on. Dick had finally managed to collect all the paperwork on Betsy Drayton and they had pieced together a likely scenario of how her death had played out.

From reading her file Colin knew that Dr. Sandler was aware of her allergy problems, especially the one for nuts. One of the items found in her stomach according to the autopsy report was peanut particles. Both her driver and her housekeeper verified that she almost always wore a fanny pack around her waist that held her allergy medications. She would have had them with her in Dr. Sandler's office as the driver said she always walked to his office wearing it. That, along with the will as the motive, was enough to pin her death on Dr. Sandler.

So far, they had four murders they could attribute to Dr. Sandler—Pete, Betsy, Henry and Jeremy. And one attempted murder, Liesel— two, if you included Shawn. There was still so much work to be done. With the exception of one patient, they had finally been able to contact each former, living patient. The only one they hadn't been able to find was Jessica Tyler. Colin had finally made the connection that it was Jessica Tyler he had seen going into the doctor's office that day when he was leaving it.

Her father, Congressman Tyler was in Europe when they had finally been able to track him down through Interpol connections. He had told them that the last time he'd heard from her had been when the Metropolitan police had dumped her on his door step two weeks ago. They'd found her passed out drunk in front of her car outside a Georgetown bar. One of his aides had driven her to her apartment and he hadn't heard from her since. When Colin asked him which Georgetown bar, he hesitated for a moment and then answered, "I think they told me it was The Bayou."

Colin spent the next two nights camped out at The Bayou in Georgetown trying to see if he could find her. It was after midnight on the second night and he was just paying his tab to leave when he thought he spotted her coming out of the alcove where the ladies' room was. She looked a little like her picture, but not a lot. If he hadn't been looking so intently for her, he would not have recognized her.

The pictures in the paper always showed a sophisticated woman in an up-to-the-minute newly styled gown, smiling at the benefactor she was posed with. The Jessica he was staring at now looked like a fashion reject from biker's week. Her way too short black leather skirt revealed the dark upper band of her black panty hose with every step she took, and those had several runs in them disappearing right into her stiletto black heels. The sheer black blouse she wore half way tucked into the skirt did nothing to soften the harsh black outline of her push up demi-cup bra. The top of one brown nipple was clearly visible as it peeked over the edge. Her hair looked like it had been up at one time because there were long strands hanging around her face with bobby pins still stuck in them.

He watched her as she very precariously made her way to a table where several punkers were sitting. As soon as she was back in her seat, the greasy-looking man sitting next to her grabbed her by the hair and pulled her head back while he jammed his tongue down her throat. His other hand freely massaged her breast over top of her bra and shirt. Colin was sickened by what he saw.

After a few minutes of watching the shenanigans going on all around the table he had an idea. He doubted that Jessica really knew these "people." They were probably just a group of leeches after anything they could take, including a free meal ticket. Colin stood up and walked over to the table. It didn't take more than a few moments for his impressive size to register on their consciousness and they all turned to look at him. "I want to talk to her," he said pointing at Jessica.

"Oh, you do, do you?" said the man who practically had Jessica in his lap.

"Yeah, I do," Colin said as he flipped his badge case out and shoved his shield out in front of him. He slowly moved his hand around the table so each person there could see it clearly. One by one you could hear the chairs scrape against the floor as the seats were moved back and everyone but Jessica disappeared.

"Now, what'd ya do that for? All my friends are gone now!" she moaned.

"Jessica, those weren't your friends," Colin said.

"How'd you know my name?" she mumbled.

"I've been looking for you for almost two weeks now," he replied.

She looked him up and down and said, "Well, I am sure glad you found me, wanna drink?"

"Yes, some coffee. And so do you." He sat down across from her and motioned for the waiter to come over.

"Yes, sir?"

"Two black coffees and leave the pot." He looked over at Jessica, "What have you had to eat today?"

"I don't remember."

"Bring us a couple of club sandwiches or whatever you have that's close."

"Can't I have something else to drink?"

"No!" he said firmly.

"But I haven't taken my pills yet," she wailed.

Colin looked at her pointedly. "What pills?"

"These," she said as she took a pill bottle out of her purse. "They help me lose weight."

Colin grabbed them out of her hand. "That's the last thing you need to do, is to lose weight!"

"Dr. Sandler says I do, says I'm getting fat! Fat, fat, fat!" she said empathically.

Colin looked at the prescription bottle. It was clearly labeled, "Do Not Take With Alcohol."

"It says not to take this with alcohol."

"I know," she said as she smiled conspiratorially. "It's not well known, but this stuff," she said as she reached over and shook the bottle, "is a great diet pill when you take it with alcohol. Dr. David told me so. Here give me two," she said as she tried to pry the bottle out of his hand.

He nonchalantly pried her fingers off the bottle and stuck it in his jacket pocket.

"Hey! You can't do that! Those are mine. Give them back!"

"Jessica, did you know that Dr. Sandler died?"

"Naw, he didn't tell me that."

It was apparent to him that until she sobered up some she wasn't going to understand a thing he said. Out of the corner of his eye he saw their sandwiches coming out of the kitchen.

"Jessica, do me a favor and tuck yourself back into your bra."

"Bothers ya huh?" She smiled as she deftly reached her hand under her shirt and repositioned herself.

"Yeah, it bothers me, but not the way you think. You come from a good family, you shouldn't be doing these things."

"I don't come from a good family, I come from no family, no family at all."

"Here, drink some of this," he said as he poured some cream into her coffee.

"I don't like it with cream. Just sugar."

"Tough, just drink it," he said sternly.

After he was satisfied that she'd eaten as much as she was going to, he asked for the bill. It was $258. He put it on his charge card and reminded himself to use the receipt as a deduction for his taxes. As a political contribution to the Congressman.

He put her in his car and drove her to her apartment. He'd already been there three times this week, he certainly knew the way.

As soon as he opened the door to her apartment he knew why she hadn't been staying there. The place smelled like sour yogurt that had been baking in the sun for days. He had never smelled a place that smelled this bad. Vomit that had not been cleaned up was most definitely the culprit. He closed the door. Now what was he going to do with her?

He drove her to a motel that was just a few miles from his place so he could come back and check on her in the morning. He checked her in using the charge card he found in her purse and then half carried half dragged her to her room. He threw her on top of the bed and removed her shoes. Then he left her a note telling her that he had her money and her charge cards and that he'd be back in the morning with breakfast. If she woke up before he got there she could call him. He left her his number and then signed it Officer Scott. He picked up the room key.

At the door he turned to look at her. What a shame. He hoped she could get the help she needed, soon. He closed the door and it locked behind him.

Chapter 108

Chantilly, VA

At nine the next morning Colin got into his car and drove to the drug store that Robert Jones worked at. It was just down the street from the motel where he had deposited Jessica the night before, or actually, earlier that same morning.

Robert took one look at the label on the prescription bottle Colin had handed him and shook his head. "Haven't seen this stuff in years. Where'd you get this?"

"From one of Dr. Sandler's patients. He convinced her to take it with alcohol like it was some kind of fantastic weight loss program. Sad thing is she probably doesn't weigh more than a hundred pounds with clothes on."

"How much alcohol?"

"Lots, she's pretty much an alcoholic as far as I can tell."

"Then these are gonna kill her, eventually. There are three refills indicated, 120 pills each. Sooner or later she's going to run her car into a tree or walk off the roof of a parking garage. Taking these with alcohol is the worst kind of punch-drunk you can be."

"Can you call over to her pharmacy and advise them not to refill them for her?" Colin asked.

"I can try. Don't know if they'll listen or not."

"Just tell them to get in touch with the prescribing doctor first. That ought to keep her from getting a refill. Either that, or I'll go by and see them myself. Let me know if you think I should."

"Okay, will do."

Colin left to go wake up Jessica. He knocked several times before he used the key to open the door. He found her exactly where he'd left her. It didn't appear that she'd moved one bit. He tried to wake her up unsuccessfully several times. She'd open her eyes mumble something and close them again. He left to go to K-mart to get her some clothes. When he returned, he told himself he'd throw her in the shower if he had to to get her up.

An hour later that's exactly what he was doing, holding her up in her leather skirt and sheer blouse letting the cold sting of the water bring her around. She sputtered and cussed and clawed at him but he held her under until in his judgment she was wide awake. She was mad as all get out but very wide awake.

He turned off the shower and watched her as she pulled the plastered hair from in front of her face.

"You son-of-a-bitch! What the hell do you think you're doing?"

"I'm trying to get you awake and sober." He looked at his watch, "And I'm into my eighth hour with this so it's getting pretty old! Take your clothes off, get a shower, and put these on!" He shoved a plastic shopping bag into her hand. "And if I don't hear you moving around in here, I'll come in here and strip you and do it myself! Now get busy!" he said as he slammed the bathroom door. "And don't forget to shampoo your hair. It reeks of tobacco and whiskey!" He called through the closed door. He found the TV remote control and sat on the edge of the bed to wait for her.

Half an hour later she timidly opened the door and stepped out dressed in the jeans and chambray shirt he'd just purchased. He'd over guessed the size a little, but it wasn't too bad.

"C'mon, let's get some breakfast. I'm starving."

Jessica grabbed her stomach and her mouth at the same time at the mention of food.

"If you're going to heave, please do it now before we get to the restaurant."

She went back into the bathroom and closed the door. Ten minutes later she came out again. "Better?" he asked.

She gave him a wan smile. "Yeah, I guess. You got somethin' for this headache?"

"Honey, the only thing that's going to help that headache is abstinence. I've had many just like it. Time and tolerance are the only things that will help it. C'mon let's go."

"What about my clothes?"

"Leave 'em. You're not going to need them anymore."

"What!"

"Where I'm taking you, you won't need them."

"And just where do you think you're taking me?" she asked belligerently.

"Home to meet Mama! You're a girl after her own heart. I'll tell you all about her over breakfast." He ushered her out and closed the door behind them leaving the key on top of the TV.

He drove to the Virginian in Vienna hoping there wouldn't be anybody who would recognize her there. He had a full country breakfast while she nibbled on some toast. He forced her to help him eat some of his pancakes and made her drink two glasses of orange juice, all the while going over everything with her about Dr. Sandler, her will and her medicine. When he had told her everything he thought she should know, he asked if she'd understood him.

"Yeah, I think so. I went to a doctor who was supposed to help me with my problems. Instead of helping me he gave me a few new ones and tried to kill me. That it?"

"Pretty much. I kept the medicine and voided the refills. You don't need to lose weight. If anything you need to gain it. So, now you need to see someone about your anorexia, your alcoholism, your low self-esteem and your mother."

"My mother?" she asked with some shock.

"Yeah, according to your file you have some anger about her leaving you. I'm going to take you to see my mother so you can see how lucky you were," he chuckled. When Jessica raised her eyebrows at this he quickly added, "No, now seriously, she's a great mother and you are going to see what it's like to be smothered to death. You'll like her and she'll like you. She's a Democrat. A very devoted Democrat, just like your father, only she doesn't run for office, she puts people into office. She's very active in the local party."

"Just why am I going to meet her?" Jessica asked.

"Because you need help and she knows how to help people."

"Just take me back to my car. I don't need any help, I can take care of myself."

"If last night was what you call taking care of yourself, you're doing a deplorable job. You're a beautiful woman and you're ruining your looks running around and partying like you're at a Roman orgy. And think about all the diseases you're subjecting yourself to. Do you even remember the guy who had his tongue down your throat and his hand up your skirt last night?"

When she just sat there looking at him, he knew that she didn't. He stood up and took her hand. "Come meet my mother, she needs a new project."

He drove her over to his mother's house in Falls Church and just as he knew she would, she recognized Jessica instantly. "Jessica Tyler! Andy's daughter! What a nice surprise," she said as she gently took her arm and led her into the living room. "I knew your mother." Colin left them alone for awhile and went to go find his father.

After visiting with him in his workshop for an hour he went back inside to see how his mother was doing with Jessica. They were in the kitchen. Colin's mother was showing Jessica how to frost a cake she'd made for the Church bake sale.

"Mom, I gotta go now. Can we talk for a second?" Colin asked his mother.

"Sure, honey." She wiped her hands on a dish towel and excused herself from Jessica. They stood and talked in the back hallway. Colin briefly told her what Jessica had been through lately and what he thought she needed. Her mother agreed with him and said she would take care of everything. Colin went back to the kitchen and gave Jessica a hug goodbye.

"You're leaving me here?" she asked incredulously.

"My mom has some pretty good connections. She's going to get you some help. Trust me, Jessica. Trust her. I didn't save you just to watch you destroy yourself. I'll come back next week and if you're not happy, I'll take you home. Deal?"

Jessica thought about it. She knew she had nothing to lose, she'd already lost everything. Maybe it was time to grow up a little. "Deal," she said as she hugged him back.

Colin's mother took Jessica to a home that was run by her Catholic Diocese, one she had co-founded and supported for many years. They took her in, gave her a room of her own and provided all the psychiatric help she needed. She had people with her when she suffered the worst of her detox symptoms and she made friends with other girls that were coming back just as she was. She even started going back to church again, only they called it Mass. A few weeks after she arrived at the home she met a Catholic priest in his late thirties who had been having doubts about his calling.

Jessica gave him reason to have even more doubts. Within six months they were madly in love and going to counseling in preparation for their marriage.

Colin was asked to be the best man, because to Jessica he really was.

Chapter 109

Fairfax, VA

For the next two years Colin worked as a consultant on the Sandler case between cases of private investigating work and golf tournaments. Tying up all the loose ends wasn't as easy as he'd first thought it would be.

An autopsy had not been performed on Leroy Dressler and the family did not want his body exhumed to see what kinds of drugs were in his system at the time of his death. They thought it was pointless since the money the victims had possibly bequeathed under duress hadn't ever been recovered. The embalming process he'd been required to have was likely to mask them anyway. There was no doubt in Colin's mind that if the money was on the table waiting to be divvied up among the victim's families that they would be quite eager to prove Dr. Sandler culpable in Leroy's death.

But it was not. Try as he might, Colin could not locate the girlfriend. And he was sure that somehow she had it or knew where it was. Going through all the doctor's checks, receipts and credit card statements the most he'd been able to glean was that she probably had a kid because Dr. Sandler had spent a lot of money on toys at Toy's R Us. Using all the restaurant receipts that indicated he'd spent enough for two, he went to all the restaurants with a picture of Dr. Sandler. Most waiters and maitre d's remembered him, some even remembered him being accompanied by a very beautiful woman, but no one knew who she was.

Collecting the doctor's mail for six months only enlightened them to the fact that he'd applied for a background check at a Pawn shop the day before the shooting. A postcard from the pawn shop he had visited reminded him that he could now come purchase the gun he desired. Boy, Colin thought, if things had played out differently, he could be dead right now. Every bad golf shot became a good one for awhile, because he remembered that at least he was still there to take the next one.

All the avenues on Katherine Cheney, and Benton Riveria were inconclusive. They had left money to him and he'd prescribed drugs to them, but nothing unusual was found in their medical files. In fact, according to his daughter, Benton Riveria hadn't even taken most of his pain medication, believing that he needed to suffer for some reason. The papers normally in the patients' files detailing their problems and treatments were missing from his file, so Colin didn't really know a lot about him.

Since Riveria was the first of Dr. Sandler's patients to die, who'd left him any money, Colin theorized that maybe he had of his own free will left money to the doctor. And since it had come at a time when the doctor was in need of it, maybe the idea to keep it coming in took hold from there. His death was around the time of the doctor's divorce and alimony settlement. Boy, if that were the case, the old gentleman's act of kindness had sure backfired on a lot of other people. Both Riveria and Cheney had been old and sickly. It was possible they just died on their own. Since he couldn't prove otherwise, that was the way it had to be.

Nancy Meridan's inheritance was still tied up in the courts. She had left money to him but she would never have taken any kinds of drugs, her religion would not have allowed it, according to all the people he talked to about her, she was a devote Christian Scientologist. Her medical records were very decisive. She died from cancer. He may have tried to steal money from her but Dr. Sandler did not kill her.

So all in all, Colin figured Dr. David Sandler killed five people. He believed Leroy Dressler was murdered, he just felt it even if he couldn't prove it. He'd attempted three others. He wrote his final report and cleared out his office.

After a year or so of tracking down check kiters, credit card thiefs and dishonest bank employees, he decided it was time to take his next career seriously. And in order to do that, he needed to consider moving south. Somewhere he could play golf almost all year long. Over the twenty years he'd been playing the sport he had made numerous trips to the Carolina coasts to play. Some watering holes in Myrtle Beach stocked his favorite brand of liquor just for his frequent visits.

He knew he could find an affordable condo somewhere on a golf course in North Carolina, South Carolina or Georgia. Florida was out, too hot, too much crime and too many hurricanes. Georgia was a bit pricey and buggy. It would have to be one of the Carolinas.

During the winter he had gone to one of the expos they had every year at the Holiday Inn at Tyson's Corner. They showcased the more prominent Brunswick County developments. He had filled out a few registration cards at several booths which had put him on mailing lists to receive offers to visit. For a very nominal cost he would be invited to come down to play some golf and stay in a luxury condo if he agreed to take a look at the property they were trying to sell him. It was a great deal for him, three days of golf and two nights lodging for the price he'd normally pay for one round of golf. He sent back every offer he got with dates filled in when they could expect him to arrive. By the following summer he had decided on the area he most wanted to check out.

He liked Sea Trail Plantation at Sunset Beach as it already had three golf courses. Ocean Ridge Plantation, close to Ocean Isle Beach, was planning to have three courses, two were already built. And finally, St. James Plantation on the road to Southport, which had one and they were working on the second with a third to follow. He decided to see if he could rent a beach house for two months during the summer. It would give him a chance to play all the local courses and it would give Adam a place to come when he could arrange his vacation so they could spend some time together. Adam loved the beach and, since he had his own car, he could come down anytime he could finagle a three-day weekend. It was just like when he was Adam's age, any road trip was exciting.

Chapter 110

Sunset Beach, NC 1994

Jenny Miller thought the major events in her life were over. Life would continue on and she'd enjoy it, but nothing of any significance would be in store for her now. The thrill of falling in love, culminating in marriage and the birth of her children were all behind her now, likewise her rather successful career. All was in the past, these stages of her life, though none were accomplished in what could be considered a conventional manner.

Yes, it would be rather boring from here on out. She'd be content, but she really didn't expect anything truly exciting would happen to her again. She'd had it all. It was someone else's turn to be the center of attention. In the next few months she would come to realize that her life wasn't as all wrapped up as she thought it was.

She stood gazing out the front of the miniature golf course shack, through the lush beds of hybrid petunias to the second hole and beyond to the rest of the course. This was the nicest little golf course she had ever seen. It was really more of an exotic garden than the image most people would connect to a little putt putt golf course.There were no windmills, no plastic animals, no spouting volcanoes and nothing with flashing lights or bells going off for a hole-in-one.

It was shady and serene with quaint little waterfalls and brooks filled with speckled round stones you could see through the crystal clear water. There were different groupings of plants at each of the eighteen holes. Right now flowering gardenias were scenting the breeze wafting over from the third hole.

It was a riot of color during the spring; the start of their season. A dense canopy of magnificent Oaks provided welcome shade through the heat of the summer and into the fall; the end of their season. She loved this place. It was like working in the garden of Eden, except, as yet, she'd found no apple tree. Serpents, yes... two snakes so far this year. Minor nuisances really, since she now knew the snake removal company's number by heart. Although the last one had been chivalrously removed for her by a customer. She gratefully bestowed free passes upon him and his family for the rest of their vacation week at Sunset Beach, North Carolina.

She could see the cars beginning to line up at the light to go over the quaint, bascule swing bridge that connects the mainland to the barrier island. The bridge was now open to boat traffic traveling the Intracoastal Waterway. You could just barely see the high masts of the larger sailboats as they glided through the opening.

This bridge, with all it's controversy, was the heart of Sunset Beach, the last beach in North Carolina before you reach the South Carolina line. In fact, you can actually walk from Sunset Beach to Bird Island, which is in both states, if you get the tides right. A shallow estuary called Madd inlet separates the two during all but low tides when people can walk or ride bikes from one to the other. During high tide the strong current rushing in at waist level can cause you to loose your footing and be pulled into the rushing waters.

It was a Saturday morning, Transition Day at the beach, people checking out at 11:00 am and a new group arriving to check in at 3:00 pm. There were four places you didn't want to be today: the rental offices, the grocery store, the ABC store, and the road to the bridge.

Usually Jenny didn't work on weekends, but being the agreeable person that she was, and since she really didn't have anything better to do, she had switched days with the owner's son, Craig. So here she was watching cars and trucks lining up, each filled to capacity with coolers, beach chairs, surfboards and kids.

Every third or fourth vehicle pulled a boat or jet skis, every sixth or seventh had a bike rack.

It wasn't bad enough that the bridge itself had only one lane, it also opened to boat traffic every hour, on the hour. So during the time it took the bridge to open, the boats to pull through, and the bridge to close again, the new arrivals would have a captivating view of the miniature golf course, the ABC store and a small souvenir beach shop, unless they chose to get out of their cars and walk to the banks of the Intracoastal Waterway to watch the boats pass by. This usually took fifteen to twenty minutes. For every third or fourth cycle of this she would have the noise of some over-cranked car radio playing rap music, ruining the tranquility of the day. In time they would all move through the light and 45 minutes later it would all begin again. Why didn't people listen to Country or Classical music that loud?

Saturday was typically the worst business day of the week since the tourists were trying to get settled in and the local people were trying to avoid the traffic. Not at all like the Saturdays she used to know.

It seemed so odd at times. Was it just two short years ago that she had been a General Sales Manager for a very large automobile dealership in Tyson's Corner, Virginia? Talk about traffic, boy she sure didn't miss that. This was nothing in comparison.

Chapter 111

Sunset Beach

Jenny was jolted out of her reverie by the sound of car doors slamming. A family was piling out of their mini van to play some miniature golf. She greeted them and made small talk about the weather, the bridge and answered their questions about how nice it must be to actually live at Sunset Beach. There were seven of them so she rang up $28 and helped them select putters and balls and sent them on their way to the 1st hole.

While counting out the money, she noticed that her nails could use a new coat of polish. There was so much down time with this job that she had learned to bring newspapers and a book, as well as her manicure kit and her Gameboy. She stripped off her polish and rubbed some cuticle remover around the nail base making her fingers all gluey and thought that now would not be a good time for a customer.

She took a lot of pride in her appearance. She was very attractive, for her age, owing to the good genes she inherited from her mother, who at 68 looked 48. She had long blonde hair that she usually wore up in a twist with a tortoise shell clip or in a French braid falling down her back. She had green eyes with yellow flecks around the pupils, long dark lashes with the help of mascara, and a set of lips that smiled into a pink cupid's bow to reveal straight white teeth.

She sported a cinnamon-toast colored tan from her small freckled nose all the way down her shapely petite 5'4" frame to trim thighs and legs revealed by her short jean cutoffs. She had an overall athletic look about her. She looked wholesome and fresh. What attracted men to her most though was her sparkle. She had a sensual energy and a pixieish quality about her that was a real turn on to men. Without her saying anything, her body communicated to them that she had what it took to give them pleasure. An abundant bosom and a tiny waistline started that conversation and her effervescence kept it going.

She walked into the ladies' room and used her hand brush to scrub the cuticle remover away. On the way back to the shack she noticed that the butterflies were plentiful today so she grabbed a chair from the shack to sit outside and watch them. She loved watching the butterflies flit around, going from bush to bush, leaving one and traveling on to the next to see what else was in store for it there. Something like her and her life lately. She filed her nails smooth and applied a coat of polish.

She kept her nails natural, she didn't like the tips or acrylics that were so popular, preferring to keep hers short and polished either light pink or a neutral color. Today they'd needed a lot of work, they'd become a bit ragged-looking with most of the polish chipped off. While they were drying she watched the gentle butterflies settling here, then settling there, but never staying very long in either place. Rather skittish they were, never really committing to any one place. Well she was committed to one place. She loved it at Sunset Beach.

She heard more car doors closing so she got up to wait on the new people coming in to play golf. It was starting to get busy now. People were coming off the beach and venturing out to the tourist attractions and restaurants. There were three restaurants within two blocks of the mini-golf course. One was just across the street above Bill's Seafood Shop. Crabby Oddwaters, a favorite restaurant for both the tourists and the year 'round locals. They had expanded two years ago so they could accommodate more people during the busy summer season, but they still had people lined up to go in and more people waiting in the lounge. Around 4 o'clock in the afternoon the smells that wafted over caused her stomach to growl with hunger pangs and she would envision herself at a table stuffing her face with crab legs dripping with butter or Mahi Mahi cooked Cajun Style.

At 5:00 her relief came. She got into her little white convertible and drove around the block into Sea Trail Plantation, her home for the past two years. She drove past the Club Villa condos and across the cart path for the golf course, past the pool, the little Chapel on the Green and the tennis courts. She drove along the winding road admiring the houses, the lakes and the landscaping. She turned into her driveway, pushed the button for the automatic garage door and pulled into the garage. Home again, home again, jiggity jig. It had been a very nice day. She wondered what the evening had in store for her.

Chapter 112

Sunset Beach

As she came in through the connecting garage door, she was immediately greeted by her one year old cock-a-poo, Taffy. She was a great dog, smart as a whip and the best behaved dog she'd ever had. Shortly after moving to Sunset Beach she had relented to her daughter, Paisley's insistent pleas of "I want a doughgie " and, after a lot of research, she bought one. It was a decision she never regretted even though she had spent a fortune getting rid of the kennel cough Taffy had when they got her.

Paisley was lying on the couch watching TV. She looked up, smiled, and said "What's for dinner?"

Jenny thought about it for a moment and said "How about going out for crab legs when Rusty gets home from the beach?"

That met with a very enthusiastic response and Paisley was up and running for her bedroom to get ready. At eight she was just starting to get those insecure feelings pre-adolescents have about their appearance, and while she could care less about what she wore around the house she was very particular about what she wore in public, just in case someone she knew saw her.

Jenny took a shower to wash off the combination bug repellent and sunscreen she always wore when working and fixed herself a drink. A few minutes later she heard Rusty turning on the outside faucet to rinse the sand from his feet then come in through the front door.

"Hi, Mom," he called. "What's for dinner?" So much for "how was your day?"

"I thought we'd go out for crab legs, what do you think about that idea?" she called as he went through the family room heading for his bathroom on the other side of the house.

"That sounds great, Mom. Just let me take a quick shower and I'll be ready."

They usually had all you-can-eat crab legs on Wednesday nights at the Tavern on the Tee Restaurant on the Plantation, which they could walk to. However Wednesday didn't work out for Rusty because he had to work. So instead they would drive to Calabash just a few miles away and go to one of the many seafood restaurants there that catered to the tourists. It was good food, they would just have to wait awhile to get served. Weekends were very busy this time of the year.

When they were all ready they piled into her convertible and she drove out of Sea Trail Plantation using the south exit. That put them on Lakeshore Drive, a meandering two-lane road that skirted the Intracoastal Waterway. There were some magnificent houses set back from the road. As you drove by you could see their long docks stretching hundreds of feet from the rear decks to the water. Each house had its own style and level of luxury, but not one of them could have been purchased without the word "million" somewhere in the price.

The views between the houses were so picturesque that it almost made you want to freeze-frame each segment in your mind to review and enjoy again later. You could see boats sailing up and down the Intracoastal and beyond the opposite shore you could see the back side of Sunset Beach and Bird Island. A mile or so of marshland was dotted throughout and there was always an abundance of wildlife that could be seen flying in and out as you followed the curves of the road. It was the kind of road that made you drive more slowly so you wouldn't miss a single vista. As the road took a very deep turn away from the water it signaled the approach into Calabash, a quaint fishing village struggling to keep its small town atmosphere despite the annual influx of tourists.

Calabash, whose sign declared it "The Seafood Capital of the World", was a haven for hungry tourists and had been for many many years. In fact, during the 1930's Jimmy Durante and his troupe dined at an inn owned by a woman who served them the best seafood he had ever eaten. He told her when they departed that he would make her famous and years later when he had his own TV show he did, saying "Good night Mrs. Calabash, wherever you are," at the end of each show.

Today, there are quite a few more restaurants than there had been back then, and due to the good service and food they all do well during the season as people keep coming back year after year. The Calabash style of cooking is a batter based method of frying and is very popular in the South, but the fresh seafood coming in from the Calabash River all day long is what really makes the difference. If you go down to the waterfront in the late afternoon you can watch the shrimp boats coming in and unloading their catch. Some of them have even set up little shacks where they sell the shrimp directly from the boats.

They went to Eastside Calabash Restaurant, right in the heart of the little city. They have a huge dining hall and sometimes you don't have to wait even during the season. They were lucky tonight and were seated right away close to the buffet tables. While they were ordering the crab leg special, Jenny watched her kids. She was proud of them. They had very nice manners and their politeness made them seem much older than they were. She could tell that Rusty was scoping out the waitresses and even though she would love to see him ask one out, she knew he was too shy.

He was working part time as a dishwasher at a restaurant called Tamer's at Ocean Ridge, another golf resort a few miles away. It had been a rough couple of years for him. This growing up thing had thrown him for a double loop and Jenny had had to go along with him on his bumpy ride. He was almost fifteen now and a great kid.

Paisley, on the other hand, was an ingenue just beginning the early stages of pubescence. One day she was so childlike and wanted to play with her Barbie's and the next she was reading teen magazine and eschewing anything that had to do with those baby things she had outgrown. It was Jenny's hope with this move to North Carolina that she would be able to be more involved in her children's lives and be able to help them to overcome some of the difficulties of growing up.

Their life here in North Carolina was a big change from the life they'd had back in Northern Virginia. It was not easy leaving a very loving family network, but they were all doing well and beginning to think of North Carolina as their home not just a place they used to go to on vacations. Although they did miss Jenny's parents, her sister Jean, and all their friends, they spoke with them often on the phone, e-mailed them almost daily and looked forward to their frequent visits. All in all, "nothing could be finer than to be in Carolina".

Chapter 113

Sunset Beach

It was a glorious Monday morning at the Mini-Links. There was excitement in the air as a new set of tourists was being turned over after the weekend. The Tourists, called "Tourons" or "Morists" by the locals, an affectionate name derived from a combination of Tourists and Morons, were refreshed from their weekend of moving in and settling down. Now they were up and about, seeing the sights and drinking in the local flavor. The locals didn't really dislike the "Tourons" that much, it was just hard to adjust to being confronted by a crowd everywhere you tried to go in the summertime.

Since most of the vacationers here at Sunset came year after year after year, even the out of the way local hangouts were overrun. There were always lines to get in for breakfast at Nell's on the road to Ocean Isle and at The Pancake House in Calabash on most weekends, but the weekdays weren't too bad.

Jenny was not having breakfast out today at one of her favorite places though, much as she'd like to. She had to work. As she opened up the little wooden hut in preparation for the day, she thought about why she was working again, so soon after she had left her other job.

Even though Jenny had carefully budgeted her money in anticipation of moving to Sunset Beach, there was one thing she had not counted on—the school system. Paisley had come from the Fairfax County school system, one of the best in the nation, to Brunswick County, one of the worst in the nation. Even though the county had some of the most expensive real estate on the east coast, once you left the coastal regions, it was a pretty poor county. The public schools reflected that.

She tried the public school for her, but Paisley did not do well there. She didn't do well with the peer pressure. In an effort to be accepted and liked Paisley seemed to lean away from her upbringing to please her friends. Luckily, Jenny was able to spot this in time and put her in a private school, where the focus was much more directed toward learning. She was doing very well there, but it did cost money to send her and next year would be even more expensive as she outgrew the grade levels this school had to offer. She would have to go on to a college prep school in Wilmington—Cape Fear Academy. Again, this was an unplanned expense, so Jenny had to get a part-time job to augment her income.

When she found the job at the Mini-Links, she couldn't believe her good fortune. It was perfect. It was only from June through August, she could work any hours she wanted, her kids could be with her while she was working if she wanted them to be, she could wear the most casual beach wear and it was only a few blocks from the house. Paisley could even ride there on her bike. And it was such an easy job; keep things clean, wait on the customers and enjoy the scenery.

She worked two or three days a week from 9 to 5 and also did the bookkeeping. It was enough to pay Paisley's tuition for the year, so Jenny was very happy. Rusty hadn't been doing very well in the schools in Virginia, but the public schools down here seemed to be doing the trick for him. Jenny was grateful for that. She couldn't have afforded two kids in private schools unless she went to work full time and that would have been a shame since the whole idea behind moving down here had been to spend more time taking care of the kids.

As she lifted the louvers for the little shack and turned on the red neon open sign she breathed in the fresh crisp air of the morning scented with the perfume of the flowers from the second hole. She opened the register and put in the bank that she had brought with her from home. She turned on the ice cream and slushie machines and checked to make sure she had enough balls in the basket. She flipped the switch for the pump to start the waterfalls and pressed the on button for the music piped throughout the course. As she was setting out the golf clubs she heard the first customers pull into the parking lot, open and close their doors and come up the front steps of the deck.

As she finished laying out the rest of the clubs on the carpet-covered counter she said cheerily, "Good morning early birds, you can have the first tee time, and there's no waiting to play through!" She spun around to face the most handsome man she'd ever seen in her life. When her eyes locked with his it was almost as if the breath had been sucked right out of her. She couldn't breathe. She just stared, drinking him in with her eyes.

He was rather tall, she wouldn't have been able to look right into his eyes if he hadn't been leaning his crossed arms on the counter, watching her. His deep blue eyes were appraising her just as hers were appraising him. Embarrassed by the sudden knowledge that she had been staring, she stammered, "One game or all day?"

That's when she noticed that there was someone with him, a young teenage boy with the same penetrating blue eyes. The man looked to the boy and asked, "All day, I think. What about you? Are you up for more than one game?"

"Sure," the boy said with a shrug, "why not?" The man turned his face back to her and smiled as he stood all the way up and reached into his front pants pocket. "All day for two, please," he said as he whipped a twenty out of his gold money clip and handed it to her.

Jenny thought she was going to lose it. Somehow, just the look of this man had unnerved her. She took the twenty from his hand and rang up the sale, counting his change back to him. "Help yourself to the putters, the scorecards are over here and there's complimentary bug spray if you think you need it."

"Do we need it?" he asked, wrinkling his brow.

"No, I don't think so, but you usually do at night. It's one of the reasons I won't work at night. The bugs just love me," she said with a smile. Inside she was screaming, "now why did I say that?"

He gave her a huge grin and said, "I can see why." He looked pointedly at her chest, lifting an eyebrow slightly.

She looked down to see strawberry syrup on her white tank top. She must have leaned too close to the flavor burst part of the ice cream maker when she switched it on. She had the grace of a buffoon. "Oh," she said mortified. "Enjoy your game. Oh! I forgot to stamp your hands for all day play." She reached into the drawer under the counter and brought out a rubber stamp. She stamped the back of the boy's hand first. And then the man's, being careful not to touch him with anything but the stamp. She felt that if she touched him in any way that she would be reduced to a small pile of ashes. The heat from his eyes was suddenly incendiary.

As they walked over the bridge to the first hole she followed them with her eyes until he turned to gaze back at her. Then she quickly turned away and headed for the ladies' room to wash her shirt.

In the safe confines of the ladies' room she clutched the sink and breathed deeply in and out several times while looking at herself in the mirror. What was wrong with her? Other than that big red splash of color between the outline of her breasts. She quickly whipped the tank top off and ran it under cold water, with a little soap the stain washed right out. She wrung it out as good as she could and then shook the wrinkles out. It was ribbed and mostly nylon so she knew it would dry fast in this heat. When she put it back on, she was aware of how it molded to her bathing suit top, accentuating that part of her. Well, that couldn't be helped. It would just need some time to dry.

As soon as she opened the door her eyes searched for him. There they were over on the third hole. He was wearing khaki shorts with a green polo shirt, his wavy silver blonde hair lifting gently in the breeze. There was a ruggedness about him that appealed to all that was female in her. His broad shoulders, his trim waist and his long legs covered with dark curling hair all contributed to his attractiveness to her. There wasn't anything about him that she didn't like. He was damned near perfect in her eyes. That meant he was probably married.

All her grown up life Jenny had been quick to assess the opposite sex. She'd heard many years ago that whenever a man saw a woman or a woman saw a man, they automatically sorted them in their minds as to whether they would or they wouldn't do "it" with them. Most people did this all the time and just weren't aware they were doing it. Jenny knew. Most men fell into the "no" category, some into the "maybe" category, but very few fell into the "yes" category. The ones that did, were invariably married. It had been a fact of her life for so many years she didn't even question it anymore.

This man was definitely a *yes*. Her whole body had responded to his presence and now that he was away from her, her eyes were trying to locate him on the course. More customers came to play and she got busy getting them onto the course.

When the man and the boy came around the 14th hole she was able to watch them play. The man had a deft touch and he looked so good standing over the ball, and almost like it was the most natural thing for him, he hit it right into the hole. She couldn't watch him on the other three holes because of the trees and bushes but she was waiting when he crested the top of the eighteenth hole.

He looked magnificent standing there, from his sandals to his full thick head of hair being tousled by the breeze. He looked confident, stunning and extremely virile. He was facing her now, but keeping his eye on the ball so she had free reign to look at his chiseled chin and shapely, sensuous lips. As he tapped the ball his head came up and his eyes met hers across the length of the hole. Embarrassed that he had caught her watching him again, she hastily turned her back and busied herself.

When they came back by the hut to get another ball after theirs had dropped into the well, she pretended not to even notice they were there in front of her.

"Nice course," he said.

"Thank you. The owners take great pride in keeping it nice."

"It has some surprising water hazards."

"Didn't fool you though. Neither of you lost a single ball," she quipped.

He laughed, "I'm an old hand at this. I've learned to walk the hole before I putt it."

She noticed he was staring at her chest again, she looked down self consciously. The shirt hadn't dried very much, if at all.

"I see you got the red syrup off."

"Yes, I'm a slob, what can I say? I don't even eat something and I can still get it all over me. It was from the ice cream machine when I leaned over to turn it on this morning."

"You have ice cream?" he asked with interest.

"Yes, we have an after golf special, it's only a dollar when you play golf. These are the flavors," she said as she pointed to a colorful display. "Chocolate, Strawberry, Butter Pecan and Cotton Candy."

"So what flavor do you recommend?" he asked.

"Well, my absolute favorite is chocolate, the woman's substitute for sex. I eat a lot of it here." She quickly realized what she had just said and blushed to the roots of her blonde hair. Now why had she said that! She berated herself and covered her lips with her hand as if she could shove the words back into her mouth.

He gave a delightful chuckle. "Well, then chocolate it is and make mine a double!"

As she made their ice cream cones she soundly admonished herself for being so stupid. She really must appear to be a bumpkin to him.

"You're not from around here are you?" he asked as she handed him his cone. Their fingers brushed each others and a tremor traveled down her arm. She had to swallow to keep from gasping at the unexpectedness of it.

"Well, I am now. I moved here from Herndon, Va."

"Small world. I'm from Fairfax, Va." he said as he licked around the side of his cone. *That tongue*. Oh God, she'd better not look. She turned to the boy.

"Are you from Fairfax, too?"

570

"I was," he said shyly, "I live in Woodbridge now."

"This is my son, Adam. My name is Colin."

"I'm Jenny. Are you vacationing here?"

"Yes. We'll be down here for two months. Can you recommend some good restaurants?"

"Of course. What kind of food do you like?"

"I don't know, I'm pretty easy. What's good around here?"

"Well, depending on how far you want to drive, we have it all, but if you don't want to drive far, there's seafood, Italian, Greek, Jamaican and you can get a really good steak right over there at the Tavern on the Tee in Sea Trail Plantation."

"A good steak sounds good. Maybe we'll do that tonight. What do you think Adam?"

"I think that would be okay. C'mon let's play another game, I want to see if I can beat you this time."

"Fat chance! But give it your best shot!"

They left to play another round while Jenny waited on more customers.

When they came back around again, Jenny was sitting outside the shack reading a book. Trying to act nonchalant, she smiled over at them and called out, "Did ya beat him, Adam?"

"Nah. He's too good for me."

Jenny sat up and said, "Here use this club." She handed him a grooved putter with guides on it. She turned to Colin, "Now, you use this club," she handed him a putter that had the head loosely turning in the hosel.

"I can't use this club, it's broken!"

"Well, don't you want to show Adam how good *you* are, that it's not just the putter? Besides it's no fun to play with someone who always wins." She gave him a wink and mischievously patted Adam on the shoulder. "I don't even think you'll need a handicap for this round."

Colin smirked at her and went off behind Adam. Jenny laughed.

They left after that last round, Adam finally proclaiming victory. He thanked her for the club and Colin thanked her sarcastically for his club. Jenny experienced a profound disappointment that Colin was no longer around.

She ate her lunch while telling herself how foolish she was being thinking about him. This whole day she had been like a schoolgirl with a crush. Mentally she kept shaking herself, telling herself how childish she was being. The man had a son, he most likely had a wife. Stop coveting somebody else's husband, even if he did have the sexiest ass and the most impressive shoulders. And those chest hairs covering the top of his chest and base of his throat, visible from the opening of his golf shirt, kept coming back to her mind all through the afternoon. Why did she think a hairy chest was so sexy? She knew many women abhorred hairy-chested men. Not this woman. Just how had this man gotten under her skin and so quickly? This was not like her at all.

She called to check on Paisley. Paisley was going to the pool with a friend and the friend's mother and Rusty was still at summer camp. He wouldn't be back until next week. The crowd thinned out around 4:30. That was the time people started heading back to their condos for a nap or to get ready for dinner. At five her shift would end and she'd be relieved.

She had everything ready for the next shift except for collecting the balls out of the well. The well was a wooden box over a three foot hole in the ground with a gray roof at the top resembling one you'd see on a wishing well. It had a hinged door on the front that opened up. If people were around she had to climb into the well to bring the basket full of balls up. If no one was around she would just kneel on the ground and lean over until she could grab one of the handles and haul it up. She preferred this to climbing down in the well because the well was home to spiders and frogs and other squishy things.

No one was around so she got on her knees and leaned into the well. She was just about able to make contact with a handle when she felt a soft breeze pass over the edge of her jean cutoffs and cool her skin at the top of the back of her thighs. Then suddenly she felt a burning sensation caress the exposed area of her uppermost thighs, the part that joined to her buttocks, and she somehow knew that someone was staring at her. She turned her head and looked under her arm and saw an upside down Colin staring fixedly at her uplifted bottom. She quickly righted herself, pushed herself out of the well and back onto her heels. She stood up and spun around both hands going to her beet red cheeks.

Colin gave her a very provocative smile out of the side of his mouth and in his sultriest deep voice asked, "Anything I can help you with down there?"

"I was just trying to get the balls up. No one was around a moment ago, so I thought I was safe," she mumbled.

"Well, you're still safe, but just barely," he said with a devastating wink.

He walked over and oh, so effortlessly reached in and pulled up the basket of balls one-handedly.

"I came back to see if you would accompany me to dinner. I have it on good authority that there is a restaurant over there that has a pretty decent steak." He gestured where she had before, toward the Plantation.

"I hope you haven't gotten the wrong idea about me. I can't go out with you."

"Why? Are you married? Engaged? Seeing somebody?" He hadn't seen a ring but that didn't always mean anything.

"Oh, no, nothing like that, I just don't know you," she said simply.

"Well, how are you going to get to know me if you don't go out with me?"

She thought about that for a moment.

"C'mon, you're on your home turf. I'll even meet you at the restaurant if you want."

Still she hesitated.

"What are you afraid of?" he asked.

"That's just it, I think I am afraid. You do things to me."

"I know." He waited a few moments before lifting her chin with his fingers adding, "You do things to me, too. Is that bad?"

573

Jacqueline DeGroot

"I don't know."

"Well, let's just take it one step at a time. We'll meet for dinner and we'll talk and get to know each other. Who knows? I may find that I don't even like you." He smiled at her and winked.

That damned wink again! He should bottle it. "Okay, but I may have to bring my daughter if I can't find a sitter. She's eight."

"That would be fine. Adam has opted for a pizza and some rental movies. Would seven o'clock be okay?"

"Yes, seven is good. I'll meet you there."

He reached up and pulled something out of her ponytail. He held up a spider by one of its legs. "Did you want to keep this?"

"No, you can have it," she said as she shivered.

She was pleased to see that he didn't kill it. He just placed it on a leaf on a nearby bush. With a wave of his hand he was down the steps and walking towards the only car in the parking lot besides hers, a white Mustang convertible.

She shook her hair out to make sure there weren't any more spiders and went to dump the balls into the basket on the counter.

Her mind was on all the things she had to do before she could meet him at seven. Finding a babysitter was at the top of the list.

574

Chapter 114

Sunset Beach

Colin knew the moment he saw her. The sensation of seeing her had created a feeling in him that was like having a frog jump from the bottom of his stomach to the top. Instantly he felt awakened and aroused and aware of her femininity just as he'd been in high school when the cheerleaders had walked by his locker. He'd felt an electrifying spark when he looked into her emerald green eyes, and he'd known. This was the woman Dr. Sandler had been talking about. This was the woman he was destined to meet. And oh, Lord! What a woman she was.

First he'd been assaulted by her vivid green eyes, and then all those alluring curves. He'd wanted to lick the strawberry syrup on her shirt between her breasts. And when she went to stamp their hands, he'd tensed against the possible brush of her skin against his. He'd been a little disappointed when she'd so carefully avoided touching his hand. It had been agony to just walk away from her then. He had felt her eyes on him as he and Adam played the course and whenever he could, he stole a glance over at her, too.

After the first round when he saw her in her wet tank top it was all he could do to keep his eyes from staying on her chest and feasting on the voluptuousness of her. The bathing suit under it had done little to hide the erectness of her nipples.

And that conversation about the chocolate ice cream. She sure blushed easily, from her throat to her ears. She'd certainly become flustered.

But what she'd done for Adam had been truly wonderful. The joy he had gotten out of beating his Dad at golf was something he hadn't counted on. He didn't mind losing if it put a grin like that on his son's face. And somehow she'd known. She'd said, "It's no fun to play with someone who always wins."

That was pretty much the exact opposite of the way he played the games in his life. He'd always played to win, no matter what.

The clincher though, had been when he had come back to ask her out. The sight of her upraised bottom, the smooth tanned thighs yielding to just a glimpse of white tantalizing cheeks poking out of her cutoffs had transfixed him.

And somehow it was all the more erotic that she hadn't meant for that view to be seen as was evidenced by her over bright cheeks. Only a true blonde could blush that shade of pink.

He had been worried there for a moment when he'd thought she might have belonged to another. But, no, she was his. He had no idea how long it was going to take to convince her of that, but she was his, no doubt about it.

He went out onto the deck of the beach house after he'd dressed for dinner. He sat in a chair at the patio table next to Adam who was scoping the girls out on the beach with a pair of binoculars.

"You sure you don't mind me going out to dinner tonight?" he asked him.

"Of course not Dad. If I had a chance to date a real looker you wouldn't horn in on me would you?"

Colin laughed. "She did look good didn't she?"

"Well, I know you Dad, you ain't gonna date no dog."

"Here," he said pulling a twenty out of his money clip. "Order a pizza on me."

"Thanks." Adam called, "Have a good time. And make sure you're in by eleven."

"Yeah, right," Colin answered.

He left the beach house that he had rented on the island to drive to the restaurant. He was waiting at a table for her when she came through the restaurant door. She looked beautiful and sexy in a short, slip-like, flowered sun dress. Her light blonde hair was pulled back from her face and piled on top of her head, secured with a tortoise shell clip. She looked elegant, fresh and wholesome.

The hostess saw her and came over and gave her a hug. Then another man who seemed to be in charge came over and took her hand in both of his. Colin felt a surge of anger but he was careful not to show it as the man led her over to where Colin was waiting. The man released her hand and helped her into her seat as Colin stood up to help her. He sat back down and raised his left eyebrow as a form of a question about all the special treatment.

As a way of explanation she said, "I'm on the Food Services Committee for the Homeowner's Association. I live here on the Plantation."

"Oh," was his simple reply.

"You look beautiful in that dress, but I miss the smell of citronella you had about you today."

She laughed. What a nice, sweet sound it was, he thought. "I scrubbed it all off and substituted it for Giorgio. I may be carried away by mosquitoes when I walk home from here."

"Boy, you live that close huh?"

"Yeah, it's one of the reasons I chose the lot I built on. It's close to the pool, tennis court and the library, and I don't have to worry about drinking and driving, I can just drink and stumble."

He laughed. What a hearty male laugh he had, she thought. "Well, now that I know you drink, what'll it be?"

"I drink champagne," she said coyly. "They didn't even serve it here when I first moved in, but now they keep some in stock for me." She smiled.

"One bottle coming right up", he turned to flag a waiter when that man showed up again, with a glass of champagne!

She shrugged her shoulders sheepishly, "They really know me well here, sorry."

He changed the subject. "So I gather you found a babysitter for your daughter?"

"Yes." Get to the heart of the matter first she said to herself. "I have two children, Paisley is 8 and Rusty is 14. He's away at camp right now. How old is Adam?"

"18, almost 19."

"They're more than 5 years apart," she observed as she reached for the glass of water that had already been poured for her. She took a few small sips before putting it down.

"Tell me about yourself, Colin. What type of work are you in that allows you two months off at a time?"

"It's what kind of work that I'm out of that allows me to be off for two months. I'm retired from Fairfax Country, have been for about four years now. I was a detective. Now, I'm working on my second career. I'm trying to turn pro so I can get on the Senior's tour when I'm fifty. I can join the Carolina's team, the Sunbelt tour now. So I guess you could say I play golf and hope someday to make some money at it."

She smiled, "I've never been out with a policeman or a professional golfer before and here I get both in the same night."

He smiled back at her. "And how is it you're here, all the way from Herndon?"

Before she could answer, the waiter came to take their order. Since they hadn't even looked at the menu, they figured they'd better get down to the business at hand before continuing on with their conversation.

"See," she said, reaching across the table to his menu and pointing with her pink-tipped finger, "this is the steak I told you about, Drunken Jack steak. It's great."

He smiled over at her, "One would get the opinion that you drink a lot."

"Naw, alcohol in food just gets cooked away. Can't get drunk that way. But you can with this," she said as she raised her champagne glass up in salute. She took a sip and placed it back down. He picked it up, turned it around to where she had just taken a sip and put it to his mouth. He drank from the exact spot her lips had just touched.

Jenny quivered as she watched him. This man was out of her league.

They both ordered the Drunken Jack steak with a baked potato and salad. He ordered a Canadian Club with ginger ale and left her to her champagne. They thoroughly enjoyed the meal and the conversation never seemed to halt unless the waiter was there.

They both declined dessert in favor of an after dinner liquor. She chose B&B and Colin chose Grand Marnier. They finally got back to the question he'd asked her awhile back about why she had moved here.

"I retired from the car business after 21 years. Retail can be a very hard life, especially on families. Fortunately I made good money and had some good investments over the years. When I felt that my children needed me to be around more, I arranged to sell my house and build one here. It didn't take too long for me to realize that Paisley needed more of a focused educational program than the public schools here could offer her, being from Fairfax County, I'm sure you understand. The schools down here just can't compare. So I put her in a private school in Shallotte and next year and the years after that it looks like she will be going to a school in Wilmington."

"I didn't realize all this before or we might not have moved here. But now that we have, I'm glad we did. Rusty is doing so much better than he was up North, he even skipped a grade. He has a lot of friends here and he just loves the beach. So the only problem was paying for Paisley's tuition, that's why I got the job at the Mini-Links."

"The children's father is nowhere around?" he asked, hoping that was true. The waiter laid the check on the table by Colin's arm and Colin, engrossed by the conversation, just laid his charge card on top of it, not even bothering to look at the bill.

"Rusty's father lives out west, we don't keep in contact. He hasn't seen Rusty since he was a baby. Paisley was artificially inseminated so there never was a father, per se. It's just the three of us and of course, our little dog Taffy. How about you? I gather that you and Adam's mother are no longer together."

"We were divorced about four years ago. Seems there was a Mr. Wonderful even more wonderful than me," he said with a wry grin.

"I'm so sorry," she said. "It can really be hard on the kids when things don't work out."

"I was very upset at the time, but now I'm actually very happy about it. You don't seem like the type to have an affair with a married man."

She looked up sharply and met his eyes. "I'm not the type to have an affair."

"You haven't had a relationship with anybody since Rusty was a baby?" He asked with incredulity.

"Well, yes, I was kind of engaged once, but we never, you know..."

"Since you and Rusty's father were separated you haven't...?"

"No. Sorry you bought dinner now?" she asked with a smirk.

"Not in a million years," he said while shaking his head and smiling.

The waiter brought back the charge card receipt for Colin to sign and thanked them for dining with them.

"Can I drive you home?" he asked.

"I can walk, it's not far," she replied.

"Well, can I walk you then?"

"Then you'd have to walk back to get your car."

"So?"

"Well, then I'd have to walk you back!" she said with a laugh.

"Okay," he said, "that'll work. We'll get our exercise walking back and forth all night and I'll get a chance to know you *better*." The word better had definitely been emphasized.

"Colin, you're not going to get a chance to know me *better*. You might as well know that now."

Oh, yeah? We'll just have to see about that won't we? he said to himself. To her he said, "I don't know what you mean, I'm not that kind of guy. I am not easy either, if that's what you're trying to infer."

She looked up at him and laughed. "Okay, how about driving me home after we've had a walk on the beach?"

He smiled broadly. "Good deal." And walked her over to his car.

"I noticed your car today," she said. I drive a white convertible, too. A Pontiac Sunfire."

"Is that the car company you used to work for?"

"Yes, A Pontiac and GMC dealership."

"I wish I hadn't bought this one," he said as he opened the passenger door for her to get in.

"Why not?" she asked.

"You'll see," He said as he walked around to his side to get in.

She watched him as he squeezed his large body in behind the wheel and lifted one knee with both hands to get it positioned right. She laughed and it sounded like music to his ears. "Didn't you test drive it first?"

"Yeah, but the only thing I noticed was the young girls on the street looking at me. Something about getting separated, separates you from your sanity."

She knew that to be a fact. She herself had been party to many such deals, she of course had been on the other side of the desk. Oh, the Firebirds she'd sold to middle-aged men looking for attention. She looked up at the sky, trying to put those days from the past out of her mind, in a small corner where she liked to keep them.

"Look at all the stars that are out tonight. This is one of the things I love the most about living here on the coast, away from the big city."

He looked over at her as she lay with her neck extended, her head on the head rest. It was hard for him to focus on his driving when all he wanted to do was to kiss her throat all the way down to her collar bone and beyond. He gripped the wheel and mentally went through the Redskins' front offensive line.

When they crossed over the bridge he debated as to whether he should just park at the main parking lot where the gazebo was or if he should park in front of his beach house where there was a beach access. Better not frighten her off, he thought. Take the slow and easy, safe and gentle approach. She was already a bit skittish.

They made their way down to the beach. It was completely dark now, but the moon and the lights from the houses illuminated the sand and the water's edge. She removed her sandals and he, his shoes. They left them by the boardwalk and they strolled down to the water. Eventually they had walked away from the thinning crowd and they were all alone.

"Adam and I rented a pontoon boat to go out on the Intracoastal tomorrow, would you and Paisley like to come with us? We could take a lunch and picnic on one of the islands behind Bird Island."

She thought for a moment. She liked him and she did want to see him again. With both kids, she could relax and enjoy getting to know him. And she loved being on the water. "Okay," she said tentatively. Then more enthusiastically, "I'll pack the lunch. I'll make some fried chicken and potato salad. Is there anything you and Adam don't eat?"

"Liver," he said with a grimace.

He reached down as they were walking and talking and took her hand. It felt warm and small in his and he loved the softness of it against his calloused palms. He took it as a good sign that she didn't pull away. They walked and talked hand in hand until she turned to him and said, "I think we should go back now." He put his hand on her cheek and leaned into her. She quickly averted her face. "No, it's too soon. I don't want to ruin it."

"Ruin it?" he asked perplexed.

"Ruin it," she repeated.

"Care to explain, how one kiss will ruin it?" He was a touch angry now and she knew it.

"Colin, I've had a really nice time. A nicer time than I've had for as long as I can remember. I'm not ready to be kissed. If the kiss isn't right, then it'll be over."

"Jenny, I guarantee you, the kiss will be right."

"I can't take the chance. What if it's not?"

"How long do you normally take before you try to find out?" he asked with a hard bite to his voice.

"Three or four dates," she said meekly.

"Three or four dates! Are you purposely trying to drive me crazy? I am aching to know how you taste. I've wanted to kiss you since I first laid eyes on you this morning."

"No, I'm not trying to drive you crazy. I don't know what it is I feel about you, but I want to stretch out this feeling. I don't get it very often."

"Trust me. It won't go away," he said softly as he put both hands on the sides of her face and leaned down to her.

She ducked her head and spun around. If she didn't let him kiss her tonight then at least she'd be able to see him again two more times before it was over.

"No! I want to wait! I'm just not ready for this."

He put both hands up, palms forward and backed away. "Okay, okay, we'll do it your way. Tomorrow counts for the second date right?"

"Yeah."

"Then I want to see you the next night, too. Let's agree on that now."

"Sure. If that's what you want."

"You know damn well what I want." Then added, "But we'll do it your way." He said softly as he reached for her hand again. They walked in silence back to the gazebo and then to the car.

He drove her across the bridge just enjoying looking at her as her hair, now loosened by the ocean breeze, fluttered around her face. She had no idea how beautiful she was. Or if she did, she didn't act like she knew.

He drove her home following her directions and stepped out to see her to the door. "Very nice house. I like the colors." It was a white house with a multicolored blue roof and blue shingles. The porch lights were on waiting for her to get home. The yard was nicely landscaped and trimmed. "A lot of work for such a little lady," he commented.

"I pay to have it done. I hate yard work."

"I'll pick you and Paisley up around ten o'clock if that's okay?"

"That would be fine. Thank you for dinner, I'll see you tomorrow."

He took her hand and pressed it to his lips. "This doesn't count does it?"

She blushed and said, "No, this doesn't count."

He spun around, went back to his car and backed down the driveway, waving his hand through the open top just as she opened the door to the house and looked back to wave at him.

Chapter 115

Sunset Beach

Jenny stayed up late that night making potato salad using her mother's recipe and then she baked some chocolate brownies. She got up early the next morning to make the fried chicken. She got a big cooler out of the garage and loaded it up with the potato salad, the chicken, some bread and butter pickles, fresh blueberries she'd bought at Holden's Farm Market, fresh baked rolls and some of the brownies. She didn't know why it was important to show off some of her culinary skills, it just was. She added some home-made lemonade and a few cans of soda for the kids.

She and Paisley were ready when Colin and Adam came to the door at ten. She invited them in and introduced Paisley and Taffy. Paisley was a little shy, but Taffy was delighted to meet any new body she could lick.

She led Colin around to the kitchen so he could lift the cooler. As he walked in he looked around and commented. "What a beautiful home. You have good taste. This looks like something you'd see in a magazine. I like that it's so bright and open and airy."

"Well, thank you. I've always like the idea of a great room, it seems so practical. When the builder and I designed it, I was looking for ways to save money. This way I've eliminated the living room and dining room and the extra furniture they would have required. The bonus I get a nice big kitchen that I absolutely love."

As he walked by the French doors leading out to the screened-in porch and deck he observed, "This looks like the view for the 1st hole of the Maples course."

She opened the doors and they walked outside. "Yes, it is, have you played it before?"

"Oh, many, many times. The Grand Strand is my home away from home. I think I can drive here from Fairfax blindfolded." He took in the cluster of Adirondack chairs facing the trees, the flower beds and the hammock strung between two trees gently swaying in the slight breeze. This was a nice home. It felt cozy here. "In fact, one of the reasons for my extended stay down here is to decide where I'd like to relocate to. With Adam out on his own, there's really no reason for me to stay up North anymore. And I need to be somewhere I can play golf all year 'round. Sea Trail was one of the places I was considering."

She didn't know why it pleased her so to hear that, but it did. She answered with a noncommittal, "Oh?"

"Yeah, I have an appointment tomorrow to check out Ocean Ridge and then next week I'll check out St. James Plantation. I prefer the developments that have more than one course."

"Mom, Adam wants to know if he can play one of my video games," Paisley called from inside the house.

Jenny turned and headed back inside, "Maybe when we get back. Colin's probably paying for this boat by the hour so we really should get going."

"Okay," she said glumly. She turned to Adam and said, "Later. They always say later. Ever notice that?"

"Yeah," Adam said commiserating with her. "But later's good. I'm anxious to get on the boat myself so I can throw you into the water!" He said giving her a big grin as he picked her up. "Let's see how much you weigh so I can figure out how far I can throw you!"

"Mom!" Paisley cried as she kicked her feet out at him.

"Okay, you two, behave," Colin said in a stern voice as he came back inside and locked the French doors. "Adam, help carry some of this stuff out."

He walked into the kitchen and looked at the cooler and the bag of chips, cups and napkins sitting beside it. "This is a day cruise you know, not a week," he said.

"Well, the Minnow was only going out for a three-hour cruise, you never know." she quipped.

"We'll be on the Intracoastal. It's hard to lose your way when there's land on both sides."

"With you driving, maybe. With me driving I can guarantee you I'd get us lost."

He bent down and lifted the cooler to his shoulder as if he was lifting a feather pillow. It had to ride as a middle passenger in the back seat as it was too large to fit into the trunk. She picked up her beach bag and the tote with the chips. Colin loaded everything into his car as she said goodbye to Taffy and locked the door.

As she got into the passenger seat beside him she said, "We have to be back by four or so. I don't like Taffy to go any longer than that without being walked."

"I don't think that'll be a problem. I'm sure we'll all have had enough fun in the sun by then," he said as he put the car in gear. "We're off! Everybody know how to swim? I've only driven one boat before in my life."

Jenny quickly turned her head and looked at him. In profile he was classically good-looking. Nice shaped eyebrows over eyes fringed with thick lashes, a straight nose, full lips and a rugged square jaw. "You're kidding aren't you?" she asked with some concern.

"No, I have some friends in Washington State that live on a lake and a few months ago when I was there visiting, Daniel showed me how to drive his new souped up motorboat. That's the only time I've ever been a captain. But how hard can it be? There are no lanes you have to stay in right?"

Jenny sighed and turned back to the kids who were playing some kind of slap-hand thing. "Make sure as soon as you get on that boat that you both put your life vests on and keep them on!"

Colin chuckled, "Don't worry so much, life is an adventure. Relax, I'll get you home safely. After all I don't want anything to interfere with tomorrow night," he said as he glanced over at her and focused on her lips.

She felt the heat course through her body as if some kind of a current had just entered it.

After a few minutes of silence, he reached over and squeezed her hand as it lay in her lap. "Speaking of tomorrow, is there anywhere special you would like to go?"

She thought for awhile and then said, "No, not really. Why don't you and Adam just come over to the house and we'll barbeque something on the grill."

"Sounds like a fine idea to me, and then after dinner we can have Adam take Paisley up to the Mini-Links for a few games of golf while we get to know one another *better*." Again that emphasis on the word better.

She looked down at his firm thighs spread wide as he straddled the steering wheel. Suddenly she wanted to run her hands over them, feel the coarse bristly hairs running through her fingertips. What was happening to her? She knew exactly what was happening. She was lusting for this man in a way she'd never lusted before. It was as if he had aroused a long dormant part of her feminine nature and it was awakening with some very strong impulses. She looked away just as his eyes met hers. He'd seen her looking at his groin area with longing, of that she was sure. The fire she saw in his eyes burned into hers, branding her as his.

They arrived at the marina in Little River just in time. Jenny felt as if she could jump in the water now, her skin was so overheated. The guys unloaded the car and put everything on the waiting boat. Then Colin went to the office, signed some papers and left his credit card as a deposit.

A man returned with Colin and went over everything on the boat with them. She noticed that Colin was listening very intently to his every instruction. She checked Paisley's and Adam's life vests making sure they were snug. Colin noticed and sneered at her. Then they were pushed off and on their way.

After they were well away from the marina and any other boats they all took a minute to remove their over clothes. When Colin whipped his T-shirt up and over his head, Jenny nearly swooned. The man was a god. His chest was everything she'd ever pictured while reading trashy romance novels, broad, tanned, well-defined and covered with dark curling hairs interspersed with a few silver ones. The silver stopped as the hairs tapered down from his chest toward his bathing suit. Those were all dark as they lined up to go under his waistband and down to his manhood. His flat stomach and visible latt muscles made her realize that this was obviously a man who exercised and kept in shape. The powerful muscles bunched on his arms were evidence that he also lifted weights.

Jenny had to sit down as she took him all in, her eyes traveling the long length of him before finding their way to his face and his twinkling blue eyes. He smiled at her obvious approval of him and winked at her. He knew how good he looked and he was dazzling her with it on purpose.

It was Jenny's turn, and if she hadn't known it, he had, as he nodded in her direction for her to uncover herself. She stood and turned her back to him as she slowly removed her T-shirt. Then she didn't know what happened to her. Something got into her head and she decided why should she be the only one agitated and uncomfortable. She unsnapped the top of her cutoffs, zipped down the zipper and shimmied out of them with a few extra wiggles than she actually needed to get them past her hips. Then she just let them drop and stepped out of them. She smiled when she heard his loud gasp. Two could play the game he'd started.

Looking down at her chest she made sure her skimpy top was covering all the essential parts of her and then she slowly turned around. The look she saw as his eyes popped wide was worth the price she'd paid for this suit. Her best asset was pushed up for maximum cleavage and although there was still plenty left to tantalize the imagination, all you had to do was follow the curving lines of the material to get the idea of the shape of her breasts. Full and high were mounds that would overflow even his large hands. He grabbed his sunglasses and a baseball cap from his beach bag and turned back to take the wheel from Adam before she could notice the way she had affected him.

For several hours they all took turns driving while Colin stood at the ready. Jenny had been on many boat rides but had never driven one herself and she found that she enjoyed it, especially when Colin put his hand on her shoulder to lean in to tell her something. Nothing he was murmuring was that essential for her to know, so she knew exactly what he was doing. His breathing on her neck as well as his eyes feasting down her cleavage was doing incredible things to the lower part of her, making her wish at times that the kids had not accompanied them. But thank God they had, or he could have taken her right here on the boat if he'd wanted to, something she had to make sure he never knew.

They found a small, mostly deserted island just before the inlet to the Ocean. They anchored the boat a hundred feet or so from the shore and carried the things they would need ashore. As the water was only three feet deep most of the way in, Colin had no trouble carrying the large cooler on his shoulder. Jenny and the kids followed with a blanket and everything else.

Jenny had finally acquiesced and let them remove their life jackets since they were no longer on the boat. Earlier on the boat, when Jenny moved to put one on herself after removing her over clothes, Colin took it from her and tossed it away saying, "First of all it's not necessary and second, you'll spoil the view."

Adam helped Jenny spread the blanket while Paisley went to find things to put on the corners to keep it down. Then they opened the cooler and spread everything out on the blanket. It was better to keep the food sand-free than themselves. They all sat on an edge and ate until they were stuffed.

"You are a wonderful cook," Colin commented, "this is the best fried chicken I've had in I don't know how long. And look at Adam, he's on his third helping of potato salad."

"Dad, you're not supposed to comment on what other people are eating. You always told me not to, remember?"

"You're right. Forgive me," he said shooting him a lopsided smile.

Everybody helped clean up and then the kids went to play in the water.

"You outdid yourself," Colin said as he reached for another brownie. "These are great. Can't eat too many though, I'll lose my boyish figure."

"There's nothing boyish about you, Colin," Jenny said as she stretched out on the blanket. "You are all man, one hundred percent."

"So you noticed, huh?"

"How could one not?"

"I started really getting into working out when Lynn, my ex, left me. It's how I spent the lonely hours passing time. Plus, I knew I had to get back into the dating scene sooner or later and I figured, what the heck? Women seem to like the big and brawny guys, why not give 'em what they want? You're no slouch in the body department either, your figure is unbelievable. You must work out too."

"I do an aerobics class two or three times a week plus I take karate."

That caused his eyebrows to lift a bit. "Really, what belt?"

"I'm stuck on brown, I don't have the discipline now to go for black, or the time really. I can only get to the class once a week most weeks."

"Is this something you do so you can fend the guys off?" he asked.

"No, it's just something I've always wanted to do. Rusty's a black belt. He took lessons in Herndon for three years. He wanted to quit, but I wouldn't let him until he got his black belt. He did it in record time and then quit."

"So, do you date much down here?" he asked as he brushed some sand off of the blanket and laid down on his side with his hand supporting his head, looking up at her.

"Everybody on the Plantation has a son or a grandson they want to fix me up with. I tell them I'm just too busy right now to get involved. I've gone out with a few to things like Christmas parties and some shows in Myrtle Beach."

"But nothing on going?" he questioned persistently.

"No." She was quiet for a few minutes before saying. "Colin, I'm sort of a weird duck when it comes to men. I've only had sex with one man, and that was my husband. I've just always thought I had to be married before I gave into that kind of thing."

"Do you still feel that way now?" he said looking directly into her eyes.

"Sometimes I do, sometimes I don't. You spend enough New Year's Eves alone and you begin to wonder about all the restrictions you put on yourself."

The kids hollered for them to join them. Colin looked down the length of her, stopping at the two pieces of cloth that concealed the parts that most aroused a man. "What a waste," he said as he got up and then her pulled her to her feet. "Let's go see if we can dunk some heads."

They played with the kids in the water until they were all tired. Then Jenny reminded everyone that it was time to replenish their sunscreens. With a groan from Paisley they all trudged back to shore to the blanket. Jenny helped Paisley and Colin helped Adam, then the kids went off to find out what was on the other side of the island. Colin called after them to be back in an hour so they could get the boat back on time. Then he picked up his sunscreen and squirted some into his hand. "C'mere, let me do you." he said aware of the double entendre.

"Not a chance," she replied. "Just do yourself, you must be used to it by now." She countered returning one double-edged statement with another.

He laughed uproariously. And she smiled over at him.

He walked over to her and spun her around smearing a generous handful of lotion on her back. "Since massaging your front is out of the question, I'll have to be content with doing your back." He gently rubbed her back and shoulders running his fingertips under the straps of her top and letting his fingertips stray slightly below the waistband of her bottom. It felt wonderful and even though it was close to ninety degrees outside, she got goose bumps.

When he handed her the lotion and turned his back on her she realized just how tall he was. She had to extend her hand all the way to reach the tops of his shoulders. His skin felt smooth and warm and his muscles were firm beneath her hands. His back was so broad that she soon opted to use both of her hands. His back was sprinkled with a few dark hairs at the top. As she coated them with lotion they laid down and became almost straight. Just above his waistband on his right side she noticed a small scar. "What's this from?" she asked.

"An over zealous Marine I arrested once. He had been frisked by my partner but apparently he missed a small knife. Luckily, I turned around when I did, or it would have gone into my gut. As it was it didn't go all the way through my belt. It was just a small cut. Couldn't golf for a month though, that was hard."

"You really like that game, huh?" she asked though she already knew the answer.

"Yeah, I do. When I get out on the course, nothing else matters. It's a wonderful sense of freedom. Ever tried it?"

"No. And I don't ever want to either. As far as I'm concerned, if the object is to hit the ball the least amount of times possible, why hit it at all?"

She had him laughing again. This time he put his arm around her shoulder and pulled her close as he kissed her near her ear. "You're wonderful, you know that?" he whispered.

She looked up at his smiling blue eyes and smiled back, "My mother always tells me so."

They walked around the small island digging their toes into the wet sand trying to follow the small clams as they buried themselves with each new wave of water on the shore. They found the kids poking at a crab with a stick trying to make it grab onto it.

"C'mon guys, time to head back," Colin called to them.

"Aw, Mom, do we have to?" Paisley wailed.

"Yes, we do. Hurry up. Those dark clouds over there look a little threatening. We don't want our novice captain to have to deal with a storm on top of everything else."

They carried everything back to the boat, the tide making it deeper than it had been before.

When they got back to the Marina, Colin collected his credit card while Adam and Jenny stowed everything in the trunk, except for the cooler. When they arrived back at Jenny's they hosed off in the driveway, trying to get rid of as much sand as possible. The kids squirted each other and then Colin grabbed Jenny by the arm as he held the hose on Jenny's cleavage and said with a raspy voice, "Show me those hard nipples, like you were showing me yesterday." Jenny pulled away from him and managed to wrest the hose away from him. Before he knew what she was about to do she jammed the hose down the front of his bathing suit and said, "I think you need some cooling off!" He yelped and hopped around as he pulled the hose out.

"You have no mercy." he said to her when he finally got his breath back.

She smiled and retorted, "Kindly remember that."

Colin carried the cooler into the garage so Jenny could empty it and then he and Adam said good-bye to Paisley and Jenny. Colin looked directly into Jenny's eyes and leaned down to whisper in her ear, "That's two down, one to go."

Chapter 116

Sunset Beach

Colin and Adam showed up the next evening around five o'clock. Jenny opened the door and Colin smiled with a little chagrin. "I forgot to ask what time we were supposed to be here before we left yesterday. And I didn't have your phone number or your last name, either. The mini-golf wouldn't give me your number, but they did give me your last name. Do you know how many J. Millers there are in the phone book?"

Jenny held her hand over her mouth and laughed.

"Well, are we too early? Should we leave and come back?" he asked.

"No, come on in. I could use some extra help in the kitchen," she said as she wiped her hands on a dish towel. "Adam, why don't you see if Paisley wants to set up that video game for you to play?"

"Okay," he called as he went off to the right side of the house towards Paisley's bedroom.

"Ah," Colin said as he pulled her into his arms, "now's my chance."

Jenny pulled away, pushing hard against his chest. "Oh, no. That's for the end of the third date."

"Really?" he asked. She nodded. "I didn't know that," he said humbly. He backed off, his hands up in the air, "But I don't want to break any rules here. What's for dinner?"

She led him around the counter to the kitchen. "Steak, potatoes, corn, and salad. Then we have a nice Orange Delight cake for dessert."

"I already have my dessert planned," he said.

She threw the towel in his face.

He looked around the kitchen and saw pieces of foil spread around and a cutting board and knife. "How can I help?" he asked.

"Well, we need to cut some potatoes and onions into large chunks. Think you can handle that?"

"Yup!"

"You're not gonna cry are ya? I hate to see grown men cry."

"I'll try not to."

"Okay, here are the potatoes, the onions are in the bowl over by the sink, there's the cutting board and knife. I believe in very sharp knives, so be careful." she admonished.

"So, how was your day?" she asked him as he washed his hands. Jenny knew he had planned to visit Ocean Ridge today.

"Oh, it was good. I had a good round of golf at Lion's Paw, courtesy of the sales department. And then I went on a tour of the Plantation and looked at a few model homes."

"Well, what did you think?"

"I liked the course and they will eventually have three, but it was more or less a links style course and I don't think that's as challenging. The homes were nice, but a bit bigger than I need. Actually, I'm thinking that a condo would be more my style."

"So, Ocean Ridge, is out?"

"Yeah, I think so. What did you do today?" he asked.

"Paisley and I went to the pool. Taffy and I took a long walk. I did some housework and then we went to the grocery store."

"Sounds like you could stand a little more excitement in your life. I hereby apply for the position." When she arched a brow at him, he hurriedly added, "Okay, potatoes and onions are done, what's next?"

"Next, we're going to put a few potatoes in the center of each piece of foil, like this." She showed him and he placed the rest of the potatoes on the other three sheets. "Then we put a few pieces of onion on top of the potatoes, except for Paisley's, she doesn't like onion." He plopped a few chunks of onion on three foil pieces. She handed him a crystal butter dish and a small knife, "A few slices on top of the onions." He sliced off eight pieces of butter. Then she handed him a jar of salsa, taking back the butter dish and knife and giving him a large spoon. "A tablespoon or two goes on top of the butter, except for Paisley, she doesn't like tomatoes." When he was finished doing that she handed him a bottle of garlic powder. "Sprinkle some of this on each one, except.."

"I know, except for Paisley's, she doesn't like garlic."

"You're really getting the hang of this."

"What's next?"

"Half a piece of corn." She pointed to the dish of corn on the cob, each piece had already been broken in half.

"Then a little salt and pepper and you're done. Except for the wrapping and cooking. She showed him how to wrap them in little bundles leaving some room for the steam and then she put them on a cookie sheet.

"Okay, now we cook these on the grill. How are you at grilling? It's supposed to be like second nature with you guys."

"I haven't grilled out since I lost my grill in the flood." he said.

"What? What flood?"

"There was no flood, that just what I call it when I'm referring to something I lost in my divorce. People ask you a lot of questions about a divorce, not so many about a flood. You'd think it would be the other way around though, a divorce being so personal and all."

"Yeah, I know. I lost a lot of things 'in the flood' too." she said.

"C'mon let's go out to the grill and you can tell me all about it."

"Want to take a drink with us?" she asked.

"Yeah, that's a good idea. But only one, I don't want anything dulling my senses tonight."

She put a bottle of Canadian Club on the counter and a bottle of ginger ale.

"Aw, you remembered. You didn't just go buy that for me did you?"

"Are you kidding?" She walked over to the pantry door and opened it. There on the floor, covering the whole floor area was every kind of liquor imaginable. "When you're in the car business, everybody thinks you drink a lot. Every Christmas, I got replenished."

He chuckled as he fixed himself a drink.

"Just what did you do in the car business?"

"I managed. I managed a.." Just then there was a loud crash from Paisley's bedroom. Jenny and Colin both ran to see what had happened.

Somehow Adam in all his enthusiasm for the game had managed to pull the game off the ledge where it was positioned on top of the TV. Sheepishly he stood, joystick in his hand, while Paisley stood there with her hand over her mouth going "Awww."

"Adam! What have you done?" Colin shouted.

"It's okay, Colin, everything's fine, Rusty's done this before, too. It's no big deal. Let's just put it back up there."

Colin and Adam put the game back on the shelf and reconnected it. Then Colin gave Adam a hard stare. "Be more careful, next time."

"Geez, Dad, it was an accident."

"I know, just try not to have any more."

Colin and Jenny returned to the kitchen and carried everything out to the grill on the back deck. Jenny let Colin start it up and place the packets on the grate before she sat down at the table with her drink. She propped her crossed feet on an empty chair. He came over, picked them up, sat down and replaced them in his lap.

"Nice feet," he said stroking the top of her instep, admiring the cute little toes covered with light pink polish. "Now, why don't you tell me about your 'flood'?"

He continued to rub her feet while she told him about R.J. and what seemed to be a life she'd lived eons ago.

"Must have been hard, the prospect of raising a kid all by yourself," he said.

"I had my parents and really, I think it was better this way. I never would have had Paisley the other way."

She went inside to get the steaks that had been marinating.

598

"So tell me about Paisley," he said as he added the steaks to the grill.

They talked about Paisley and how she was conceived until the steaks were done.

"Does she know?"

"Sort of, as much as an eight year old can understand. She knows she's special and that I wanted her so badly that I had a doctor help me have her. When she's older I'll explain it in more detail."

Jenny went to get the salad and the dressings, then called the kids. They ate out on the screened-in porch and Jenny beamed at Colin's lavish praise. After the meal Adam took Paisley up to the Mini-golf. Paisley got all her golf free and so did her guests. Adam had brought his own car and Jenny thought that Colin had probably suggested that. The man didn't miss a trick. Together they cleaned up the mess and were sitting outside enjoying the night when the kids returned.

Adam said something about hanging out at the video game concession at the beach and excused himself after thanking Jenny for the meal. Paisley was sent to get a bath and then to bed.

Both of them knew what was coming, and Jenny had to admit that she was a little tense.

"Is it the end of the date, yet?" Colin asked.

"It is if you're leaving," she replied.

"Well, I'm leaving, then."

She walked him to the door and they stood in the foyer looking at each other.

"What are you so afraid of?" he asked her.

"I don't know."

"Come here." She walked into his arms. He wrapped his arms around her and slowly lowered his head to hers, keeping his eyes locked on hers. Then he gently placed his lips on top of hers and crushed them under his. The kiss was sweet and gentle as his lips moved over hers and then he held her tighter as his passion took control and he changed the kiss into a searing, torrid kiss

599

that melted away all of her resistance. Her arms reached up and went around his neck as she opened her mouth to his. His tongue thrust into her yielding mouth with a driving insistent wildness. When she groaned, he shuddered and devoured her honeyed sweetness as if his very soul needed it to survive. She had been waiting for this kiss forever and her body viscerally tightened as his tongue repeatedly plunged into her. When he released her it was only because they both needed to breathe. The kiss had been perfect, and they both knew it.

"I've changed my mind, I'm not leaving now," he said as he bent down and put his hands behind her knees. He picked her up and carried her over to the sofa. He sat down and sat her on his lap. Then he put a hand on each side of her face and kissed her again, his fingers tangling in her hair as he pulled her closer to him. He kissed her over and over again until they were both breathless and she was quaking. He rubbed the side of her neck with his thumb while he pressed his forehead against hers.

Panting, he managed to breathe the words, "What do we get to do on the fourth date?"

She laughed a delightful little laugh, "I don't know, it's been years since I ever had more than one."

He kissed every part of her face, her eyelids, her brows, her nose, her chin and then he moved her hair away from her ears and languorously labored over them, licking all around her ear lobe breathing fevered hot kisses into them, all the while groaning and gasping and telling her that she tasted so good.

When he trailed kisses down her throat to the beginning of her cleavage his hand joined his lips there and he cupped her fullness over her shirt, brushing his thumb over her already distended nipple as it pushed up against her bra. Deftly he unbuttoned the front of her shirt and opened it, moving it away so he could feast his eyes. He was already rampart hard and probing up against her bottom, he could imagine what the sight of seeing her was going to do to him. He pulled his lips away from the rising swell of her breasts and looked down at her in her lacy demi-cup bra. "Aw, Jenny, if you're going to make me stop, you'd better do it now while I still can." She slowly sat up and pulled her shirt back together. She moved to get off his lap, but he held her there. "No, don't get up, stay here." He looked into her eyes. "Oh, what you do to me. I've got a hard on that's like iron. Tell me, what's it like for you? Are you as turned on as I am?"

"That expression, that one you said. When a man is aroused and ready he says, 'he's hard' or he 'has a hard on.' What's the expression for a woman to use?"

He thought for a minute. "I don't know. She's ready? She's hot? She's horny?"

"Why not I'm soft? I have a soft on? We are the exact opposite that way."

"No. How about I'm wet, ready and yielding?" he suggested. "She could say, I'm ready to yield to your hardness," he joked.

"So, I don't get a hard on, I get a *yield field*?" she asked.

"Yeah, so yield your field baby!"

He kissed her deeply and then pulled away and asked softly, "So when are you going to 'yield your field' to me?"

"I don't know. I guess we'll have to talk about that, but not tonight. I can't even think straight."

He bent to kiss her again, this time softer and more leisurely, trying not to get his passion out of control again.

Twenty minutes later she walked him to the door, her lips swollen and her breasts aching from the engorgement of being aroused by his kisses.

"This is where we started about an hour ago," she said.

"Yeah, and it's nowhere near finished. Count on it. Good night. I'll call you tomorrow. I got the number off the phone." He stooped down to taste her lips one last time before leaving.

She watched him walk jauntily to his car and then closed and locked the door. She went into the master bathroom to get ready for bed, she looked into the mirror as she brushed her teeth. There was a light in her eyes that sparkled. As soon as the toothpaste was gone from around her mouth she noticed that her lips and the skin around them were red and chafed. She rubbed them with Vaseline. Wouldn't do to get chapped lips now. Not now when she'd finally found someone whose kisses were perfect.

Chapter 117

Sunset Beach

Jenny had to work at the mini-golf the next day so she took Paisley to keep her company and to help her fish the balls out of the pond by the first hole. They really were getting low on extra balls but Jenny kept wondering if her real reason for being over by the first hole was so she could see Colin's car if he drove past. She had forgotten to tell him that she was supposed to work today when he'd said he'd call her. When she had pulled into the lot this morning she had purposely pulled her car into the first slot so her car would be visible from the road whenever he came off the island. Then he'd know she was at work. All this worrying about missing a phone call was beginning to make her feel like she was in high school again.

The morning dragged by as she tried to keep busy and not think about what had happened last night. Last night she had wanted Colin to touch her. Everywhere. The feeling was so foreign to her that she kept trying to reject it and dismiss it as being caused by something else. But she hadn't been drinking. She hadn't had any provocative dreams lately and she hadn't been reading any particularly torrid romance book. She was just a single mother, spending time with an absolute hunk of a man, who desired her as much as she desired him. Maybe that was the key.

That Colin wanted her and made no bones about it was certainly thrilling. That he had intimated that he was in fact going to have her, electrified her and made her feel defenseless against the sensual power he had over her.

He said they'd talk. He was going to make an assault on her common sense. Just what approach he would use would be interesting to see. Would it be the "I'm a man, you're a woman, let's do what comes natural approach?" Or would it be the "You want me, I want you, let's just do it baby", approach. That it would feel so right she had no doubt. That it was so wrong for the way she'd led her life she was certain. So why did she want to be with him so much? Why did she shudder when she remembered being in his arms? Why did the very center of her fill with a hot, restless need when she remembered him opening her shirt last night? She could feel the flush on her face as she recalled his kisses. Just where was he, anyway? She thought impatiently. Why does the man always get to be the one who sets the timetable? If he didn't call 'til 11:59 tonight, he'd still be keeping his word about calling today. And she'd be a basket case.

She and Paisley were just cleaning up the mess from their outdoor picnic lunch. They were sitting at a picnic table under some trees in a small clearing near hole 16, when Jenny recognized the sound of his car. That was one thing about the car business that would never leave her. She could almost always define a car by its sound or a glimpse of its fender. Her heart immediately started to race in anticipation of seeing him. But she didn't turn around. She willed herself to face forward, hearing him walking up behind her until she heard Paisley exclaim, "It's Colin and Adam!"

Even then she didn't turn as she felt him take her long braid and move it over to her shoulder. He then bent and placed a kiss at the base of her neck close to her collarbone. She almost fell off the bench backwards, and probably would have if he hadn't grabbed her shoulders. "Surprise you, did I?" he asked in a sultry deep voice.

She looked up at him as he stood close behind her. "Yes you did, in fact," her voice unintentionally coming out as a soft purr.

He came around and sat on the bench opposite her. "Forget to tell me something last night?" he asked as he clasped her hands in his in the center of the table. Out of the corner of her eye she saw Paisley drag Adam off to play golf.

"Yes, I was pretty flustered when you left last night, if you'll recall. It didn't dawn on me until I was in bed setting the alarm that I hadn't told you I had to work today. I'm sorry."

"That's okay, I knew where to find you." He added softly, "Same place I found you the first time."

They looked into each other's eyes for several minutes, neither saying anything. God, he looked good, she thought.

God, she was so beautiful, he thought.

The slamming of cars doors alerted her to the fact that pretty soon she'd have new customers to tend to. She gently removed her hands from his and stood up, collecting the trash and depositing it into the trash can by making a perfect arcing toss.

"Whoa, the lady's an athlete," he said with admiration.

"Only with a paper bag. Can't seem to do it with a basketball," she said wryly.

"Yeah, I saw that basketball hoop on the side of your driveway. Does Rusty play?" he asked.

"No," she smiled, "Paisley does."

"Like mother, like daughter."

They walked over to the hut and he leaned on the counter with his arms crossed just as he'd done the very first time she'd seen him. Her heart actually ached at the sight of him there and yet it seemed natural for him to be there, coming to see her.

He watched her as she waited on the customers, smiling and teasing the kids, bantering with the adults. She had a natural beauty that didn't require makeup. He took his time analyzing all he could see of her while she assisted a large family reunion group. Her hands were elegant and dainty with her own nicely manicured nails polished a pale pink. She wore absolutely no jewelry, though he could tell that her ears were pierced. She had nicely shaped ears and he remembered lingering over them with his tongue last night. Her flaxen hair had several strands of different colors blended throughout which were interwoven into a smooth even braid that went just to where her bra strap was visible through her shirt. He wondered if it was similar to the one she'd been wearing last night. Just the thought of her and the way she'd looked last night in her lacy bra caused a generous amount of blood to begin flowing through his veins in response to his body's command. He was glad he had the counter to shield him.

Her white sleeveless shirt had a wide collar that came to a deep vee, with only three buttons starting at her cleavage and ending in a knot tied just above her waist. If she stretched or lifted her arms he got a fleeting glance at her midriff. She wore cuffed jean shorts that made her tanned legs look long, even though he knew they couldn't be. She was way shorter than he was, probably by almost a foot. She had well-formed calves and nice knees, the thighs were firm and sleek but they had just the barest jiggle when she walked. Following the shapely line of her legs were her slim ankles and small feet tucked into backless sandals. You wouldn't know this woman had borne two kids. Her trim figure didn't show any signs of stretch marks or extra fat. She must have always taken good care of her body.

He was standing at the end of the counter now, near the scorecards and bug spray, trying to stay out of the way of the people paying and the people picking out their putters. A group of tired golfers with their own putters in hand came up to the register and started chatting with Jenny. He heard one say "So, if I get a hole-in-one on number 2 or number 18, I get a free game and another chance to come see you. Honey, you know I'm gonna get one, just fill out the ticket right now." He was hitting on Jenny and Colin didn't like it, not one bit. Colin was about to vault the counter and smash his face in when Jenny said in a sweet syrupy southern voice, "Now sir, golf is a game of honor. Only fishermen tell lies." The other three golfers guffawed and one slapped him on the back. "She sure put you in your place, Charlie! Golf doesn't seem to be your game today." They moved away and selected their balls. As they walked by Colin gave "Charlie" a look that told him Jenny was off limits.

Jenny saw the angry look on Colin's face as he turned back to her. "Low lying scum!" he said out the side of his mouth.

Jenny laughed. "Colin, it's only a group of guys out having some fun after a game of golf and a few beers, lighten up. I'm sure you've done a lot worse after a game of golf."

That he had. The drinking that accompanied some of his golf trips down here had often incapacitated him for the next day's game. "Yeah, I guess you're right. I just don't like the idea of another man even looking at you. What have you done to me Jenny?" he asked with a grimace on his face.

She laughed again. "It's been years since another man has been jealous over me."

"And just why is that Jenny? You're absolutely gorgeous. Why have you been alone all these years?"

"Just busy I guess. And the fact that I drag two youngsters around with me everywhere I go does tend to limit my prospects, you know."

"You could have ten kids and I'd still want you. You do know that I want you don't you?" he asked as his eyes bored into hers.

"I know. What I don't know is what for?" she answered with a sugary smile.

"How 'bout when you get off I show you," he said with a leer. Then he added, "And of course, I'm willing to feed you first. You and your ten kids."

"It's still just me and Paisley until Saturday. I promised her Sharkey's pizza if she was good today, and she's been excellent, so I can't let her down."

"Well can we get two pizzas? Or is this strictly a mother-daughter thing?"

"No, I'm sure she'd be delighted if Adam came. Are you paying him to keep her *occupied*?" she asked with a raised eyebrow.

He laughed. "Not so far, but I will if that's what it takes."

"I notice you're not wearing your bathing suit under your clothes, are you wearing the same bra you wore last night?" he asked huskily.

Her cheeks flushed instantly. "It was still wet from when I washed it out last night, and no, it's a different one."

"What size do you wear? You look like you could be a 38C or D."

"Colin! Stop that!"

A customer came to the counter and told them that the soda machine took his dollar. Jenny grabbed the key, opened the machine and gave him the bottle that was stuck in the chute. Noticing that it could stand to be refilled she enlisted Colin's help carrying the racks from the storage shed.

"Getting the balls out of the well, restocking soda machines, pretty soon you're gonna have to put me on the payroll, lady," he joked. "Either that or let me take it out in trade."

"And just who should be paying who for that?" she asked trying to feign a scathing reply.

"Honey, I'm so good, *you're* going to want to pay me," he said with an exaggerated air of confidence.

"And who says I'm not any good?"

He put the rack of sodas he'd been carrying down in front of the machine, reached into his front pants pocket and pulled out his money clip. He grabbed her hand and pulled it in front of her chest, palm up. Then he put the money clip in her palm. "That's all I have with me right now. I'll use it to pay you or you can use it to pay me. When we're finished we'll decide who gets to keep the money." She looked down at her palm. The clip was full, there was a $100 bill on top.

"Let me see what you think I'm worth," she counted it. There was $1300 there. "So you think I'm worth $1300?" she asked.

"No, I think you're worth millions, but that's all I have. You're missing the whole point though, the money will be coming back to me. I'm that good."

"We'll see," she said, "In the mean time you'd better hold onto that, it could be a long time before we find out who gets to keep it."

"Damn!" he said as he put the money clip back in his pocket and began refilling the machine.

Jenny took one of the empty trays back to the shed and got another full one. Damn! is right, she thought. Of all the

608

approaches she'd considered he'd use, she never thought he'd offer to pay for her!

After they finished with the soda machine and Paisley and Adam finished their game, Colin took Adam home so they could shower and change for dinner. It was agreed that they would all meet at Jenny's at 6:30. That would give her time to freshen up too.

They ate pizza and drank Bloody Mary's at Sharkey's and then went back to Jenny's for a game of Mille Bornes, a French card game that challenged two teams to outdo each other getting a thousand miles. Jenny and Adam were one team and Colin and Paisley were the other. They played twice, both sides winning once.

Then Colin pointedly asked Adam to go play fish or war or something with Paisley in her room for a few minutes. They had obviously discussed the possibility of this happening because Adam said, "Of course, Dad," with a knowing smile and quickly ushered Paisley out of the room.

Jenny cleaned up the mess from the table and straightened the chairs. Colin came around to where she was fidgeting and turned her to him as his arms went around her waist meeting at the base of her spine, where they locked. He held her close. She could smell the maleness of him. The musky masculine scent of him blended with the woodsy pine scent of his aftershave in her nostrils. Imperceptibly she breathed in deeper trying to capture his scent forever.

"Jenny, I couldn't sleep last night, thinking about you." He bent his head at an angle and placed his lips oh so gently over hers. He moved them lightly over hers savoring the soft fullness of her lips. When he deepened the kiss she was ready. She moved into his hardened body and put her arms around his neck. When she threaded her fingers through his hair and pulled his head closer to hers he groaned and the sound of it made her knees weak. She lapped at his lips and limned her tongue all around the inside of his lips brushing against his teeth with her tongue. He became almost savage then, thrusting his tongue in

609

and out with fevered persistence, trying to feed on the essence of her.

When he finally loosened his grip and eased himself away from her it was only for an instant. He pressed his lips back to hers, taking first her top lip between his and then the bottom one. Then he kissed the sides of her mouth and plundered her all over again, bringing her back into the fold of his powerful arms, molding her against his hard chest. He swallowed the soft moan that came from her lips.

When finally he gripped her shoulders and set her away from him, his breath was ragged and his eyelids were heavy over eyes burning with desire. "Jenny," he gasped. "I don't know about you, but I can't take much more of this." He took her hand that was against his chest and pulled it down to feel the hard bulge that was between them. He was unprepared for the torture that brought as she gently wrapped her fingers around him and squeezed him. "Oh, my God!" he said as he laid his head down on her shoulder. After a few moments he moved his hand down to where hers was and gently removed it. "As good as that feels, I can't believe you want me to walk out of your house with the front of my pants wet."

"If we're going to keep seeing each other, we're going to have to have some guidelines here. And, we *are* going to keep seeing each other," he said adamantly.

"Do you work tomorrow?" he asked.

"No," she answered.

"Then can you meet me for breakfast? We have to talk. Without the kids. And there needs to be a lot of people around."

"Why a lot of people?"

"So I can't get distracted from what we need to discuss. You can bring Paisley to the beach house. Adam can watch cartoons with her and then take her for a walk to the beach stores. Okay?"

"Okay. What time?"

"Say, eight o'clock, eight thirty. Whenever you get there."

He put one arm around her waist and walked her towards the door. "Adam!" he called. "You ready to go?"

"Coming!" was the reply they heard.

"I hope you get a good night's sleep," she said softly.

"Yeah, me too. Although I kind of doubt it. My problem is getting worse, not better. Now if I could sneak back and sleep with you, I'm sure everything would be all right by morning, I'd be refreshed and oh so satisfied."

"And so broke," she teased.

He laughed. "It would be more than worth it, I'm sure."

"Good night," he said as he kissed her on her forehead. "Sweet dreams," he said to Paisley as she came and hugged his leg while he tousled her hair.

Chapter 118

Sunset Beach

The next morning Jenny drove over the bridge with Paisley, timing it so she'd catch the bridge open to vehicle traffic and arrive at Colin's beach house shortly after 8:00 am. The beach house he had rented was on the more desirable west end, right on the ocean just about at 32nd Street. The name on the colorful carved wooden sign was Family Tides.

It was huge and very nicely decorated in mauves and teals. Jenny knew houses like these rented for close to $2,000 a week during peak season. They were in peak season. Had he really spent close to $16,000 just on accommodations for his vacation?

Paisley had to go to the upper level to drag Adam out of bed. He reluctantly stumbled out of bed and down the stairs, dragging his comforter behind him. When he plopped on one of the sofas and wrapped himself cocoon-style in the comforter, Paisley settled in beside him. Rug rats was on, a cartoon Jenny didn't particularly care for but could really find no reason to censure, other than its true to life crudity.

"He doesn't look done yet," Jenny said, "he looks like he needs to go back and cook a little while longer."

Colin laughed. "He had a late night last night. There were some kids on the beach who asked him to join them for a clam fest on the east end."

They left the two of them snuggled side by side, Paisley enraptured with the antics of the Rug rats, Adam snuggling in for a few more minutes of shut eye.

Jenny and Colin got into his car and drove over the bridge to the mainland. Jenny suggested Nell's for breakfast so that's where they went.

When they were settled into a booth and served some coffee, Colin reached for Jenny's hand. He stroked it tenderly. "I missed you last night. I went from one side of the bed to the other all night trying to find you."

Jenny blushed and smiled slightly. "I missed you, too. But I slept like a baby. You know, I've often wondered where that expression came from. Baby's generally don't sleep all that well, at least not at first."

"I guess that's true. I wasn't home at night very much with Adam. I was working the third shift when he was born."

"It must've been very hard on your wife not having you there."

"I guess she got used to it. When she got tired of it, instead of telling me, she found a replacement," Colin said with some bitterness.

"Weren't there any signs that the marriage was in trouble?" Jenny asked.

"If there were, I sure didn't see them. I think that was the hardest part for me to accept. Someone I trusted, living with me, sleeping beside me every night, being so deceitful. And me being oblivious to it all. It makes me think that it could happen like that again and that scares me."

"Were you still being intimate with each other?" Jenny asked quietly.

"Yes, but there wasn't the same passion that there used to be. I didn't want her like I want you, I never wanted her as much as I want you." His eyes met hers and she could see the heat in them.

The waitress came and they gave her their orders. Then Colin took both of her hands in his and leaned part way over the table. "Have you ever noticed that within ten minutes of our being together one of us always turns the conversation to sex?"

Jenny laughed. "Yes and that one of us is usually you!"

He laughed too. "That's because we have this chemistry between us and it's drawing us together."

"What a line! C'mon Colin, you can do better than that. Besides I almost flunked chemistry. I never could understand it. Chances are I won't now."

"Jenny, don't tell me you don't feel the way I do, That you don't feel aroused every time I'm around. It's in your eyes. It's in the way you breathe and the way you look at me. At least admit it. You want me as much as I want you, and you know it." He stared at her intently challenging her to deny it.

"Okay, I admit it. I want you. Now what?" she whispered softly, conscious of the public arena they were in. Nell's was THE local's hangout. She'd already seen several people that she knew walk in.

His insides clenched at her words. He knew she wanted him, it was just exhilarating to hear her actually say it.

In answer to her question he gave her a little smile as he squeezed her hand. "We give in to it. We let our passions take control."

"Just like that. We just go hop in bed and get passionate."

"Yup. Best thing to do, feeling the way we do."

"Tell me something Colin. Have all the women you've ever dated just fallen into bed with you?" she asked with just a touch of anger in her voice.

"Yes," he said as he shoveled a bit of omelet into his mouth. Somehow their food had shown up and Jenny hadn't even been aware of it. She looked down at her pecan pancakes and started putting butter and syrup on them.

"Well, I'm not like them!"

"I know. We'd have already done it by now if you were."

"This conversation is over!" she said imperiously.

"No it's not!" he said putting his fork down loud enough to call attention to them.

"Colin, please don't make a scene," Jenny implored.

"Okay. Then talk to me. What worries you? Why are you trying to talk yourself out of doing something you obviously want to do very much. You're an adult, you're allowed to enjoy adult pleasures. You're a luscious woman, you should have a rutting man. And I hereby apply for the job."

"It's not that easy. At least not anymore," she said as she put a bite of pancake in her mouth. "Now you have to know your partner and every partner they've had for at least fifteen years back." After another bite, she added, "You have to be worried about so many kinds of diseases. And I'm not on any kind of contraception. I don't want to get pregnant. I worry about my reputation, what will people think? And the kids. Is this a good example to set for them?"

He looked over at her and reached for her hand. "I'm sorry Jenny, I guess I wasn't thinking about all those things. I meant what I said though, I want you and I mean to have you. I will do anything and everything you tell me to do. I'll get tested right away. I'll get some condoms. And I promise we will be very very discreet."

Jenny took another bite and then put her fork down. Suddenly she just wasn't all that hungry, at least not for food. The concern and caring expression on his face had done something inside her, caused her to open a door that had been long closed to her heart. Thoughtfully she said, "I don't think condoms are good enough, maybe I'd better see my doctor and get on the pill. I'll get tested while I'm there so you'll know I'm safe."

"Jenny, I'm not worried about that."

"Well you should be! Colin, you've known me less than a week. Maybe we should slow down a bit, take more time to get to know each other."

"How much time?"

She thought for several minutes while he kept his eyes on her face watching her expressions.

"How about a month?"

"Too long."

"That's too long?"

"Yeah. A month is too long. How about a week?"

"I don't think a month is too unreasonable."

Just then the waitress came to their table for the third time asking if everything was alright. They were getting very busy and she was trying to move them on.

Colin was not in the right frame of mind to be interrupted just then and he responded with a curt, "Do you mind? We are arguing about when we're going to have sex."

"If!" Jenny almost shouted.

"When!" Colin hissed back.

Jenny stood up and grabbed her purse. Leaning down to him she whispered ferociously, "Is this your idea of discreet?" She spun around and headed out the door.

Colin stood up and threw money on the table instead of taking the bill to the register. He ran out the door after her.

When he finally caught up to her she was walking down the road heading towards home. He grabbed her arm and turned her around to face him.

"Jenny, I'm sorry, so, so sorry." The tears streaming down her face caused his face to cave in in anguish. He pulled her to him and hugged her tightly to him, running his fingers through her long silky hair. They stood there for several minutes while he held her and kissed her brow.

The traffic on 179 was whipping pretty close to them so he pulled her away from the street side, and with his arm around her waist, he led her back to the car. Amazingly she had gotten almost two blocks away before he had caught up with her. When they got to the car he leaned her up against the side and looked down into her face as he brushed a few stands of hair away from her face.

"Maybe you're right. Maybe we are going too fast. If it's a month you want, a month it'll be. Just be patient with me. I don't think I've ever wanted anything as badly as I want you. Except maybe that time when I was eight and I wanted those Roy Rogers six-shooters for Christmas," he said with a tender smile. He lifted her chin with his finger tips and bestowed a sweet, soft, lingering kiss. Even though he was trying to keep the passion out of it, it was still there for both of them.

"Those kids are probably sprouting roots on that sofa by now. What say we all spend the day at the beach and I'll fix my very special spaghetti sauce for dinner?" he suggested cheerfully.

"Sounds wonderful," she said. "Let's stop at the grocery store for some salad ingredients. And I'll make some garlic bread guaranteed to keep you away from me for at least a week."

"There's not a chance of that, especially if I eat some too," he said as he opened the car door for her. She slid into the seat and he eyed her shapely legs. A whole month, how was he going to do it?

Chapter 119

Sunset Beach

They spent the day at the beach watching the kids on the recumbent bicycles they had rented for the day and helped them build a sand pueblo village that Paisley had constructed in her mind. She was really quite a creative kid and pretty soon everyone around stopped by to admire their work.

They played in the waves, Colin and Adam surfing with their body boards and Jenny and Paisley floating on rafts. At lunch time Jenny and Colin went up to the beach house to fix sandwiches for everybody. While Jenny was washing some lettuce in the sink, Colin came up behind her and put his hands around her resting them on her bare stomach. Jenny felt the heat of his palms on her and nearly fell back against him. When he started kissing the back of her neck she did lean back against his naked chest. The hairs brushing against her back were just one of the many sensations she was trying to cope with as she shivered from his touch.

"Cold?" he asked in a sensuous, thick voice.

"No, far from it," she replied dreamily.

When his hand roved up and cupped her bikini-clad breast, her knees did buckle and he had to grip her tightly with the hand still around her waist to keep her from falling.

Gently he turned her around to face him. Their feet were touching, their thighs were touching and his hands around her waist were bringing their lower bodies together. When they connected, he brought his hands down to her buttocks and pulled her to him grinding his hardness into her soft warm flesh.

Just then they heard somebody running up the back deck steps. They jumped apart just as Paisley ran into the room and then into the bathroom.

"I guess she waited too long again!" Jenny laughed.

"Why doesn't she just use the ocean?" Colin asked.

"Are you kidding, I've trained her better than that!"

"Jenny, everybody does it. Where do you think the fish go?"

"A lady just doesn't do that," she retorted.

Paisley came out just in time to hear them discussing one of Jenny's weird peccadilloes. "You should hear the one she has about spitting out chewing gum. And Mom's got very peculiar ideas about where you can or cannot kill a bug." Then she ran out the door slamming the screen door behind her.

"Much as I'd like to continue where we left off when we were interrupted, I think it's probably safer if we finish making lunch. Then you can tell me about these idiosyncrasies your daughter thinks you have while we eat," Colin said as he reached for a piece of celery. He popped half of it into his mouth, bit it and put the other end in her mouth careful not to touch her lips. If he touched her lips he'd have to kiss them and he wasn't sure how he'd stop.

They sat in beach chairs in a little circle eating their sandwiches and munching on grapes, chips and some vegetables. Colin and Adam were indulging in a few afternoon beers and Jenny was drinking a wine cooler from a sipper cup. "Okay, Paisley," Colin said. "Tell me about your Mom's problem with spitting out gum."

"You gotta get her to tell it. It's a hilarious story that she made up. Actually she makes them up all the time, this one's just her best."

Colin looked at Jenny with lifted eyebrows. "Okay, Let's hear it. You've got center stage."

Jenny was suddenly self-conscious. "It's just a story I tell the kids, you wouldn't like it."

"Yes, he would mom, so would Adam, c'mon," Paisley prodded.

"Yeah, c'mon," Colin mimicked.

"Okay." She relented. She took a long sip of her wine cooler and sat back in the chair.

"Once there was this very poor black family who lived in North Carolina, a man and a wife with four children. Their youngest son played basketball in high school and one day a scout came and saw him and invited him and his family to Chapel Hill so the young man could try out for the team at Duke University. It was such an exciting time for them and they pinned all their hopes for getting out of poverty on him and his up and coming successful basketball career. With the money they had saved all winter they bought him a brand new pair of basketball shoes. They were the first new pair he'd ever had. They borrowed a car from some friends and they all piled in to drive the young son to Chapel Hill. Wouldn't you know it, on the way there they had a flat tire. While the young man was out helping his father put on the spare he stepped in some chewing gum that someone had spit out their car window. He tried to scrape it off, but with all the ridges in the tread it was almost impossible to do. When they arrived at the gymnasium where he was to try out, he eagerly approached the coach and introduced himself. Right on the spot they threw him a basketball and told him to show them what he could do with it. He took lay up after lay up and missed them all as his shoes went *thump, clomp, thump, clomp, thump, clomp.*" With each clomping sound she made her lips smack like something sticking to them. Paisley and Adam and Colin laughed uproariously. Paisley and Adam mostly at the story. Colin mostly at the way she was making the sound effect. "He didn't get the scholarship that he wanted so badly. So, the moral of this story is, throw your gum where it belongs, not out the window where some poor kid will step on it and lose his whole future over it."

"That's a good story, you can bet I'll think about it every time I get rid of my gum," Colin said with a grin.

"Now tell them about the bugs, Mom," Paisley said.

"That's not so weird, honey, a lot of people don't like to see bugs killed," Jenny said.

"But you do kill them."

"Only if they're inside. If they're outside and not on me, they get to live. If they're inside, they're dead meat."

"If they're close to the door, she'll shoo them out and give them a chance, but if they come back in, she smacks 'em!" Paisley said hitting her fist against her opened palm. "She's pretty deadly with a fly swatter."

"Dad can catch flies in his hand," Adam piped up.

"Really?" Jenny said amused. "What a talent," she said facetiously.

"You try it sometime," Colin said. "It's not that easy."

"You'll have to show me."

"I will when we get back to the beach house, there are plenty down by the trash cans."

"I'll look forward to it. Apparently it's all down hill after the fourth date," She said with a smile.

"There are other activities I had planned but you kaboshed them, remember?" he said teasingly.

"I remember. Boy, that wine cooler's going to my head. Suddenly I'm sleepy, I could use a nap."

"You can use my bed," he said suggestively, then added. "I'll stay here and entertain the kids."

"Okay. Is it all right if I use your shower too? I don't want to get sand in your bed."

"Of course," he said. "I don't want you to get sand in my bed either."

She picked up their lunch things and her beach bag and went back up to the beach house. Finding the master bedroom on the top floor she looked out the sliding glass door to the beach. Colin was throwing a frisbee back and forth to the kids. He looked so tanned and so well built as he flexed his muscles catching and throwing the disc. She felt the heat coursing through her and when she turned and looked at his bed she felt a melting desire between her thighs. No more wine in the hot afternoon she told herself as she made her way to the bathroom.

The shower felt so good on her slightly sunburned body. She had been so concerned about everybody else's sunscreen that she'd forgotten all about hers. She used Colin's Pert Plus shampoo and conditioner to wash her hair, knowing that without a separate conditioner she was condemning herself to comb through many tangles. She toweled off with the towel hanging on the towel rack, still damp from his last use of it, instead of grabbing a fresh one. The slightly abrasive feel of it against her smooth skin was somehow erotic, just knowing he'd used it to rub against his bare skin. She was even finding something sexy about a few stray body hairs she'd seen on the floor. She was definitely losing it, she thought as she went into the bedroom.

She had only one change of clothes with her and she didn't want to wrinkle them by sleeping in them so she slid between the sheets with nothing on. She nuzzled into his pillow on the queen-sized bed. Had there ever been another man who had smelled so good? She drifted off to a marvelous slumber, the kind you get when you steal a nap in the middle of the day, your body all tingly and clean, your mind at complete peace with everything.

When she awoke it was because she heard a soft masculine sigh. She slowly opened her eyes and turned over to find the source of it. Colin was leaning against the doorframe, his eyes staring at her with profound desire.

He'd come up to check on her and found her asleep in his bed with her long blonde hair spread out behind her, fanning her shoulders and the pillow she lay upon. The beauty of the sight of her lying there had taken his breath away. As she turned to face him he noticed that she had the top sheet tucked under her arm and that her shoulders were bare.

"Are you in my bed naked?" he asked almost choking on the question.

She nodded slightly.

"Arrgghh!" he groaned as he gripped the doorframe behind him with his fingers, turning his knuckles white with the effort. After a few moments and several deep breaths he pushed off from the doorway and walked into the room. He sat on the bed, his hip close to hers. "Would you scream if I were to slip in there beside you?"

"I wouldn't scream, but I wouldn't be very happy," she replied.

"Give me a few minutes and you would be." He leaned down to stroke her hair. "You're hair is so beautiful, so soft and so silky."

"I used your shampoo and your hairbrush, I hope that was all right."

"Oh no, now I'm gonna get cooties. Of course it's all right. The kids took a walk to the Beach Mart. When they get back, dinner should be just about ready."

He leaned down and placed a kiss on her shoulder. Then he followed it with several more going up the side of her throat and ending with her lips. He kissed her with infinite tenderness careful not to brush her lips too harshly with his five o'clock shadow. He pulled away and looked at her upturned face. Then his hand joined hers at the top of the sheet and he slowly pulled it out of her hand. At first she resisted slightly, then she didn't resist at all. When it fell to her waist, his eyes followed it. God, she was exquisite. Her full rounded breasts, poised high on her chest were bared to his view and he eyed their creamy whiteness, contrasting against her deep tan. Her rosy-colored aureoleas were the size of half dollars, the nipples sitting in the middle of them like pencil erasers. They were jutting out to show their hardness, reacting first to the cool of the air-conditioned room and then to the heat of his eyes.

While his lascivious eyes feasted on her breasts, his hands slowly made their way to touch them, cupping and hefting the weight of them in his palms. He gently kneaded and felt their firm texture. "Ahh, Jenny. When a man dreams about a woman's breasts, ones like yours are what he envisions." He rubbed her nipples with his thumb and his slightly bent forefinger, gently tugging and massaging them.

Jenny felt heat in the deepest part of her body and a weighty feeling settled into the bottom of her womb. Her body was internally making itself ready for him and the certainty of it scared her. Her mind warred with her body telling her to make him stop while her traitorous body wanted her to urge him on. Everything he was doing felt so good. When he dipped his head to suckle one turgidly hard nipple, she groaned from the pleasure of it. Reaching her hands up to grasp his head, entangling her fingers in his hair, she pulled him closer to her.

The sound of the kids opening the front door and running up the stairs to find them made them pull apart. "Damn!" Colin swore as Jenny grabbed for the sheet. He stood up and Jenny could see his bathing suit tented out in front of him. He left the room and closed the door behind him so she could get dressed.

They finished fixing dinner together in silence, each dealing with their own inner turmoils. They sat around the chrome and glass dining room table listening to the kids talk about everything under the sun, but neither of them was really listening. They were in their own little world and couldn't seem to pull themselves out.

The spaghetti was delicious and Jenny complimented Colin on his cooking. He mumbled a half-hearted thank you and smiled sheepishly at her. It was obvious to everyone that there had been a significant mood swing in the beach house. Jenny solicited Paisley's help in the kitchen and pretty soon they made short work of the incredible mess Colin had made making his home-made sauce. After the kitchen was back in order Jenny turned to Colin and said, "I think we should be going now. I think we're all getting a little tired. Paisley and I have to get up early tomorrow to drive to Charlotte to pick up Rusty from camp."

Colin had completely forgotten about Rusty. "So will we be seeing each other tomorrow?" he asked.

"No," she replied. "I won't be getting back until late. It's parent's day at the camp. We'll leave after dinner."

He walked over to her and took her shoulders in his hands. "I don't care what time it is, I want you to call me, okay?"

"Okay," she said, "I need the number." He gave it to her and walked them and all their gear down to her car. After she was settled behind the wheel of her convertible he put both hands on the door sill and leaned in to give her a kiss. "I was sorry we were interrupted, how about you?" he asked.

"Yes, I was sorry, too. But I really think we should wait a month," she said looking up at him.

"So, counting from the day we met which was Monday to today, Friday, we can subtract 5 days from 28 and we've only got 23 days to go," he said.

"I meant a month from today. And a month has 30 or 31 days," she countered.

"Not February. It's a month and sometimes it only has 28."

She laughed. "Okay, 28 less today then. That's 27. Four weeks from today."

"Four weeks," he groaned. "We'll never make it you know." He leaned in to kiss her and she passed her cinnamon flavored gum from her teeth into his mouth. "Now don't spit that out on the ground!" she called as she backed out of the driveway.

Chapter 120

Sunset Beach

Jenny and Paisley left early the next morning to make the five-hour drive to Charlotte. When they got there, Parents Day was in full swing and Rusty was anxious to enlist her for his team. They did the three-legged race, sack race and egg throwing contest and placed very well in each one. Jenny nixed the pie eating contest so Paisley competed with him in that one. For lunch they feasted on hot dogs and hamburgers cooked by the camp counselors.

Jenny met all of Rusty's friends and his favorite counselors. After an afternoon of paddle boating and watching archery tournaments, a dinner of barbequed ribs was served, accompanied by corn on the cob and baked beans. They left shortly before six to make the long drive home.

Jenny was nearly exhausted by the time they arrived home and she supervised Rusty's unpacking. But nothing would have kept her from calling Colin as promised. She'd been looking forward to it all day, between all the activities. She quickly took a hot shower and settled into bed, propping the pillows up behind her. She dialed Colin's number and was thrilled when he answered on the first ring. He'd been anxious to talk with her too, it seemed.

"Hello," his husky voice drawled.

"Hi," she said almost timidly.

"I've still got your gum in my mouth," he said

"You're kidding!"

"Nope. You want it back? You can come over for it now if you want." He made some chomping sounds so she could hear he was chewing gum.

"You are nuts!"

"Just about you. How'd your day go?" he asked.

626

"It was exhausting, I'm beat." She told him about Rusty and all the games they'd played together.

"Sounds like fun. Are you in bed now?"

"Yes," she said coyly.

"Tell me what you're wearing."

She looked down at herself. For a brief moment she was tempted to lie and tell him she had a sexy teddy on, but she couldn't. "I have a white T-shirt on that has a crane standing in a marsh with a frog halfway in his mouth. The frog has his hand wrapped around the crane's throat so he can't be swallowed. At the bottom it says, 'Don't ever give up.' Under that I have a pair of man's boxer shorts on."

"Whose?"

"Mine."

"No, I mean whose were they before?"

"Mine. I bought them for me. They have little smiley faces all over them."

"Oh. A real slave to fashion I see."

"I like to be comfortable when I sleep."

"Sleep? What's that?" he joked.

"What did you do today?" she asked.

"I went golfing at Oyster Bay and then I came back and counted the girls on the beach that had tattoos."

"Really? What was the final tally?"

"The number got so high I had to give up, somewhere in the hundreds," he said.

"It's a pretty big thing down here, especially with the college kids."

"You don't have one do you? I haven't seen one on you, but then I haven't seen all of you yet."

"No, I don't have a tattoo. I don't like them. You don't have one do you?"

He hesitated for just a few seconds.

"Yeah, I do."

"You're kidding aren't you?"

"Nope, I got one."

"Where?"

"Someplace you have touched but not seen."

"Now I know you're kidding. Nobody has a tattoo there."

"I do."

"Naw, they wouldn't do it there. And besides you couldn't stand the pain there."

"They numbed me."

"I don't believe you. What's it of?"

"A butterfly."

"A butterfly!"

"Well actually it depends. Sometimes it's a small gentle butterfly, sometimes it's the gigantic pulsing *Mothra*. C'mon over, I'll show it to you. It's *Mothra* right now."

Jenny laughed. "You are impossible!"

"Does that mean you're not coming?" he asked, sounding hurt.

"Entomology really doesn't interest me all that much, and once you're seen one butterfly, you've pretty much seen them all," she quipped.

He laughed. "Okay, some other time, maybe. What are you doing tomorrow?"

Jenny thought for a minute. "Church at eight, brunch at either Tamers or the Surf Club and then laundry. You would not believe all the dirty clothes Rusty brought home."

"Can we join you for brunch? Then Adam can take the kids to the pool while we do the laundry together."

"Sure, don't you want to go to church with us, too?" she asked.

"No, I think it's way too soon to meet your pastor, don't you? Besides all he'd have to do is take one look at me and know I'm planning on making you sin with me in exactly 26 days."

"Don't you and Adam go to church?"

"Not very regularly, I'm ashamed to admit."

"Oh," she said.

"What's that mean?"

"I don't know, I just never thought I'd be dating a man who chews stale gum, has a butterfly on his penis, and doesn't even go to church. I'm not sure this is the man my mother's been praying for me to meet."

He laughed good naturedly, causing her to smile on the other end.

"Your mother's praying for a man?"

"For me, not for her, she's already got one. A really good one."

"How do you know all this?" he asked.

"She tells me all the time. It's part of her bedtime prayers that she says for everybody, 'And please, Lord, find a nice man for Jenny.' I don't believe she's ever once asked for a tattooed, used gum-chewing atheist. But I can't be sure, maybe I should phone her, they could be running out of the other kind."

"Mothers always approve of me. Sometimes even a little too much," Colin said.

"Oh? They've come on to you?" she asked, getting his drift.

"Oh, yeah. I almost had my own Mrs. Robinson story when I was in high school."

"What happened?"

"At the time I was worried that the daughter was pregnant, if I'd gotten the mother pregnant too, the babies would have been sisters, aunt and niece and daughter, grandchild. It was a pretty sobering thought. Besides, along about the same time my Spanish teacher, Miss Rodriguez, thought I needed a little private tutoring after school."

"So what happened? Was the daughter pregnant?"

"No, thankfully. But I did learn some pretty interesting Spanish phrases."

"Colin, you are amazing," Jenny said.

"She told me that, too," he said smugly.

"I think we'd better call it a night. I may need to get to church extra early to say some prayers for you."

"Just pray that I have the strength to last 26 more days."

"Good night."

"Good night, sweetheart."

Jenny hung up the phone and curled into her pillow repeating the last words he'd said over and over again. He'd called her sweetheart. And it made her feel like somehow she belonged to him.

Chapter 121

Sunset Beach

Jenny dressed with painstaking care early the next morning. This would be Colin's first time seeing her really dressed up. Heels, hose, matching purse—the works. She selected a dressy business suit that she'd always received lots of compliments on, a blue and gray herringbone design that had a short pleated skirt that showed off her legs. The double breasted jacket was meant to be worn over a frilly white shirt but Jenny wore it over a lacy gray camisole. Navy blue stockings, shoes and purse completed her chic, elegant look. She wore her hair in a fancy French chignon, pulling a few wavy strands loose around her face And for the first time in ages she actually put some earrings in her ears, smooth pave pearls with a braided gold rope border.

After church Jenny drove to the beach house to get Colin and Adam. Colin's initial reaction to her attire was a low whistle then he asked, "Did you say The Surf Club, or The Watergate?"

"The Surf Club is the southern version of The Watergate," She said knowledgeably.

"Are we dressed all right?" Colin asked, indicating him and Adam in their matching khakis with collared golf shirts tucked in at the waist. Colin had a belt, apparently Adam had forgotten one. Both were wearing Docksiders with no socks.

"You're fine. I'll admit I'm a tad over dressed but I never get a chance to wear my good clothes anymore, it's always jeans, cutoffs and bathing suits. Can you imagine a life with that dress code?" she said trying to make fun of her lifestyle.

After introducing Rusty they all piled into her car since it was the only one with five seat belts. They decided to go to the Surf Club because Colin and Adam had never been there. Paisley was in the mood for their strawberry crepes, and Jenny had obviously dressed for it. They would do Tamers, a favorite of both of theirs another time.

Adam and Rusty hit it off surprisingly well even though there was five years difference in their ages. Video games being what they were, hours of play distinguished the novice from the expert, not years of age. They both had a passion for the games. Rusty had subscriptions to all the trade magazines and Adam belonged to a local Nintendo club.

Paisley took Adam's lack of attention to heart and glommed onto Colin, asking him question after question and reaching up through the opening above the console for his hand whenever it was idle.

They arrived at the Surf Club looking like a well-to-do family having brunch at their favorite country club after church. Colin kept his hand on the small of Jenny's back in a proprietoral manner as they were led to a table by the big glass window overlooking the golf course. As soon as they were seated and placed their drink order, the kids left for the buffet and omelet station.

Colin, sitting next to Jenny, picked up her hand and seductively brought it to his lips. He kissed each knuckle in its turn as he looked into her eyes. There had been a two-fold reason for this, first, he wanted to, second, he wanted all the men who had eyed Jenny as they were ushered to their table to know that she belonged to him.

When the kids came back they were all talking at the same time, excited about the day ahead of them and all the plans they had with each other. Jenny laughed and reminded them that half the day would already be gone by the time they got home and changed their clothes. Better save some stuff for tomorrow.

"Adam has to leave tomorrow to go back to work on Tuesday, but I think he's going to try to get a four-day weekend in two weeks." Colin said. Well, that put a damper on everybody. Jenny and Colin left to go to the omelet and crepe station.

"Well hello there! Long time no see," she was greeted by the chef.

"Hi Gregg. I've been incredibly busy and too lazy to drive this far. Gregg, this is Colin. Colin, Gregg. Gregg makes the very best strawberry crepes. He knows that lots of whipped cream is absolutely essential!"

"Absolutely!" Gregg agreed. Jenny laughed with him. "I guess I'll start with one, you know me, dessert first before I get too full."

Gregg fixed a crepe for her and a loaded omelet for Colin. Then they headed to the buffet to load up on all the other breakfast foods offered there.

When they got back to the table there was a glass of champagne at her place.

"Does everybody in the Carolinas know about your passion for champagne?" he asked dryly.

"Yes, I try to make sure of that," she said with a delightfully wicked laugh.

They all ate their fill, stuffing themselves with bacon, sausage, corned beef hash, grits, biscuits, waffles and pancakes. Jenny had a record four crepes along with everything else, in addition to three glasses of champagne. Colin was enjoying watching her eat with such enthusiasm. He put his hand on her thigh to pat it tenderly and was astonished to feel a garter belt clip. His eyes widened and he looked over at her face, questioning her silently with his eyebrows raised as he plucked on the clip. She nodded and discretely slid her skirt up until he could see where the stocking ended just a few inches above the hem of her skirt. He drew in a deep breath and slowly expelled it as he rested his forehead on his open palm, his elbow propped on the table. The woman was just too sexy. Over and over he muttered, "25 days."

"What happens in 25 days?" Paisley asked.

"I become sane again," was Colin's only answer.

They all went home to Jenny's house to change their clothes, the kids into swim suits, the adults into shorts and tank tops. While the kids were at the pool, Jenny and Colin were going to watch the golf tournament on TV and do laundry. At Jenny's suggestion Colin brought some of their own washing. She tackled the huge pile that had amassed, sorting it into five loads.

After Jenny started the washer she grabbed a deck of cards and she and Colin played gin while he watched the golf tournament. After awhile he took the cards from her hands and placed them on the table. "Time for a make out break," he stated and pulled her into his arms. He kissed her passionately running his fingers through her hair and up and down her back as his lips slanted first one way and then the other over her full lips. After many heated kisses, where their tongues entwined over and over again, she found herself prone on the couch, his gyrating body grinding into hers. He used his hand and positioned his engorged shaft up against her pelvic bone and moved against her just as if he was actually in her causing them both to groan and gasp for air as they continued, frantically kissing each other's lips.

The fire between them was intense, the passion on their faces unmistakable. Jenny was running her hand up and down Colin's outer thigh when she accidentally slid her hand up underneath his shorts almost touching his hip. The groan that was wrenched from his lips caused her to shudder and her hand continued searching for him. When her fingers closed around his fully aroused erection, he keened with the sweet ecstasy of it. She could hear the agony in his low pitched sob as he struggled to maintain control. Suddenly she knew what she had to do. What she *wanted* to do. He had to have some relief. He was actually in pain. She pulled away from him and looked into his tortured face. Her eyes met his and she saw the hunger, the longing to have her and to lose himself in her. She leaned up on her elbow and whispered, "come into the laundry room with me."

"You want to fold laundry, now?" he asked incredulously, his voice dry and cracked.

"No, it's just the one place nobody else ever goes, but me."

She eased him off of her, then took his hand and led him to the laundry room. Shutting the door behind them she pushed him back against the closed door. Kneeling on the floor she unbuttoned and unzipped his shorts and let them fall, then she hooked her thumbs under the waist band of his jockeys and eased them over his incredibly hard erection. The sight of her looking unabashedly at him caused his erection to throb and pulsate almost as if it were doing a dance for her.

"No butterfly. No Mothra either," she said as she leaned into him and let her tongue touch the very tip. He groaned like a man dying, "Oh, God, Jenny. Jenny, Jenny." When she opened her mouth and took him into her she felt his thighs tremble. Slowly she started licking and sucking on him exactly as she had learned from a book R.J. had made her read many years ago. First it was a lollipop, a huge delicious sucker, then it was an ice cream cone quickly melting and dripping everywhere as she tried to catch and lick each side, careful not to loose any. She tried to take as much as she could into her mouth but she couldn't close her lips anywhere near the base of it so she wrapped her hand around the part she couldn't swallow, gently agitating it up and down as she licked the length of his shaft over and over again. By the sounds he was making she could tell that he was thoroughly enjoying the tongue lashing and sucking action. When she gently cupped his swaying balls and stroked them with her fingertips while at the same time frigging and sucking on his straining cock, she felt him jerk and then spasm as he jettisoned his load into her warm, welcoming mouth. She took it all and swallowed it, never taking her mouth away from his hardness until it softened in her mouth. Then she eased her lips over him careful not to hurt him while he was still in such a sensitive state.

As he stood still leaning against the door, his pants around his ankles, she stood up, went over to the wash tub, rinsed her mouth and washed her hands as she warmed a washcloth for him. Then she knelt back down in front of him and washed him with tender strokes using the warm cloth.

He reached down and pulled her up by the elbows drawing her close to him and giving her a deep kiss that made her heart sing. When he finally released her he said, "You've got some explaining to do. Where did you learn how to do all that?"

"I read a lot. And I was married to a hedonist once, remember? He was very precise in his instructions."

"Well, thank God, for that!" Colin said with a smile.

"C'mere," he said picking her up and depositing her on top of the dryer. She felt the heat from the dryer on her thighs then she felt the heat from him as he inserted his big hands into the stretch waistband of her shorts and underwear, lifted her momentarily off the dryer while he pulled them both down and off in one quick movement.

"Hey!" she screamed. But he was quick to silence her as he pushed her down against the back of the dryer and the wall and spread her legs bending them at the knees. His head ducked immediately down and he started kissing her and tonguing her, his face buried deep into her womanhood. Jenny's hands fell to his head as she tried to steady herself against the back of the dryer. When Colin lifted her up by her buttocks and brought her to the edge of the dryer, she moaned as his tongue entered her even deeper. He was sucking and lapping frenziedly, milking the essence out of her and into his mouth when they heard the front door slam.

"Hey, where is everybody?" they heard Rusty ask as he and Adam walked around the family room and the dining room, right past the laundry room door.

Colin slowly eased away from her and lifted her off the dryer, quietly setting her feet on the floor. He whispered into her ear, "Honey, I'm so sorry." He kissed her gently on the mouth and she tasted the muskiness of her own arousal.

They both reached for their clothes and quietly donned them, starting to laugh at themselves as they heard the kids tromping around trying to find them.

"It's been years since I played Hide and Seek," he said in a low voice.

"I've never played naked Hide and Seek before," she said with a giggle.

They had just finished adjusting their clothes when the door opened. "Here they are! Mom, what's for dinner? We're getting hungry," Paisley said as Jenny and Colin pretended to be folding towels.

Jenny looked over at Colin and smiled, "You owe me $1300."

"Hey! That's not fair! It was the kids who interrupted me. I'd of had you and you know it, just a few more minutes and you would have come all over my face. I want another chance."

"Oh, you'll get one. In 25 days."

There was silence for a minute while they actually started folding the clothes from the dryer. "We'll never make it 25 days and you know it," he said.

"I'm going to the doctor's tomorrow to get started on the pill and to be tested."

"I'll go get tested tomorrow, too."

"It's a little late now, I swallowed your semen, that's gotta be worse than absorbing it through the walls of the vagina. You're already on your way to my blood stream, so there'd better not be anything bad in there!"

"Well, at least we know you're not pregnant," he said with a smile as he kissed her deeply and with great care, like he'd just discovered a treasure he hadn't even known existed.

Chapter 122

Sunset Beach

Adam returned to Virginia the next day and Colin went to play golf with some of his Fairfax County buddies who were staying in Myrtle Beach for their vacations. On his way south he stopped at the Calabash Medical Center and had blood drawn for the tests he requested. He was told he could pick up the results at the end of the week.

Jenny had to work at the Mini-Links so she enlisted Rusty's help as a babysitter. Even though Paisley was quite capable of staying by herself during the day, Jenny felt better if Rusty acted as an overseer.

While walking around the course enjoying the beautiful landscaping, Jenny's thoughts reverted to Colin. Always when she was alone these days her thoughts strayed to him and what he might be doing. She knew he was golfing with his friends from Virginia and that there was a pretty good likelihood that he wouldn't be back to Sunset until late.

As she walked the pathways from hole to hole she admired the pampas grass gently swaying in the breeze. She pulled down a flowering branch from a crepe myrtle to see what it smelled like, it sure didn't smell like much for such a beautiful blossom. She had always loved this peaceful place. To her this was more of a garden than an amusement attraction, but today everything looked brighter and more lush. The Jasmine was a treat for her nostrils as she rounded the curve to the 12th hole. The huge leaves of the phatsias were a more vivid green than usual and the purple blooms of the snapdragons where like miniature jewels all clustered together. She couldn't have asked for a nicer place to be while she was thinking such warm thoughts about Colin and marveling at how well they had gotten to know each other in one short week.

Had it really been just a week ago today that they had met? It didn't seem possible to her that she could already have such deep-seated feelings for him, and such a hunger for his touch. But she did and it was both exhilarating and scary all at the same time.

At ten o'clock she walked back into the hut and phoned her doctor to make an appointment. That was one of the things she really loved about living down here, they said they could take her the next day. Up North she would have had to wait at least two weeks or sit in a waiting room for half a day. Twenty-four days to go now and she was a little nervous. What had she agreed to? Had they actually made an appointment to have sex? When he wasn't around it all seemed so stupid and she didn't know why she had been pressured into agreeing. When he was around, she didn't even know why they were waiting.

She enjoyed being alone for most of the morning, being introspective and collecting her thoughts. The afternoon became very busy as she went from one task to another, trying to keep up with the customers and the need for more balls, more clubs, slushies and ice cream.

She was very tired when she got home but the smell of the pot roast dinner that had been cooking all day in the crock pot and a nice cool shower revived her. After dinner she watched a video with the kids and then retired to her room to read before going to bed.

Long after everyone had been asleep the doorbell rang. Jenny lifted her head off of her pillow and looked over at the clock. The large red numbers indicated it was 11:30. She'd only been asleep for about an hour. Instantly she knew who it had to be. She hit the touch lamp twice illuminating the room and jumped out of bed. A quick glance in the mirror and a shake of her tousled hair was the only thing she allowed herself time for. She didn't want him to ring the bell again and chance waking up the kids.

When she opened the door to him, he looked every bit as tousled as she did.

" 'Lo," he said with a wave of his hand. "Just wanted to stop by on my way home to say good night."

"Colin! You haven't been drinking and driving have you?" she questioned as she opened the door wide to let him in.

"I had some beers this afternoon, but I haven't had a drink since about seven or so. I'm just bushed. We played 36 holes and God was it hot today!"

"Yeah, I know. There wasn't even a hint of a breeze after lunchtime," she concurred.

"Were you asleep?" he asked with an apologetic sound to his voice.

"Yeah, but it's okay, I haven't been sleeping too long. The prince hadn't come to rescue me from the dragon yet."

They walked arm in arm over to the sofa and sat down cuddled next to each other.

"I went to the doctor's today," he said.

"I made an appointment today. I go tomorrow morning."

He reached down to pick up her hand from her lap and put her fingertips to his lips. Softly he kissed them and then equally softly he licked them and then one by one he put them in his mouth lightly sucking on each one. It caused a shiver to go up her spine and she wondered about this erotic sensation that she had never enjoyed before.

He placed her hand back in her lap and leaned fully back into the cushions on the couch stretching his arms out on either side of him. Letting his head drop back against the back of the couch he let out a deep sigh. "I wish I was home now, I'm so tired, I don't think I have the energy to even get up."

Jenny looked at his face, his eyes closed and his face slack. He would be sound asleep in a matter of minutes and she knew it. It was either send him on his way right now or let him fall asleep on the couch. She grazed his face with her fingertips, smoothing his hair away from his brow.

"C'mon, come get in bed. You can sleep with me tonight, but you can't touch me and you have to be up before the kids are."

640

"Can I sleep naked?" he asked with a small grin as she pulled him to his feet.

"No, keep your underwear on and everything in them, in them!" she said. "C'mon, I'm trusting you to be good 'cause I don't want you to drive off the bridge and into the Intracoastal in your sleep."

She helped him into her bedroom and he looked around for a few seconds before collapsing on the bed. "Nice digs," he said referring to the faux marble neo classical bedroom set, just before he slipped out of his shirt and pants and fell onto the bed. He was sound asleep before she could remove his socks and get him under the sheet.

She went to turn off the family room lights and to make sure she'd locked the door and then she checked on the kids.

Heaven help her if they woke during the night from a bad dream, they were both accustomed to coming right to her bed and climbing in. Upon entering her bedroom she walked over to the clock and set it for seven o'clock. That should be early enough to beat both the kids out of bed. But somehow, she just knew she'd be awake earlier, if she slept at all.

Colin's first thought, when he awoke early the next morning and saw where he was, was that he'd finally slept with Jenny and now he couldn't remember a thing about it. Then he slowly recollected walking with her from the family room to her bedroom and removing his shirt and pants before falling exhausted into her bed.

Sleep. That's all he'd done, a part of him was relieved that nothing had happened and a part of him was a little disappointed. But now all parts of him were becoming aroused as he lay next to her sleeping form watching her scantily-clad body rise slowly with each breath she took. She had on a long T-shirt that came to the top of the back of her thighs. From where he was it didn't appear that she had anything on underneath unless it was just a pair of underwear. Her angelic face was just inches from his and he could hear her even breathing and smell her honeysuckle shampoo. If the alarm hadn't jolted him at that precise moment, he would have reached for her and pulled her to him, smothering her with breathtaking kisses and covering her body with his hard, powerful one.

But the alarm had sounded and the din it made had darn near stopped his heart. Jenny's eyes opened and she crawled over his chest to get to the offending little black box to silence it. They were surrounded by a restless quiet now as they both looked into each other's eyes.

"Good morning," he ventured.

"Mmmph," she muttered. Putting her face down into the middle of her pillow.

"Not a morning person, are we?" he questioned jokingly.

"Not unless I can get to the morning with some sleep under my belt," she said a little irritably.

"Sorry, I slept great," he said with relish.

She picked up her pillow and flung it at him just as he reached for her around the waist. He took the brunt of the soft blow against his cheek as he pulled her to him, sliding her across the sheet and pulling her T-shirt up in the process. She was wearing underwear, he could feel the elastic of the waistband. Their thighs connected and their legs entwined. He rubbed his coarse-haired legs up and down her smooth-shaven ones. "Oh, you feel so good," he said as he massaged her back and then let his hand stray to cup one of her buttocks.

"Colin, our agreement for you sleeping in my bed was that you wouldn't touch me. You're touching me."

"That was for last night. You didn't define what I could and couldn't do this morning."

"Yes, I did. I said you had to be up before they were."

"I am up. See?" He took her hand and pressed it to him.

He was definitely up.

"Colin, please don't make this any harder than it is. Wait a minute that's not what I meant to say." They both started laughing at her unintended pun, and Colin released her just enough so she was able to scramble out of bed and run into the bathroom.

When she came out of the bathroom the bed was empty. She noticed that his clothes had been picked up from the love seat where she had discarded them last night. A deep sense of loss came over her as she realized that he had probably gone to the beach house to shower and get ready for whatever he was doing that day. She didn't even know what his plans were.

She dressed in a pair of cutoffs and a tank top over her bathing suit and went out to the kitchen to start some coffee. She was shocked to discover Paisley all curled up next to Colin on the sofa, both of them engrossed in a Yosemite Sam cartoon.

"She heard me in the kitchen trying to find the coffee pot. I told her you invited me over for breakfast this morning and that you were still sleeping when I got here. How rude! Coffee's brewing. She showed me where everything was."

Jenny smiled, pleased that Paisley was none the wiser about her sleeping partner of last night. She got straight to work fixing a big breakfast for everybody. Pancakes, sausages, bacon and lots of fresh fruit. Rusty woke up right when everything was ready, carrying a sleepy Taffy in his arms. Taffy liked to take turns sleeping with everybody. Jenny was silently thoughtful that last night had not been her night even if Taffy couldn't tattle on her.

The only touchy moment was when Colin got up to leave so he could make a tee time and his shoes were nowhere to be found. At the same moment they both looked across the room and met each other's eyes. They both realized where his shoes were, and there was no way he could just walk into the bedroom to get them and then walk out carrying them. Both Rusty and Paisley were helping in the search.

"Oh, you know what?" he said as he hit his open hand against his temple, "I forgot. I didn't wear any. I mean we're at the beach and all, so who needs shoes anyway?" He kissed Jenny lightly on the lips and then walked out the front door barefoot. This was when Jenny realized that she was falling in love with Colin.

Chapter 123

Sunset Beach

The next two weeks were filled with swimming, dining out, entertaining the kids and trying to keep their hands off of each other. Paisley and Colin had become good TV buddies. Colin liked to watch the golf tournaments on TV and Paisley liked to watch anything on TV. It was not unusual for Jenny to look over at them from the kitchen as she fixed dinner to find them playing "Go Fish" while the golf infomercials were on.

After dinner Colin would take Rusty out to one of the lakes on the Plantation and they would fish together, always coming back with some outrageous tale about an electric eel or a twenty-foot alligator. Each backing the other one up no matter how ridiculous the story.

They went swimming at the pools and Jenny marveled at Colin's athletic form as he effortlessly did the butterfly stroke back and forth across the pool as if it was just a common breast stroke, not the grueling and strenuous exercise that it was. His powerful arms and strong back moving through the water so gracefully were very erotic to her. They took long walks on the beach, often going all the way to Bird Island to read the latest mail in the Kindred Spirit mailbox. Anyone wishing to express themselves was free to leave their thoughts in a spiral notebook that was always kept there. Sometimes the messages were sad and sometimes they were joyous, like the ones they left there.

A couple of times Jenny accompanied Colin as he played a round of golf. She would drive the cart and admire some of the most beautiful real estate in the world while he worked on perfecting his game. Usually they were paired with another couple and Jenny would listen to their comments about Colin's incredibly long drives. If it weren't for the other golfers, Jenny would have had no idea how good Colin was. She just knew he sure looked good doing it.

Late one afternoon, when they were all at the beach flying one of the many kites Jenny had collected, she watched as Colin removed his shirt and went in for a swim. After he waded out past the breakers she watched him swim parallel to the shore, taking powerful strokes to propel him. His arms came out of the water curving over his head and pushing the water behind him. It looked like he was gliding through what she knew to be rough currents. Colin looked absolutely magnificent, a force working with nature, not just existing but excelling in the Earth's bounty. When he finished his workout, which she knew was a futile exercise in libido control, he walked out of the surf toward the shore.

Then it hit her. She'd seen this exact scene before. It was from a daydream she'd had years before when she'd vacationed at Carolina Beach and was walking on the beach. There was no doubt that this was the same image she'd seen, a tall muscular man coming out of the water, his chest glistening with wet dripping strands of hair, streams of water running down his hairy legs. He had a big smile for her that was lighting up his face as he walked out of the water and onto the sand and reached out his hand to her.

Mindless of her long summer dress she ran to join him, being swept up into his arms and into the surf by a force she could never have resisted. Jenny was in love. Whether it was the answer to the years of her Mama's prayers or the long awaited destiny that had been ordained for her, she didn't know. All she knew was that she loved this man.

When they got back to Jenny's house they ordered some pizza as a special treat for the kids. While they were waiting Colin and Jenny walked out the back door to the golf course. Homeowners and their guests could walk the course after 5:00 pm with three clubs so Colin frequently went out to the first hole behind her house to work on his putting and driving. Sometimes Jenny accompanied him, ostensibly to watch the egrets coming in to roost in the trees that bordered the Calabash River. What she really watched was Colin. She didn't know that much about golf, but she knew she loved watching him play it. He hit the ball a long way and even though she could never seem to follow it with her eyes, he always managed to track it and walk right to where it landed.

He was so athletic that it was a joy just to watch him swim, golf or play basketball with the kids in the driveway. It wasn't just that he had the physique for it, which he surely did, he had a certain natural grace and coordination to go with it. He must have really been something to contend with as a policeman, she thought, and a part of her regretted that she had never known him when he was in the prime of that career.

While they were walking the course to the second hole Jenny asked Colin if he knew what was going to happen in ten days. He gave her a look that said, are you kidding? Of course I know what's going to happen in ten days. But his words were simply, "Did you think I'd forget?" When she didn't say anything he stopped walking and faced her.

"Jenny, of course I know what happens in ten days. I think about it almost every single waking moment."

Jenny looked up at him. "Me, too." she said simply, regret making her eyes cloud. "Sometimes I get mad at myself for being the way I am."

He was silent for a few seconds before he said, "It won't make any difference in the long run. I want you to be sure. Ten more days isn't all that bad. But I am not waiting any longer!" he said as he scooped her up against his side and kissed her on the nose.

A part of her was thrilled that he wanted her so much that he would be patient and wait for her. The other parts of her wanted to mutiny with her common sense. Her body was not her own these days. She was wanton in her thoughts, shocking herself with some of the erotic thoughts she was having about her and Colin.

"My parents will be here tomorrow," she said. "They're going to stay for a few days and then they're going to take the kids back with them for two weeks. We've been talking about it for a few weeks but Mom didn't know when Daddy could get away from work. They found out yesterday that the section his crew was working on is finished and they don't start a new section of the building for a few more days so he's off until then."

"Great!" he said his eyes twinkling. "I'll have you all to myself soon." He bent down to kiss her lips and decided that he wanted more so he dropped his clubs on the ground and wrapped his arms around her, lifting her up against his crotch so she could feel his desire for her burgeoning. He was kissing her cheeks and then her neck when he turned away and spat. "Ugghh! Bug spray! Can't say I care for your new cologne!" She laughed and rubbed her neck. "Sorry, but I can't go out this time of day without it unless you want to see red welts all over me."

"I only want to see my hands all over you! C'mon," he said as he grabbed her hand, "we'd better head back, I'll bet the pizza's there by now. And knowing those two, they won't save any for us."

As they were walking through the back yard, Colin told her that he wouldn't be coming over for a few days. Jenny was absolutely crushed, even when he explained why. He thought she needed some time alone with her parents and that it would also be a good opportunity for him to spend a few days at Porter's Neck playing golf with his old mentor and former partner. He'd been putting him off ever since he got here and he was beginning to feel guilty about it since it was his beach house Colin was renting at a remarkably reduced rate. That appeased Jenny a little, knowing that he would have had to spend some time up there anyway. I guess it's just as well that he go while I'm entertaining my folks rather than when we'd have the opportunity to spend some time alone during the next two weeks, she thought.

After dinner they went up to the pool and played water volleyball with the kids. It was always nice to go to the pool in the evenings. Usually they were the only ones there, as was the case tonight. The underwater pool lights were eerie and at the same time romantic. It was during one particularly energetic save that Jenny became separated from her bikini top. As she covered herself with her hands she looked around for it floating on the water. It was nowhere to be seen. She looked over at Colin and saw a huge grin on his face, his twinkling blue eyes telling her everything she needed to know. "Colin! Give it back!"

"This?" he asked innocently as he waved her top in the air. "It'll cost ya," he whispered over to her. Meanwhile the kids had begun to see what was happening. Rusty, coming to his mother's rescue, made a grab for it but Colin held it up just a little too high for him to reach. Paisley scrambled out of the pool to bring her a towel.

"What'll it cost me?" she asked him directly, getting a little angry.

"Remember the laundry room?"

"Yeah," she said slowly. Apparently he wanted her to go down on him again. Typical male.

"I want to finish what we started." he said.

Well, she was wrong, he wanted to go down on her.

"Next week, as soon as I get back and we're alone. Deal?" he said dangling her top by a strap and acting like he was going to throw it into the Calabash River behind the pool if she didn't agree.

"Okay, I agree," she said.

He walked over to her and kissed her on the lips. Then his lips went to her ear. "Can I help you put it on?" he asked. She grabbed it out of his hand and dove under the water to put it on. He was already at the bottom of the pool watching the show when she noticed him and quickly spun around. She could hear the sound of his laugher even under the water. Next time she thought, I'm wearing my one piece when I'm in the pool with him!

When he left that night they stood on the porch unable to pull themselves away from each other. "I'm going to miss you like crazy," he said.

"Ditto," she said stealing a line from the movie "Ghost" that they had watched together just the night before.

"You remember what you promised. That taste of you that I got before was just enough to tease me unmercifulessly. I can't wait to taste you again."

Every bit of blood that was coursing through her body instantly changed direction and started heading for her center, creating a heavy feeling in her lower pelvic area. "Oh, Colin," she moaned as she ran her hand up his thigh and clutched at his swollen shaft.

"Careful," he murmured. "The neighbors. Don't forget your reputation," he said with a laugh as he removed her hand, kissed it and trotted down the front steps to his car.

Chapter 124

Sunset Beach

Jenny had a very nice visit with her parents. Her Dad went golfing while she, her Mom and the kids went shopping, to the pool or the beach. Jenny had to work two of the days they were there so it was nice to have her mother home entertaining the kids. Jenny and her mom gave Paisley her first cooking lessons. They made toll house cookies together, a huge casserole dish of lasagna and real southern fried chicken. Whenever Jenny's mom came down they cooked every meal as if they were feeding the whole neighborhood. By the time they left Jenny always had a restocked freezer.

Late one night, after everyone was asleep except Jenny and her Mom, she told her about Colin. Her mom said she had known something was going on because the kids had spoken of him each time she called. But she told Jenny that even if they hadn't she would have known anyway. There was an inner glow coming through her eyes now, a look of contentment that she'd not seen before.

Her children were part of the reason that Jenny was in Sunset Beach enjoying the sunshine and peacefulness of this coastal community. It had been a chance to start a new life with a greater appreciation for all she had. Now those things were becoming overridden by a longing for someone special to share it all with. And she really thought that she'd finally found that special person in Colin.

When Jenny's parents left and took the kids back with them to Virginia, Jenny realized that she had the entire place to herself for one whole night. She decided it would be a make-over beauty night. Colin wasn't due back until the next evening so Jenny got out a bottle of champagne along with a facial mask, an oil treatment for her hair, special clay emollients for her body and all her manicure stuff. By the time Colin got here tomorrow she would be soft, poreless, pedicured and manicured and with long shiny, silky tresses. Popping the cork, she added another adjective, hung over, if she didn't limit herself. She really did have a weakness for the golden bubbly stuff.

Colin said goodbye to his host and hostess. They were a remarkable couple, so much in love after so many years and so concerned and generous to all the friends they cherished. Colin would never have been able to afford the level of luxury that he was enjoying on Sunset Beach if it hadn't been for Steve and Jessie. He knew they were losing a lot of money by renting the place to him instead of letting the rental agency lease it all summer.

They were truly good friends and he'd enjoyed the time he spent with them, just as he enjoyed the time he spent with Daniel and Liesel. It was relaxing and fun and nice to be a part of family life again. When he thought about Daniel, it brought a smile to his lips. Daniel had been so sure that their baby was going to be a boy. Well, the doctors were wrong, and Daniel was teaching his adorable little girl to hunt and fish and sail, much to the consternation of her mother. Well, Liesel was due again in November, maybe this time it would be a boy that Liesel could teach to cook and sew. He grinned again.

The idea of family life immediately brought a picture of Jenny to his mind. Wouldn't she be surprised when he arrived home a full day early.

He pulled into the carport under the beach house at around 7:00 pm. Instead of calling Jenny he decided to surprise her, so he showered and shaved, shaving extra closely as he had an idea of where his chin would be tonight. Her silky thighs and tender folds would need no stimulation from whiskers, he could do it all with his tongue and lips. And for really the very first time in his life, he was actually looking forward to doing cunnilingus on a woman. This wasn't a chore he was dreading, it was a delicacy he was going to savor.

At 8:00 pm he pulled into her driveway and rang the bell.

The doorbell was ringing. Jenny was all the way on the other side of the house in the master bedroom bath. Her hair all slicked back and clipped to the top of her head. Her face was a putrid pea soup green, the mask just beginning to do its work of caking and cracking. Her arms and legs were covered with a purple slimy jelly, guaranteed to make her skin baby soft, and her toes had cotton wedges stuffed between them. Between the mask on her face and the mask on her legs she was wearing a blue tube top and an old orange bikini bottom.

Who in the world could that be? She asked herself as she hobbled to the front door on her heels, careful to keep her toes up. She could see a Buick in the driveway through the kitchen window, but she didn't recognize it.

She opened the door and thought she would die. "Colin? You're not supposed to be here til tomorrow!" She slammed the door in his face and ran back to the bathroom.

"Was that Jenny?" He asked himself as he stared at the closed door. After a few minutes he rang the bell again and again. Finally he left to go somewhere where he could call her.

She was just stepping out of the shower when she heard the phone ring. Wrapping a towel around her she went over to the nightstand and picked it up, tentatively she answered, "Hello?"

"Jenny, it's me? Are you okay?"

"Only mortified beyond anything I could have ever conceived!" she blasted him.

"I'm sorry, Jenny. I was just so anxious to see you. What were you doing anyway?"

"Trying to make myself sexy for you. Did it work?"

He laughed. "Honey you don't have to try, you are sexy." He waited a few seconds. "Is it safe to come back, is that sea creature gone yet?"

"Yes, I just showered the creature down the drain."

"I'll be right there. And don't bother putting any clothes on, it's just me."

She smiled as she hung the phone up. If she'd had more time she would have put layers upon layers of clothes on just to make him suffer for surprising her like that.

A few minutes later she heard a car pull into the driveway. She looked out the kitchen window. It wasn't Colin's car. Who's Buick was it this time or was it the same one? A great night she picked for a make-over night.

As it turned out, it was Colin. He was driving a silver blue Buick LeSabre. She opened the door and was not at all ready for his foot in the door.

"Just making sure you don't close it on me again," he said as he walked inside, grabbing her around the waist and pulling her to him. The kiss was bliss. There was no other way to describe it. His possession of her mouth left no doubt that she was his woman and that he definitely had plans for her tonight. As he thrust his tongue in and around her mouth, she was gently pushed back over his arm and before the kiss was over, he had kicked the door closed and was carrying her over to the sofa.

"Let's get your clothes off, I've been thinking about this all day long."

"Colin, please. Can't we talk for a minute first?"

"Talk?" he asked like he'd never heard the word before.

"Yeah. Like where'd you get the car? What happened to yours? OhmyGod! You didn't have an accident did you?"

"No, nothing like that. It seems my friend Steve had always wanted a Mustang convertible and was even thinking about trading his Buick in on one. When we realized that our payments were about the same and that we had close to the same amount of time left on them, we just switched cars. Now I am the proud owner of a car I can fit into!"

Jenny laughed. Her smile was dazzling and it almost hurt Colin to look at it. God, she was so beautiful.

"Are we finished talking yet?" he asked.

"No," she replied, pushing him off of her so she could get up. "Would you like a drink? Something to maybe soften the mood."

"Shows what you know, hard is the operative word. Not soft."

"Canadian Club and ginger ale?" she asked.

"Oh, sure. But just one. I want to deliver a peak performance tonight. I want no complaints to deal with in the morning."

She poured him a drink and then fixed herself another glass of champagne.

"Colin?" she asked as she walked back into the family room.

"Yes?" he said in a skeptical voice.

"Would you mind it we changed the game plan a little tonight?" she asked.

"Depends. What are you talking about? You don't want to go bowling do you?"

"No, I want you to make love to me."

"What?" he asked, certain he hadn't heard her right.

"You heard me." She walked over and put one knee on the sofa cushion, took his hand and slid it up the open leg of her boxer shorts, directing his fingers to her warm, moist folds. He slid a finger into her so easily, he couldn't believe how wet she was. "Ohhh, Jenny, good God, you are so wet. Why are you so wet, sweetheart?"

"I believe my *yield field* is yielding to *your hardness*. Care to go for a ride?"

"Jenny, just how much champagne have you had?"

"On my second bottle. It's no problem though, I decided hours ago while I was stone sober that this is what we were going to do tomorrow when you got back. I'm on the pill now and all the tests were negative, so we've got nothing to worry about. Now you're back and I want to feel more than your tongue inside me. So, please, please, take me tonight."

"Don't you want to see my health certificate?" he quipped as he plunged his finger deep inside her. "Ah Jenny, I hope you're not kidding because I'm getting pretty close to the point of no return here."

"I'm sure. Only one more thing you should know."

"What's that?"

"I don't think I can come tonight, I've already had too much to drink. Tonight's for you."

"Then forget it, I don't want one-way sex. We'll wait until you're sober."

"No! Can't we do it more than once tonight? I'll probably be fine by midnight." She squirmed on his finger, gently bobbing up and down. He shoved two fingers up inside her and she shivered. Keeping his hand where it was he leaned up and with his other hand he grabbed her by the waist pulling her down beside him, laying her beside him on the sofa. He kept his fingers moving inside her until he could see her eyes glazing over and then he pulled her boxer shorts off and her T-shirt up over her breasts.

"Never would I ever have agreed to this with any other woman, but I just can't stand it anymore Jenny. I just have to have you. Now." He unzipped his pants and pulled down his shorts and underwear. He stared at her heaving breasts as he positioned himself at her entrance. Later he would not remember exactly how it had happened, but it had almost felt to him that he had been sucked inside her. And as soon as he felt the warm walls of her vagina around him he could do nothing but encourage and enjoy the sensations. He thrust himself deeply into her, thrilling with the tightness and slipperiness.

Nothing could have made him stop once he'd entered her, his urgency was so strong. His hands went to her breasts, grabbing as much as his hands could hold and running his thumbs over the raised nipples. As he pushed her down and into the sofa he bent down to suckle on one. He knew he didn't have much longer before he would explode a part of himself into her. He looked into her face falling deeply into her eyes and then with a loud groan he gave one final thrust and pumped his essence deep into her.

He was jettisoned way out into a deep black space before falling and spinning among colorful comets as he came back to earth to settle on top of her. Nothing in his life had ever felt quite like this. He felt whole and contented as well as completely satisfied. Then he remembered with a smile that she had said they would do it again later.

Chapter 125

Sunset Beach

Colin lay beside her on the sofa softly stroking her long wheat-colored hair. He had shifted his weight off of her and was snuggled up against her side. She had fallen asleep. She looked so peaceful and breathtakingly beautiful as she lay there, not seeming to notice as his fingers traced the curve of her lips, the line of her jaw and the gentle slope of her nose.

He wrapped his arms around her and held her close. Then he closed his eyes and slept.

Jenny woke up to an almost suffocating feeling. She felt like she was in an iron vise and was having trouble breathing. That's when she fully woke up and found that she was being held tightly in Colin's arms, a little too tightly. She reached around her back and tried to pry his interlaced fingers away. Sometime while they had been sleeping he had tightened his grip around her and now he was quite loathe to let her go.

She managed to relax his hold a little, but he wasn't letting go. Her face was turned into his warm chest and she could feel his chest hairs tickling her face. With an impish smile on her face she tongued his dark nipple, causing a delightful little moan to pass through his lips. As she continued licking and sucking on it his hands came to life and started stroking her back side and buttocks. She felt a stirring in his groin area and something pressed up against her hip. Her lips turned into a small smile against his chest as she moved on to tease the other nipple.

Soon he was wide awake and looking down into her eyes. She smiled up at him, a mischievousness about her signaling trouble. "You know what I was thinkin'?" she asked.

"No. What were you thinkin'?" he asked as he touched his finger to her nose.

"Wouldn't it be nice to go to the beach house, make love in your bed and wake up in the morning to the sun coming up right

657

there at the foot of the bed? We can watch the whole glorious show from the bed while we make love again," she said as she felt the fullness of his bottom lip with her fingertip.

He kissed her finger as it made its circuitous route around his lips. "Let's go," he said simply, easing away from her.

"Give me a few minutes to take a quick shower and get a few things together. Why don't you gather up some food for us to take, I think we're going to need some fortification by morning and I know there's nothing at your place but beer." With a huge smile, she turned to go back towards her bedroom.

They drove over in separate cars because Colin had an early tee time. Jenny was going to sleep in a little and then spend the day at the beach relaxing after coming back to walk Taffy in the morning.

It was shortly after midnight as they unloaded their cars and trudged up the steps to the beach house. While Jenny put the food away Colin followed her around the kitchen nibbling on her neck and ears and running his hands the length of her inner thighs each time she had to reach up to put something away. "You brought four boxes of cereal, but it doesn't appear that you brought any milk," she said as she leaned back against his chest.

"You use milk? I've always just used beer," he said as he kissed the top of her shoulder.

"Yuck!" she said.

"You don't like what I'm doing?"

"No, I wasn't commenting on that. I like what you're doing very much."

"Then you're really going to like this," he said as he ran his hands up her sides and around her midriff to caress her breasts under her sweater.

"Pull your neckline down. I want to see what my hands are doing," he said with a husky deep voice.

She obliged by pulling all the material from the neckline of her over-sized sweater forward giving him an unencumbered view of her breasts, his hands already causing the nipples to harden under his touch.

"Mmm, mmm. You sure do have great tits." He pulled on the tips of them making her writhe with pleasure. Then he spun her around and whipped the sweater over her head, bending to take one hardened peak into his mouth. The connection between his mouth and her nipple caused an electric current to pass through her body sending messages to her nether regions, preparing for the inevitability of a friendly invasion. Colin lifted her to the counter and, enjoying the more straight forward view of her from this angle, he groaned her name as he pressed kisses all over her exposed flesh.

While he was tonguing the underside of one breast he reached for the button and zipper on her jeans. He set her onto the floor while he pulled them down past her hips, delighted that she wasn't wearing any underwear. Then he lifted her back onto the counter as he pulled them off of her legs and let them drop to the floor. There she was sitting on the counter completely naked, a feast for his eyes and a feast for his mouth. He had thought about this and practically nothing else for weeks. He placed his hands between her legs and opened her up for his inspection.

Her curly light brown hairs made a fuzzy vee pointing the way to her womanhood and, as he spread her thighs, he was tantalized by her glistening pink gash. He instantly felt all of his redirected blood rushing through his veins hurrying to even more fully engorge his member than it had been before, making himself ready for her. Lifting her bottom he scooted her closer to the edge of the counter and spread her legs wide. Bending to cover her with his mouth, he positioned her legs over his shoulders. With a moan of ecstasy first from him and then from her he set himself to the task of pleasuring her. His tongue and lips surrounded her as he tried to taste all of her at once, sucking on her deep folds and pulling her nether lips completely into his mouth. He was tonguing her and licking her and sucking on her in such a frenzied state of passion that he almost didn't hear her when she begged for him to take her into the bedroom and pleasure her with his now rampart hard cock.

Jacqueline DeGroot

He removed his mouth reluctantly from her wet steamy core and undid his pants, dropping them right there on the floor. He pulled his T-shirt off and flung it aside. Then he scooped her up, each hand caressing a warm, firm buttock and settled her over his pulsing hardness. With one well-aimed thrust he was inside her. Then he shoved himself all the way into her, burying himself to the hilt. She cried out her joy of finally having that void filled and bit on his shoulder as he carried her up the stairs and into his bedroom.

He gently laid her down on the end of the bed and standing above her, he continued thrusting into her warm velvety shaft. He could feel her clamping around him as he retreated and plunged over and over again, determined that this time it would be for her, even if it killed him, which it was definitely threatening to do. When she roughly jerked on his upper arms and forced him to fall on top of her while she desperately dug her fingers into his buttocks, pulling him up hard against her clitoris, he felt the beginnings of her orgasm. Rythmetically her vagina started pulsing and throbbing in a way Colin knew no woman could ever deign to control. He watched as her face contorted into an almost painful grimace as she sobbed his name and then relaxed as the release washed over her and she was racked with convulsive shudders. The sight of her in such ecstasy caused him to begin his own spasmodic release and he yelled out her name as his own delightful pleasure swept him away.

As the waves of after shocks gradually seeped out of his body he gently pushed off of her and rolled onto his side keeping himself buried inside her. He stroked her brow trying to ease the tension he saw in her face.

For Jenny this orgasm was the undoing of her in more ways than one. Physically her body had never responded to pleasure quite this way before. The strength of her climax had taken her breath away. But immediately following the sensations was an awareness that she hadn't had before. Suddenly she knew things she hadn't known that she knew. An overwhelming feeling of

660

dread washed over her as she turned to Colin who was rubbing her eyebrows and trying to smooth out the frown lines between them.

"Colin, you killed David," she said accusingly.

"What?" he asked, just beginning to get his own senses back. He felt himself reluctantly sliding out of her.

"You killed David," she repeated, simply stating a fact that she now knew to be true.

It took him a few seconds to realize who she was talking about. "How do you know David?" he asked with a completely shocked look on his face.

"I was engaged to him."

"You're Sandler's fiancé!" he said hoarsely, almost screeching.

"Well, not anymore, thanks to you!" she retorted.

As her words started to penetrate his fuzzy mind, he began to feel like he'd been betrayed. Why had she never mentioned this before now? His thoughts were reeling back, reaching for connecting pieces to this shocking news. His distress was clearly marked in his face as he tried to make sense of what was now happening between them.

"Just why are you bringing this up right now?" Colin was angry that this special time was being spoiled and also because he didn't want Jenny to be the woman Sandler had been engaged to, the woman he had tried to find for over two years.

"I just found out."

"What? You just found out? Were you reading a newspaper while I was fucking you?" he shouted, very angry now.

"No," she said almost calmly as she tried to remember exactly how it was that now she did know, minutes ago, she hadn't. "Something happened just now."

"Yeah, I know," he smiled sarcastically. "I was there."

"No, I mean something happened besides that, something triggered my memory. I think it was my orgasm."

The word "triggered" brought back all the words he'd learned researching hypnotherapy. A feeling of incredible misery washed over him.

He looked her in the eyes and asked, "Jenny, did he ever hypnotize you?"

"Once," she stated.

"Shit!" he spat out as his fist hit the mattress between them. "The man reaches beyond the grave again!" he said furiously.

"How come you never talked to me about him?" he asked.

"I did. I told you I was practically engaged before," she said, hurt that he was questioning her so harshly.

"That's right you did. You just never happened to mention his name," he said snidely. "What about my name? How come you never connected me to him? Didn't you read the newspapers or watch the news on TV. My name was announced over and over again and my picture was plastered everywhere. Surely you must have recognized me?" he accused.

Feeling his anger towards her was unjust, she became defensive and pulled the sheet up between them, covering herself. "I was out of town. I was in Detroit," she said with fire in her eyes.

Something clicked in his memory. "That's right. I remember now. Just before he took the officer's gun he shouted that he had to take his fiancé to the airport."

She hadn't known that and it saddened her to think that David had resisted arrest because of her. Had his determination to see her off caused him to stupidly challenge the officers and ultimately end his life?

"It was days before I knew why he hadn't shown up to drive me to National. That's when I learned about his death. My friend Tammy, who worked with me, just happened to talk to our Service Manager one afternoon. A policeman had called him trying to figure out why our number was on David's speed dial at home and at work. The Service Manager had no way of knowing that David and I had been seeing each other, he assumed it was because of his obsession with his cars."

Colin inwardly groaned. He had been that policeman. He had been so close. "You worked at Royal?" he asked incredulously.

"Yes. I told you I was in the car business. I sold cars there for almost fifteen years before I became the General Sales Manager. I met David when I sold him his first Pontiac. He was one of my best customers. After his divorce we sort of started dating. One thing led to another and we became pre-engaged. We were going to formally announce it to everybody at Thanksgiving."

"God, it never even occurred to me when the Service Manager asked if I wanted to speak with his salesman that the salesperson was a woman. Do you have any idea how hard I tried to find you?"

"Why?" she asked.

He didn't want to get into the question of the money yet. He didn't want to think that she'd had it all along, that she'd dirtied herself with the victims' money. So he put her off, reverting back to where they'd left off.

"Wait, back up a minute. So you were in Detroit. Your friend from the dealership called you. Continue from there."

"When Tammy heard about David she tried to track down a newspaper, she finally found one in her parents' recycling bin. She read the article over the phone to me. Nothing made any sense to me. In fact, it still doesn't. I remember the man's name who they said shot David. It was Master Police Officer C.G. Scott. I only know you as Colin, how would you expect that I would ever have made the connection?"

"I guess you wouldn't have. Obviously you didn't," he stated.

Her mind went back to the day David made her meet him at his office. Softly she spoke out loud as she recollected her thoughts. "David said he had to hypnotize me. There were things he wanted me to know, but he didn't want me to know them then. He told me you were going to kill him. Apparently, he was right. You did," she said flatly.

Colin instantly felt the distance grow between them as she hunkered under the sheet.

"Jenny, let me explain, it's not like you think. I didn't kill him like he wanted you to think I did. He made me kill him. He was trying to kill me!"

Jenny got up, ran down to the kitchen and quickly put her clothes on. Then she grabbed her keys and purposefully ran down the steps and out of the house.

"Jenny, wait! Please... Let me explain." He ran around the room grabbing clothes out of the dresser. Trying to jump into a pair of shorts he practically fell down the stairs in his eagerness to catch up to her. He ran through the kitchen and down the steps to the beach house. She was already in her car pulling out of the driveway by the time he made it outside. He hollered after her, but she didn't stop. He ran back up the steps and inside the beach house. He finished dressing as he frantically searched for his car keys. He finally found them in the pants he had left on the kitchen floor. He ran back down the stairs and out to his car.

He saw her car way ahead of his on the long causeway and as luck would have it, he got stuck at the bridge, just as it opened to boat traffic—and not to just a fishing boat either, but to a barge, two-blocks long. As the immense commercial vessel was ushered through the narrow canal, pulled by a slow-moving tug, he banged his fists on the steering wheel as he cursed the fates, his luck and his stupidity.

Chapter 126

I-95 Corridor North

As Jenny drove north she tried to sort things out in her mind. Learning that Colin had been the policeman who shot David had been crushing enough, but the way that it had come to her continued to unnerve her. She remembered the day David hypnotized her. It had been just before she had left for Detroit. In fact, she seemed to recall something about having to hurry home to finish packing. It had been late at night and she had come directly from work to meet him. How did he know so far in advance who would shoot him? And why did he go to all the trouble to make sure she knew all this before the fact? Did he expect her to avenge his death in some way?

The strange turn of events was causing her mind to tumble over information at a remarkable speed, rejecting and sorting all the things that had happened over the last few years trying to make sense of it all. The coincidence of her meeting Colin, all the way down here at Sunset Beach, was almost too much to fall for. But he had looked genuinely shocked when she told him she had been David's fiancé. And what would have been his reason for never bringing it up if he'd known all along?

He mentioned that he had been looking for her for over two years. She wondered why. Why would he have been looking for her? Unless he suspected she knew something about the reason David was being brought in for questioning in the first place. What had been the reason, anyway? She tried to think back to the only link she had to David's death, that newspaper article Tammy had read to her. Something about a patient was all she could put her finger on.

Maybe when she got to Virginia and went to the man David had told her to see, it would all start to come together. She hadn't told Colin about everything her orgasm had brought to light. Suddenly she didn't trust him anymore. The idea that Colin could have any complicity in all this, that he hadn't been himself all the time that she'd known him, brought tears to her eyes. Could he really have set all this up? She was beginning to feel like the world's biggest fool, and a lovesick fool at that. She was just beginning to think that maybe Colin was falling in love with her, the way she had fallen for him. She hated the thought that she could have been so wrong about him.

After returning from his beach house in the wee hours of the morning she had hurriedly thrown a few things in her suitcase and grabbed Taffy. From the time she had pulled into the driveway 'til the time she had pulled back out and closed the garage door behind her, tears had streamed down her face. Tears of sadness, frustration and confusion all blending together to drip off her chin as she had run around securing the house and packing for her and Taffy. She knew by the way she was feeling that only one person could make her feel better and help her figure out this mess; Momma.

So here she was again, going home to Momma, a week and a half sooner than she was supposed to. She leaned over and patted Taffy's belly as she lay sprawled out sleeping on the passenger seat. She set the cruise control for five more miles per hour, anxious now to get home.

Colin rang the doorbell several times. There was no answering bark from Taffy and that caused him to panic. Quickly he ran to look through the glass windows across the top of the garage door. Her car wasn't there. Where had she gone? It was almost three o'clock in the morning, nothing was open. Since she'd obviously taken Taffy with her, he could only figure that she'd gone away, maybe home to Virginia, maybe not. He realized that he really didn't know all that much about her friends or her family or what her tendencies would be when confronted with so much inner turmoil. He only knew that he loved her and that now he had to find her... again.

He went back to the beach house and dialed her number, leaving a message in case she came home. Then he sat on his deck drinking some coffee waiting for the sun to come up over the ocean. This isn't how he had envisioned it would be this morning, remembering her enthusiasm about making love and watching the sun come up from his bed. He put his fingers to his temples and rubbed in little circles.

Something was nagging at him. He wished he could put a finger on it. The beauty of the sunrise was greatly diminished by having no one there to share it with. So, hoisting himself up out of the deep Adirondack chair, he went in to shower and shave and get ready for his early golf game.

After he made the turn on number ten, he gave up. His concentration was shot and he was playing the worst round he'd played in years. He apologized to the couple he had been paired with, saying he just wasn't feeling all that well.

He drove over to Jenny's and looked in the garage windows again, still no car. If she planned on being away for a few days than she would have had to ask one of the neighbors to collect her mail and to look after the house for her. She'd left way too early to talk to them before she'd left, but maybe she'd call them from wherever she was. It was worth a shot. He walked over to her neighbors on the right. He'd seen them a few times when he and Jenny had grilled outside and they had been in their back yard. He knew that they had a key and occasionally came in to take Taffy out for a walk in the middle of the afternoon when Jenny couldn't get home from work.

He rang the bell and a few moments later a smiling, friendly face appeared behind the glass storm door. "Hi!" he said, recognizing Colin from his comings and goings, even though they had not been formally introduced.

"Hello," Colin said, forcing a smile to his face. "I'm looking for Jenny. We had a bit of a spat last night and now it looks like she flew the coop," he said sheepishly. "Did she go to Virginia do you know?"

"She called not even an hour ago, asking if we could get her mail and take out the trash can on Wednesday. She didn't say where she was, just that she had to get away. But I could hear the kids in the background, if that helps you any."

"Yeah, it sure does. The kids were already in Virginia at her parents. You wouldn't happen to know where they live, a phone number or their name would you?"

"No, I sure don't," the neighbor replied. "Somewhere in Northern Virginia is all I know, sorry."

"Well, thanks anyway." Colin called as he turned to walk back down the path to the driveway.

"Wait! I think it was somewhere in Fairfax County."

"Thanks." Colin murmured as he turned away again. He knew just how big Fairfax County was.

As Colin started walking back down the driveway he almost turned back to ask to be let into her house. Surely he could find something there with her parents' address. But he thought better of it. This man didn't know him. It would be awkward for both of them if he asked him to breech Jenny's confidence.

Mulling things over in his head, he sat down on Jenny's front porch and tried to think of all the things he knew about her that would clue him to her exact whereabouts.

Her name was Jenny Miller. Miller had been her first husband's name, not her maiden name, so that wouldn't help. She had worked at Royal. Christ! She had been David's car salesman! How had he missed that? Damned stereotyping! He'd sure missed all the clues on that one. But maybe there was somebody there who knew her parents, or at least their last name if not their address. He could always get an address if he had a name or a phone number from the police dispatcher's office. What was that friend's name she'd mentioned? He'd start there. He got up and went to the beach house to pack a few things.

Driving back up to Virginia he kept having that nagging feeling pulling him back from his thoughts about Jenny. It was like he had a puzzle piece in his hand and the puzzle on the table had no hole left for it to go into. The puzzle had long ago been completed, and now he had an extra piece to try to fit in. Then it occurred to him what was missing. The money.

If Jenny had been the fiancé then she had the money or knew where it was. But he really didn't want to believe that. If she knew about the money then wouldn't she have to know how Dr. Sandler had come by it? He answered his own question. No. What reason would the doctor have had for telling her? None. So maybe she didn't know it was misappropriated funds. He felt better rationalizing that she didn't know that Dr. Sandler had committed murder for it. And if she had the money then surely she wouldn't have had to go to work to pay for Paisley's tuition. Maybe she didn't know about the money. The word "yet" came out of somewhere and suddenly his head jerked.

Then the puzzle piece fell into place. He hit his head with his open palm. The orgasm! Of course. It had been the trigger for her memory. He'd hypnotized her before he died. He knew Sandler had told Jenny that Colin had killed him, so the doctor had known all along that Colin would be forced to shoot him. He remembered the gun check Sandler had done through the pawn shop. Without a doubt Colin now knew that Dr. Sandler had been planning on shooting him and expecting him to shoot back. Dr. Sandler thought he was going to take Colin with him when he checked out. He had been so sure of it that he told Jenny before the fact that Colin had killed him. What else had he told her during that hypnotic session? What was it Jenny hadn't told him before she ran away from him?

That nagging feeling made its presence known again, stronger this time. The man was reaching over the line from death to life to do something. He just knew it. What was it this time? Why did he get this overwhelming feeling that Jenny was in danger? He'd learned over the years to trust his instincts. They were rarely wrong. He wanted to convince himself that they were wrong now, but he just couldn't take the chance, not if Jenny was involved. He had to find her. He had to find her right away.

It was curious how Dr. Sandler had devised the idea of her orgasm to trigger her memory. Why had he chosen that? It seemed to Colin that it would be very unreliable and that it possibly would never have been activated. Oh My God! He knew. Jesus! He knew! He floored the pedal. His giving Jenny sublime pleasure, was going to cost her her life!

No! He wouldn't let that happen! His loving her was not going to kill her. He would find her in time. He zig zagged through the traffic as he came through Fredericksburg and drove like a banshee when he got to the beltway. There wasn't a cop who would dare pull him over, he wouldn't have allowed them to.

He pulled into the parking lot of Royal Pontiac GMC at 9:30. Everything was dark and locked up. He went to a phone and punched in the special number and codes to be connected to the police information officer at the dispatch center. He asked for Mr. Royal's home phone number. After a quick computer search they gave it to him. He dialed the number. After ten rings it was finally picked up by what sounded like a teenager. Mr. and Mrs. Royal were out of town and were not expected to be home until next week. He took a shot and queried the teenager about Jenny. Yes, she did remember Jenny and knew that she had retired and moved to North Carolina, but no, she didn't know her parents' last name but she thought that they lived in Sterling.

As he hung up another thought crossed his mind. Jenny had lived in Herndon. She had told him that Rusty studied Karate for three years. Surely he could track down the karate school that was in the vicinity of either Sterling or Herndon. If Rusty had been a student they would have had a file with emergency phone numbers in case he got hurt. Since her parents watched the kids while she worked the school would have to have her parents' number in that file. He grabbed a phone book and looked under karate schools.

There were several listed but only one that would have been convenient for them to take Rusty if they lived in Sterling. He dialed the number. There was no answer after twenty rings. He called the police information number again and was given the phone number of the karate school's owner. The police kept all this information in their computer data banks in case an alarm was set off or if there was a burglary or a fire. He wrote the

670

number on the phone book page and, after disconnecting with the dispatcher's office, he dialed it.

A man answered in what Colin assumed was Korean. Colin identified himself in English and asked if the man spoke English. A few minutes later another man came to the phone. "Hello?" he asked.

"Hello. My name is Officer Scott with Fairfax County Police, I'm trying to track down the mother of one of your former karate students. Her name is Jenny Miller, the student was Rusty Miller. Do you by chance remember him and his grandparents?"

"Ah, yes. I do. Mr. and Mrs. Fleming. Very devoted grandparents. She brought cupcakes for all the kids after each ranking test. I do not have their number here but I believe I have it at the office if you can wait til tomorrow."

"Do you remember Mr. Fleming's first name?"

"No, I don't. I don't think I ever knew it. Call me tomorrow and I'll look it up if you'd like."

"Thank you, I should be able to find them by the last name." He hung up and flipped the pages of the phone book.

Sixteen Flemings. Three in Sterling. Gerald, Martin and Phillip. Rusty's middle name was Martin. He remembered Jenny, when she was piqued with Rusty, calling him Russell Martin. He ripped out the page and went back to his car.

It was almost ten o'clock. He drove to the nearest 7-11 and looked up the address in one of their area map books. He made it from Tyson's Corner to their house in Sterling in less than twenty minutes. As he drove by the house he noticed the garage door opening and a man wheeling out a trash can. In the garage were two Pontiacs. He was pretty sure he had the right Flemings. He went to the next block, turned around and came up to park on the street in front of the house. As he walked up to the open garage door he saw someone bent over a recycling bin. It was Paisley. She was tugging it toward the driveway.

"Need some help with that?" he asked.

"Colin!" She screamed running into his arms. "What are you doing here?"

"Trying to track down your Mama. Is she here?" he asked as he hugged her back.

Just then an older woman came out into the garage, saying over her shoulder, "I can't believe you left her out here by herself, Martin. Paisley! Where are you?"

"Here, Nan! Look who's here! It's Colin!"

"Colin? Jenny's Colin?" It delighted Colin to hear himself being described that way by Jenny's mother and he smiled brightly for her.

"Not according to her if the way she left me this morning is any indication. Is she here?" he asked.

"No, she left early this afternoon to go see an attorney in Fairfax and then she called to say she needed to get away by herself for a few days. She said she'd call to check on the kids."

"Any idea where she went?" he asked as he bent down to pick up the recycling bin.

"None at all," Jenny's mother said shaking her head.

Colin carried the bin down to where the trash can sat at the end of the driveway, then walked back to where Paisley stood and tousled her hair.

"She didn't come back here to get any clothes or anything?" he asked.

"No, I asked her about that. She said she'd always wanted to go to the airport with just a toothbrush and a charge card and that's what she said she was going to do."

Well, it sounded like she found the money and was anxious to start spending it.

"Do you know who the attorney was? Or what she was going to see him about?"

"No, I was at the grocery store when she left. Maybe she told her dad something. Come on in. Is there something wrong? You look awfully concerned over a silly little spat."

"Is that what she told you?" he asked.

"No, actually she said she had a lot she wanted to tell me but first she had to make a few calls. I ran up to the grocery store for more bread and milk and the next thing I know, she's left to go see this attorney. Martin, look who's here. It's Colin, Jenny's friend from Sunset Beach."

He certainly was getting demoted quickly. He walked over to shake the man's hand who was just standing up from his reclining chair.

"No need to get up. I can't stay. I have to see if I can find Jenny."

"Is she in trouble?"

"I'm not sure. Do you know the name of the attorney she went to meet or why she was going to see him?" Colin asked Jenny's dad.

"No, she ran out the door saying she had to drive all the way over to Fairfax and that she wanted to get there and back before she got tied up in rush hour traffic."

"Can I take a look at the phone book she might have used? Maybe she underlined or circled the name or number," Colin asked.

Jenny's mother quickly went to the foyer closet to get it. "Here, have a seat at the kitchen table. How about something to eat? If you drove straight from Sunset Beach, you probably haven't had any dinner."

"That's okay. I'll eat later," Colin said.

But Jenny's mom pretended not to hear as she emptied most of the contents of the refrigerator onto the table and started making sandwiches and spooning out potato salad, coleslaw and apple sauce.

Colin scanned the yellow pages under Attorneys. It didn't appear that Jenny had marked on any of the pages. If she was going to see an attorney in connection with Dr. Sandler, maybe it was the one he had talked to shortly after Sandler had died. What the hell was his name? He scanned the pages but nothing looked familiar. He took a bite out of the sandwich Jenny's mom had put in front of him. Paisley was pouring him a glass of milk. He leaned over and gave her peck on the cheek. "Thanks, babe. Where's Rusty?"

"He's sleeping over at my cousin's house in Laurel," Paisley said.

Suddenly Colin had an idea. "Has anybody made a phone call since Jenny used the phone?"

Everybody thought for a moment. Nan was the first to respond. "No, I don't think anybody has. Martin? Do you remember calling out this afternoon?"

"No, I'm sure I haven't. We've had a few calls come in though."

"That won't matter. Do any of your phones have a redial or last call feature?" Colin asked.

"Yes, they all do," Nan replied.

"Great! Then I should be able to get connected to the attorney's office that she called. The only problem is that it won't do any good until there's someone there to answer it, so I'll know who it dialed. I'll come back at nine in the morning. In the meantime can you make sure nobody calls out on the phone she used? Do we know which one that was?"

"No, I was in the basement playing pool with Paisley," Jenny's dad answered.

"Then we'll have to try each phone. Can you avoid making any outside calls tonight?" Colin asked.

"I guess so. If you think it's that important, we'll have to," Nan said. She pulled a chair out for herself and sat down across from him. "Why don't you just stay here tonight so you don't have to come back in the morning and how about telling us what you think is going on. There's something you're worried about. Let's have it."

Jenny's dad came over to join them and Paisley went out to the family room to watch TV.

Colin took a long swig of his milk and then picked up a fork to attack the chocolate cake in front of him.

"How well did you know David Sandler?" Colin asked after swallowing the first bite and loading up another. A half hour later Colin was absolutely stuffed and Jenny's parents were absolutely wide-eyed with shock.

Chapter 127

Sterling, VA

The next morning at 9:15 Colin punched the redial button on the kitchen phone. After it rang twice it was picked up by a woman who answered, "John Marshall's office. May I help you?" That was the name he'd been trying to remember!

"Yes, is he in?"

"He's over at the courthouse, but I expect him shortly. Can I take a message?"

"No, I have to speak with him right away. I'll be right over."

"He has appointments all morning sir. Can I schedule you for tomorrow?"

"He'll see me. I'll be right there." He hung up and grabbed his car keys. He thanked Jenny's mom for the hospitality and this morning's breakfast, gave Paisley a hug and promised to call as soon as he found Jenny.

He drove to John Marshall's office and waited in the reception area while he finished with a client.

As soon as the client walked out, Colin walked right in. John Marshall stood up and put his hands on his hips.

"What's the meaning of this? Who are you anyway?" he demanded.

"You don't remember me? He said feigning a hurt look. "I'm the cop you lied to two years ago when I came to see you about Dr. Sandler's estate. You lied to me."

A glimmer of recognition came to John Marshall's face. He sat back down in his leather chair with a loud thump. He indicated one for Colin with his outstretched hand. "No, actually I didn't."

"When you first came to see me I had no knowledge of anything regarding Dr. Sandler's affairs, other than a will he had drawn up many years earlier leaving everything to his ex-wife. But then one day I was sitting in a stadium chair watching a

Hoya's game, listening to my alma mater's fight song, when I suddenly knew instructions about the disposition of some other property of his."

Colin looked at him with disbelief. "He'd hypnotized you?" Then he remembered his first conversation with him two years ago when John Marshall told him that he'd met with David, but that he didn't remember anything they'd talked about except for their alma mater.

"Apparently so," he said with a slight smile. "He knew I was an avid Hoya's fan and I guess he figured I'd eventually end up at a game since I have season tickets. They play the fight song several times a game, so it was only a matter of time before I got his message. Even when we were in college together he was always doing things like this to other people as a lark. He'd just never tried it with me before, so needless to say I was quite shocked."

"What were the instructions?" Colin asked as he tried to absorb all this.

"That a woman named Jenny might show up asking about a key. The key was taped under my desk and that I was to give it to her along with the number 60186. Sure enough, when I looked, there was a key in a small white envelope taped under my desk. The name and address of a bank were on the underside of the envelope, the number I assumed was the number to a safety deposit box."

"What bank?" Colin asked.

"First Union, right around the corner from here. When I checked with them I was told the box had been paid for in advance for twenty years."

"So, you've just been waiting for her to show up?" Colin asked skeptically.

"Well, actually, no. After two years my curiosity got the better of me and I took the key and went to go see what was in the box."

"And?" Colin prompted.

"It was full of money, I didn't count it but it had to be several hundred thousand. There was also a letter addressed to Jenny and a letter addressed to me. I guess he figured sooner or later I'd have to look. I also saw something that I thought was a little odd, a bottle of vitamins, Centrum capsules, I think it was."

"Capsules?" Colin said as he came up out of his seat.

"Yeah, why?" Mr. Marshall asked.

Colin paced the office banging his head with his hands. Those vitamins he'd found in a baggie in Dr. Sandler's desk, they hadn't been for Liesel! They'd been for Jenny! "What did the letters say?" he barked.

"I didn't read the one to her, but the one to me said that if Jenny didn't come to claim the key by June 1st, 2004, that I was to see to it that the money went to his daughter, Paisley for her 18th birthday. I was given an address in Sterling where her grandparents lived. Paisley could read the letter to Jenny but I was to throw out the vitamins. He said they were a private joke between him and Jenny."

"His daughter, Paisley? Are you sure it said his daughter?"

"Yes."

"Do you know where she went from here?" Colin asked.

"No, we didn't talk much. I assume she went to the bank. She just took the envelope with the key in it and said thanks. I can see why David was so taken with her. She sure is beautiful."

"Yeah. I know. Now all I have to do is find her before she takes those vitamins."

"Why?"

"They're filled with poison or a lethal concentration of some kind of drug. He's trying to kill her so nobody else can have her again."

"What! Are you crazy? I know David. He's not capable of anything like that!"

"When you get a chance, go over to the Criminal Investigations Bureau, ask for Major Ryan, tell him you want to see the Sandler file, then you'll find out how well you knew him."

With an abrupt turn Colin walked purposefully out the door and to his car.

He drove to First Union bank and asked to see the manager. Within a few minutes it was confirmed that Jenny had been there yesterday afternoon. She hadn't talked to anybody and no one knew if she left with anything more than she had come with or not.

He went to find a phone. While updating Jenny's mom he racked his brain for an idea. He was at a dead end. He had no idea where to go next. He asked her mother to name all the places Jenny had flown to over the last several years. She had won lots of trips with Pontiac and Nan admitted that she'd never be able to remember them all. She remembered Detroit, Cancun, Hawaii, Las Vegas, Denver, the Bahamas and Bermuda.

"When you think about where her favorite place might be, what comes to mind?"

"I always thought she liked Carolina Beach the best, but you don't fly there. Maybe Tammy would know?"

"Tammy? That was her friend from work, wasn't it?"

"Her best friend at work. She would probably know. So would her sister. I'll call Jean and see if she's heard from her."

"Okay, I'll run over to the dealership and track down Tammy."

Driving down route 123 towards Vienna, Colin thought of nothing except Jenny. His mind was racing with thoughts of her dying alone somewhere and never being found. Shaking his head he forced himself to have constructive thoughts. He had not let on to her parents how dire Jenny's circumstances could be right now. He hadn't told them about the vitamins Jenny now carried, believing them to be healthful not harmful.

Tammy came out to the showroom to meet him when he had her paged for him. Instantly he liked her, something about the genuineness of her smile broke through to him. She was trying to place his face as if she should recognize him even though they'd never met. Just as he reached out his hand to shake hers she whispered, "Colin!"

"How the heck did you know that?" he said staring wide-eyed at her.

"You match Jenny's description exactly. She's told me so much about you," she said with a slight tither.

"Oh, really? We'll have to get into that later," he said with a smile. Right now I need your help trying to find her. You haven't heard from her recently have you?"

"Not since last Sunday. Is she here?" she asked, excited at the prospect of seeing her good friend.

"She was until last night. Is there some place we can go to talk?"

"Sure." She spun around on her chunky heels and led him back to her cubicle.

He sat down and folded his hands in front of him on top of her desk. "Without going into a lot of detail right now, let me just say that Jenny has received some shocking news lately about me, Dr. Sandler and something I haven't quite figured out about Paisley. She told her mom that she needed to get away by herself for a few days. She mentioned something about going to the airport with just a charge card and a toothbrush. Do you have any idea where she would have gone?"

Without even the slightest hesitation she blurted out, "Paradise Island. That's where she'd go, without a doubt. It's like a cathartic spa for her, always has been. Check with American Airlines, she had a free voucher with them because she gave up her seat on an overbooked flight last year."

"You're sure it would be the Bahamas?"

"Not the Bahamas. Just Paradise Island, Merv Griffin's place. I think it's the Britannia Towers that she always stays in. She just loves that place."

"She gambles?"

"Oh no! She never gambles. She loves the beach and there's a cheeseburger shack that she swears makes the best cheeseburgers in the world. She just loves a good cheeseburger," she said fondly.

Colin knew exactly what Tammy meant. He'd been in attendance on one of her reverent cheeseburger hunts. They'd traveled all the way to Southport to The Provision Company on this particular quest. But it had been worth it watching her smile with delighted pleasure as she munched away on her burger.

"American Airlines connects in Miami doesn't it?" he asked.

"I think so. I know she's never flown directly into Nassau from here. And I can pretty much guarantee you that there's no way she would have left out of National. She won't go there unless somebody else is driving."

"Can I use a phone somewhere to make a few calls to Paradise Island?" He whipped out a fifty dollar bill and handed it to her. "This should take care of the charges."

Tammy waived away the money, "Believe me, if this concerns Jenny, Mr. Royal would not even consider you paying for them. She has a special place in his heart."

"Mine, too," he said with a smile and a wink.

Tammy walked him back to an unoccupied office and whispered the access code he would need to call long distance. The man unnerved her, he was so good looking and so buff. She pulled a phone book out of the desk drawer and plopped it down in front of him. As she shut the door behind him she said, "Call me if you need anything."

It was just past noon when he confirmed that she had checked into the Britannia Towers. They rang her phone several times for him but there was no answer. He asked to be connected to the security officer. Fifteen minutes later he was told that her room had been checked and she was not in it. They refused to go through her things looking for a bottle of vitamins. Who could blame them? It was a very odd request, he had to admit. He left a message for Jenny with the answering service and hung up. Then he called the airline and booked a flight. He had an hour to get there before it took off.

He called Jenny's mom and gave her the phone number of the hotel and Jenny's room number, instructing her to call her every half hour until she reached her. "Don't ask any questions," he said, "just tell her not to take any pills of any kind until I get there, especially vitamins. I should be there by five this evening, so if you haven't reached her by then, I'll find her."

He ran out of the office almost bumping into Tammy. He bent down and gave her a hug, lifting her off the ground in his exuberance. "I found her! You were right, that's exactly where she was. I'm on my way to the airport right now."

"Give her a kiss for me," she called after him.

"You can bet on it!"

He arrived at Nassau airport at 4:45 and was at the hotel by 5:55. He went straight to her room and knocked several times. There was no answer. He went back down to the lobby and at the front desk he asked for the security officer he had spoken to earlier. The man was summoned from his dinner, and after glancing at the badge Colin flashed at him, he accompanied Colin back upstairs where he opened the door to her room after getting no answer from his knock.

Colin went inside and straight into the bathroom. There was only a toothbrush and toothpaste, a hairbrush and lipstick on the counter. There were no clothes or luggage anywhere and he remembered with a smile that she had arrived with only a charge card and a toothbrush. He didn't even have a toothbrush.

Colin went over to the window that looked out over the pool and beyond that to the ocean. He pulled the drapes back as wide as they could go then he went out on the balcony and tied a small white hand towel to the railing. He came back in, closed and locked the sliding door and turned out all the lights, leaving the drapes open. He thanked the officer and then closed the door behind them as they left the room.

He went down to the pool, grabbed a chair and sat by the pool on the ocean side, facing her balcony. This way he could watch for her coming up from the beach and still know the minute she arrived back at her room if she was returning from someplace else. He watched the towel fluttering in the breeze marking her balcony for him. Probably went shopping he surmised. A woman's gotta have some clothes he thought, remembering just how good she looked out of them.

The room lights clicked on around seven and he jumped out of his chair so quickly he caused it to flip over. He ran to the other side of the pool and through the terrace doors to the bank of elevators. He punched her floor number as soon as he cleared the door and waited as they slowly closed and the elevator began its assent. He ran his fingers through his hair, suddenly nervous but very much relieved that he'd found her in time. When the door opened again he had to dodge around a large group of people waiting to go down. His anxiousness to get down the long hallway to her room overrode his normally polite nature. He sidestepped his way around them, not bothering to excuse himself. His long, quick strides brought him to her door in seconds. He knocked sharply and waited to hear her voice.

"Who is it?"

"Colin."

Immediately the door opened. He looked at her as she stood there dressed in a colorful sarong and sandals, her long blonde hair loose down her back, secured with a colorful headband with miniature cloth reggae people glued to it.

"Colin!" she gasped from the shock of seeing him there and the thrill it caused her to feel in her stomach.

"Don't say anything. Just kiss me." He stepped into the room letting the door bang behind him. He reached for her and pulled her into his arms, canting his head over hers as he roughly covered her lips with his, smothering her mouth as he took possession of it, driving his tongue in and out in wild thrusts lighting a raging fire in her veins.

"That was from Tammy," he breathed harshly.

"Now can I have one from you?" she asked breathily.

He gathered her up against his chest and joined his mouth to hers again, more than happy to oblige her.

Chapter 128

Paradise Island, Bahamas

Colin's kisses were possessive, coaxing her to respond to his potency with a passion equal to his. As his lips left hers to scorch a pathway down her neck her heart thundered in her ears. Her common sense exchanged with her need for him and she forgot all about the doubts she had been harboring. As her hands reached up to his shoulders to pull him closer she could feel the heat thrumming through her to join with the warmth emanating from him. The fire that had started as a tingling sensation in her stomach was out of control now and as his gaze bore into hers, she knew that the magnetism between them could not be denied a moment longer. Abruptly he bent down and picked her up, holding her close against his chest as he laid her on the bed.

He pulled his shirt over his head and undid his belt and zipper as he kicked off his shoes. Within seconds he was gloriously naked. He laid down beside her pulling her close while one hand untied the knot at her hip. The sarong fell open and he ran his hands between the folds trying to find her delicate warm skin with his flat palm. Her agitated breathing caused by their fevered kisses was causing her chest to rise tantalizingly in front of his eyes. His hand moved upwards to peel the sarong away from her breasts, the turgid hardness of her peaked nipples causing his own breath to come in gasps.

As he bent over her to capture the fleshy part of her breast with his mouth she moaned and restlessly moved against him. The melting softness of her willing body met up against the firm hardness of his and the agonizingly hard shaft of his desire sought to find recourse with her flesh. A sheen of sweat broke out on his forehead and across his chest as he fought the driving insistence within him. He tried to match her passion with his, holding back until she was ready for him. He suckled her breasts as she arced against him searching for that part of him that could satisfy the yearnings that were filling the deepest part of her, making her tremble with desire. When his hand spread her thighs apart he climbed on top of her and with his thighs between hers, his elbows on either side of her supporting his weight, he positioned himself in front of her smooth, wet cavity. Both of his hands caressed her face as he gently kissed her and with a practiced ease, entered her. She whispered his name as he took possession of her giving her the best that living and loving could be.

He matched his frantic downward rhythm to the upward thrust of hers and then he watched as her face and throat flushed with her release. She moaned as she careened outside of her body and then floated back to earth on an invisible slow slide back to him. As he watched her writhing and then spasming up against him he took her hands in one of his and braceleted her wrists above her head as he wildly thrust into her, repeatedly filling her core with him. She felt him shudder as his powerful body emptied itself into her. He smothered her lips with a torrid kiss as he groaned her name into her mouth.

He collapsed on top of her and then quickly rolled with her onto his side. When he could catch his breath he whispered into her ear, "You didn't trigger anything that's going to have you running away from me again, did you?"

She looked up into his face and smiled, "No, just your average, everyday, run-of-the-mill orgasm."

He swatted her bottom with the hand that was resting on her hip. "I think not, darling. That was extraordinary and you know it. Admit it. I'm the best you've ever had."

"I'm not sure I can tell by just one or two liaisons. I think I'll need a bit more time to decide about your sexual prowess," she teased.

"Honey, you can have all the time you want. I'm not going anywhere."

"How did you know where to find me?" she asked as she propped a pillow up against the headboard and leaned back against it.

"It's a long story, let's order room service while I explain it all, but before I do, where are the vitamins you found in the safety deposit box?"

She looked at him in shock. "How did you know about them?"

"I know it all. I know some things that are really going to shock you, but first answer my question," he demanded.

"I threw them out at the airport. The date had expired," she said as if it had no significance to anything at all.

He laughed heartily. "The bastard didn't think of everything after all."

Then he somberly said, "Those pills were meant to kill you Jenny. The fact that you knew to go to John Marshall to get the key to that box was only because you had had sex with somebody. He was willing to let you live as long as nobody else could have you. As soon as I took you and pleasured you, you were in a destruct mode that he had orchestrated just before he died. The man was powerful in his own way, bending people's minds to his bidding. We have a lot to talk about, but first you need to call your Mom. I'm afraid I've had everybody in a panic trying to find you." He handed her the phone as he leaned down to kiss her. Then he walked into the bathroom and turned on the shower.

A few minutes later Jenny pulled back the shower curtain and stepped into the tub to join him. "Did you get through?"

"Yes, I told her you were here and that you were going to be proving your prowess to me all night."

"What did she have to say to that?" he asked.

"Don't forget to take your vitamins," she quipped.

He grabbed her around her hips and pulled her up against him, laughter rumbling in his chest.

Under the steady spray of the warm water he lifted her face so he could gaze into her eyes. "Marry me, Jenny." The love he had for her was reflected in his eyes and she had to blink back tears as her head fell against his chest.

"I take it that's a *yes*?" he asked as he stroked her hair and back. She was so overcome with emotion that all she could do was nod her head up and down against him.

"So, I guess that means you won't be needing any more chocolate," he said, not exactly forming a question. She remembered the conversation they'd had the first day they'd met.

"That's not part of the marriage contract is it?" she asked.

He laughed and hugged her even tighter. He was still laughing as he pressed fevered kisses to the base of her throat, murmuring, "Chocolate indeed. Believe me, you won't be needing it anymore!"

His hands went around her and he lifted her by her buttocks into his arms, wrapping her legs over his hips. He leaned her back up against the tile wall and plunged himself into her moaning, "Jenny, I love you."

Chapter 129

Paradise Island

Later that night as they sat in bed eating cheeseburgers and drinking champagne, Colin asked about the letter Jenny had found in the safety deposit box.

Jenny explained the part of the letter that David had written about Paisley's parentage and how he had substituted his sperm for the donor's each time she had been inseminated.

"Life is really quirky. For years I've wondered about Paisley's father, imagining what kind of person he was and how he looked physically. Now I find out that I knew him all along. It was the shock of discovering that David was Paisley's father that sent me here to get a handle on all my thoughts about it. I always wondered why her hair wasn't the light blonde color it should have been." She bit into a pickle, shivered and stuck her tongue out. "Champagne and pickles, not a good combination."

"What else did the letter say?" Colin asked as he wiped some ketchup off of Jenny's cheek.

"There was a small vial of blood in a separate little envelope with a note that said it was his, in case I doubted any of what he was saying and wanted proof. Then there was the explanation about the vitamins." She got up and walked over to the dresser where her purse was, pulling out a single sheet of paper. She unfolded it and read: "I got these vitamins for you, since you are apparently having sex with somebody now, (and I hope he's worthy of you). I figured you'd need a little extra energy. I know how you always throw yourself wholeheartedly into any endeavor you undertake. As you take one each day, remember me and know that I am wishing you were with me instead. My love always, David."

As she walked back to the bed he looked at the swell of her breasts as they pressed against the material of his shirt. She looked incredibly sexy in it as she flashed him her bare thighs with each step she took. "The man was obsessed with you, and I can't really say that I blame him." Jenny had not done well with the idea that David had wanted her all to himself, to the exclusion of all others, even if it meant her death, so he didn't mention it again.

She walked over to his side of the bed and brushed a kiss on his shoulder. He ran his fingers up and down the outer curves of her thighs. Her eyes fell to the sheet covering his groin area. The fabric that was covering his lap was now becoming a tent with a large center pole holding it up.

As he plunged his fingers up inside her and felt her wet slipperiness he groaned and with one motion pulled the sheet off of himself and pulled her on top of him. She rode like a woman mounted on a great steed, coming off the saddle slightly and landing back down with abandonment until he could no longer contain himself and, grabbing her hips firmly in his hands, he quickened the pace, thrusting up against her as she pounded into him. She collapsed against his chest just as he jerked and pressed her buttocks firmly against him for one last stroke. They came together and then spiraled off on their own separate journeys fighting the blissful abyss to get back to each other as their union was celebrated by their trembling bodies.

Afterwards as they lay side by side staring at the ceiling Jenny turned her face to Colin's and asked, "If a man and woman had to climax simultaneously, as we just did, to conceive, how many babies do you think would have been born on this earth?"

"You really mean how many wouldn't have, don't you?" he said with a smile.

"Yeah. Frankly I'm not sure I would have been one of them."

"Now, why would you say that?"

"I guess most people can accept the idea that their father had an orgasm, but their mother...well, she's beneath that sort of lustful behavior," she mumbled.

"I think you'd be surprised. Maybe they didn't always come at the same time but women rule. They usually get what they want," he said with a smile.

"Well, I still think it's unfair, women have the periods, the labor and childbirth process and then the menopause thing. For all that, they get an occasional orgasm while the man gets one each and every time."

He rolled to his side and gathered her in his arms. "Honey, you don't need to worry. I'll make sure you get yours, each and every time."

They stayed at Paradise Island for a few days while Colin slowly unraveled the story of his investigation of David, starting with his meeting with MaryAnn, his undercover work as a patient and ending with his search for her. When he was relating the part about Jeremy, Shawn Vanscoy's lover, Jenny remembered the day in the grocery store when David had panicked after reading the tabloid pages. Up to that point she really hadn't wanted to believe the bizarre story that Colin was relating, but now she acknowledged that she had to. It was the truth and she had to accept it.

That night she cried and sobbed in his arms. Colin asked her if she had loved David and she looked up into his face and said, "I don't think I really knew what love was until I met you. But he was my friend and I cared about him."

"Would you really have married him?" he asked.

"I don't know, probably not. I always had doubts, that's why I delayed the announcement so long. I thought by giving myself time to get used to the idea that everything would be all right. It never was. I was never comfortable with the idea of sleeping with him."

Colin held her close until she was all cried out and then he tilted her head so he could look into her eyes. "You are mine aren't you? You're sure about us forever, right? 'Cause I couldn't go through what I went through again. If I lost you, I just know I wouldn't survive it."

"I've finally found the man with the perfect kiss. You don't think I'd ever give that up do you?" she said as she looked into the depths of his smoldering eyes. He bent down to join his lips with hers, murmuring against them, "It's only perfect if it's your lips on mine."

The next day they rented a catamaran and Colin took them far enough away that the island was only a tiny speck in the water. He coaxed her for the better part of an hour before he finally persuaded her to sunbathe nude for him. The erotic sensations of being completely naked in front of him on the boat sent shivers up and down her spine and every time he stared at her with that transfixed look in his eyes she shivered all over again. "I like seeing you like this," he breathed into her hair as they enjoyed the wind whipping past. "I like the reckless abandon you have for us and our love."

She had to admit she would never have imagined herself doing such a thing before, but it seemed so natural now to be like this with Colin.

When a sea plane came close to passing overhead he lowered his body over hers on the deck of the boat saying, "These sights are for my eyes only, you belong to me now." He bent to kiss one sun-kissed nipple with his fevered lips. "And I will cherish you always."

Epilogue

Sunset Beach

Two years later

With the Labor Day holiday came the last of the season's summer tourists and the end of Jenny's part-time job at the mini-golf. It had been a hectic summer and Jenny was beginning to look forward to the fall. From here her days would be centered around car pool runs to Wilmington and back.

For the residents of the local beaches it was an almost magical time of the year. They got their beaches back, and their roads, their grocery stores, restaurants and pools. They not only got them back, it was almost as if they were put there for their own private use. Not only were they not crowded, they were practically deserted. It was nice after the fast pace of the summer to slow down and truly enjoy what living at the beach was all about. Come spring they would all gear up again for the invasion, and actually look forward to the onset of summer and the arrival of excited house guests and tourists. Right now, though, it was the beginning of September and everyone was ready for the last hurrah and for the golden doldrums to begin.

Jenny drove home to find Paisley watching TV on the couch with Taffy in her lap. "What's for dinner?" were the first words out of her mouth when Jenny leaned down to give her a kiss.

"I thought we'd go to Calabash and get some crab legs. How does that sound?"

"Oh, that sounds great, Mom! I'll go get ready," she said as she jumped up to go to her room.

"We have to wait for Rusty you know. He should be home soon."

Just as she said that she heard his car pull into the driveway. A few minutes later he came through the front door. He walked right up to her and gave her a kiss on the cheek. "Hi Mom. What's for dinner?" he asked. "I'm starving."

"How 'bout some crab legs?" she asked as she poured herself a glass of champagne.

"Sounds great! Let me take a quick shower and I'll be ready," he said as he left the kitchen and headed for his bathroom.

"You're driving," Jenny called out after him.

They feasted on crab legs for almost two hours and then Rusty drove them all home. After walking Taffy around the neighborhood, Jenny decided to go for a walk on the beach. It was just too beautiful not to.

As she drove over the bridge the sun was just beginning to set. Everything was bathed in a blue-gray glow with rosy highlights. She parked right in front of the gazebo and walked down to the beach. This was the hardest time of the day for her, the kids helped keep her busy but by the fourth day she was always miserably lonely for him.

Colin was finally getting himself established on the tour and most tournaments kept him away four days. She had to stay home to take care of the kids and Taffy and besides, he said that he couldn't take the distraction of her being around anyway. He needed to concentrate and get into his own world of nothing but golf. Usually they didn't even talk by phone until it was all over. He'd probably call tonight. The tournament had ended today.

She thought about all the things that had happened in the last few years and smiled as she walked down by the water's edge. She and Colin had been married in Fairfax by a female judge Colin knew as soon as they returned from Paradise Island. Together they retrieved the money from a safety deposit box that Jenny had rented at a different bank. They took $100,000 and gave it to MaryAnn Riddel and then donated the rest to different mental health agencies around the beltway. Jenny figured that the patients who had left the money had ultimately wanted it to be used to help others to deal with their problems, so she carefully chose the agencies she thought would put the money to the best use.

Then she and Colin collected the kids and Taffy and drove back home to Sunset Beach where Colin had ceremoniously carried her over the threshold.

Now she was waiting for him to come back home to her. She turned around to start making her way back to the walkway that crossed over the dunes and led to the gazebo. The sky was quickly darkening, pretty soon it would be completely dark. She glanced up towards the walkway and saw a man silhouetted there. He was waiting there on the walkway, leaning against the railing, just watching her. As soon as she saw him she started running up the sand. He met her halfway, grabbing her up in his arms and spinning around with her in them. The light in his eyes conveyed the joy he was holding in his heart for her.

There was something special glowing in his face, something ready to burst from him and she thought she knew exactly what it was. "You won the tournament, didn't you?" she asked breathily.

"Yes! Yes, I did! I won $40,000! I'm a part of the tour now!" he shouted.

"Oh, Colin!" she said as she hugged him fiercely, "I knew you could do it!"

He took both of her hands in his and kissed them tenderly, "I wouldn't have pursued it if it hadn't been for you. You believed in me when even I didn't." She squeezed his hands and felt the ring on his right hand. She looked down at the ring that she'd had made for him. It was a massive ring with chunks of little gold nuggets framing a smooth carved out center. In the Florentine finish a gold golf club was superimposed and right beside it, ready to be hit, was a large blinking diamond representing the golf ball. The diamond had come from David's engagement ring.

They started walking back up the walkway and towards the gazebo with their arms linked around each other's waists. She was smiling up at him, he was smiling down at her.

"I have a *yield field* for you," she said in a sultry voice.

His eyes smoldered with passion as he captured her lips with his, "Let's go find a place to take care of that for you, and for me."

CPSIA information can be obtained at www.ICGtesting.com
Printed in the USA
BVOW01s1130271013

334772BV00001B/1/A